YOUR NEW
pregnancy
BIBLE

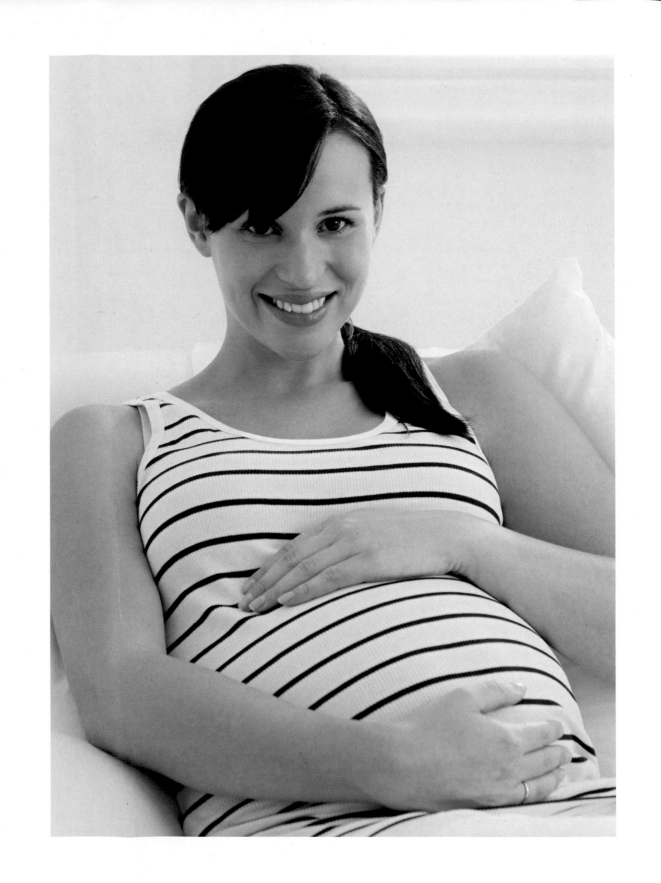

YOUR NEW
pregnancy
BIBLE

CONTRIBUTING EDITORS
Joanne Stone, MD
Keith A. Eddleman, MD

hamlyn

An Hachette UK company
www.hachette.co.uk

First published in Great Britain in 2003 by
Carroll & Brown Publishers Limited
Second edition 2007
Third edition 2010
Fourth edition 2013

This edition published in 2015 by Hamlyn,
a division of Octopus Publishing Group Ltd
Carmelite House
50 Victoria Embankment
London EC4Y 0DZ
www.octopusbooksusa.com

Distributed in the US by Hachette Book Group
1290 Avenue of the Americas, 4th and 5th Floors,
New York, NY 10020

Distributed in Canada by Canadian Manda Group
664 Annette Street, Toronto,
Ontario, Canada M6S 2C8

ISBN 978-0-600-63159-0

Printed and bound in China

10 9 8 7 6 5 4 3

Managing Art Editor: Emily Breen
Photography: Jules Selmes

Contents

CONSULTANTS AND CONTRIBUTORS

Chief Consultants and Contributors

Joanne Stone, MD
Professor of Obstetrics, Gynecology, and Reproductive Science at Mt. Sinai Medical Center, New York, is also Director of the Division of Maternal-Fetal Medicine and Perinatal Ultrasound. She also has a clinical and consultative practice and is active in cllinical research and education.

Keith A. Eddleman, MD
Professor of Obstetrics, Gynecology, and Reproductive Science at Mt. Sinai Medical Center, New York is also Director of Obstetrics and Professor of Genetics and Genomic Sciences. He is an expert and educator in maternal-fetal medicine and clinical genetics, specializing in reproductive genetics, ultrasound, and diagnostic procedures.

Other US Consultants and Contributors

Lenore Abramsky
Genetic Associate, North Thames Perinatal Public Health Unit, Northwick Park Hospital, London.

Patricia M Barnes, PNNP, MS, CNM
Certified Nurse-Midwife at Nativiti Women's Health and Birth Center, Houston, Texas.

Jane Butler, RN, CNM, BS, MPH
Certified Nurse-Midwife at Maggee Women's Hospital, Pittsburgh, Pennsylvania.

Kathleen Capitulo, DNSc, RN, FACCE
Director of Maternal-Child Health Care Center and Associate Hospital Director, The Mount Sinai Hospital, New York.

Eve R Colson, MD
Assistant Professor of Pediatrics, Yale University School of Medicine, Director, Well Newborn Nursery, Yale-New Haven Hospital, Connecticut.

Marilyn Graham, PhD, MD
Associate Professor of Clinical OB/Gyn, Indiana University, Indianapolis, Indiana.

Christine Obremski, CNM, MS, RN
Director of Midwifery at The Mount Sinai Hospital, New York.

Gayla Vanden Bosche, MA
Writer and Assistant Director, Magee Women's Hospital National Center of Excellence in Women's Health, Pittsburgh, Pennsylvania.

Other Consultants and Contributors

Stuart Campbell, DSc, FRCP, FRCOG
Professor and Associate of Create Health Clinic, Center for Reproduction and Advanced Technology, London.

Anne Deans, DCH, MFFP, MRCGP, FRCOG
Specialist in Obstetrics and Gynecology, Frimley Park Hospital, Surrey.

Wendy Doyle, SRD, PhD
Dietitian, London Metropolitan University, London.

Gavin Evans
Journalist, writing with Duncan Fisher, The National Childbirth Trust, and with the support group Fathers Direct.

Kate Harding, MRCOG
Specialist Obtetrician, Guys and St Thomas' Hospital, London.

Peter Hepper, PhD, FBPsS, CPsychol
Professor of Psychology, Head of School of Psychology and Director of Fetal Behavior Research Center, Queen's University, Belfast.

David K James, MA, MD, FRCOG, DCH
Professor, Division of Feto-Maternal Medicine, Academic Division of Obstetrics & Gynecology, The University of Nottingham, Nottingham.

Michelle F Mottola, PhD
Associate Professor and Director, R Samuel McLaughlin Foundation – Exercise and Pregnancy Lab., School of Kinesiology, University of Western Ontario, Canada.

Penny Preston, MB ChB
General practitioner and writer on pregnancy and child care.

June Thompson, RGN, RM, RHV
UK Health Visitor and freelance health writer.

James J Walker, MD, FRCP, FRCOG
Professor, Department of Obstetrics & Gynecology, St James University, Beckett St, Leeds.

Richard Woolfson, PhD, FBPS
Writer, journalist and psychologist who works with children and families.

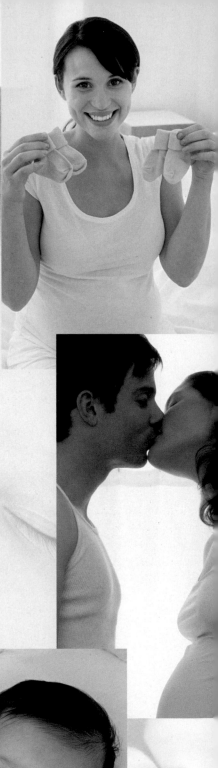

Introduction

Since it was first published in 2003, *The Pregnancy Bible* has proved to be invaluable to the expectant mothers and fathers who acquired a copy. Pregnancy is a unique experience and one that you will want to enjoy while doing what's best for your baby. Today a great deal more is known about the risks to a baby's normal development, and also what a woman needs to do to successfully meet the challenges of pregnancy, labor, and delivery than was possible in the past. However, all the information that is now available, particularly relating to situations that may be, evenly remotely, out of the ordinary, is rarely known in total to a single doctor, no matter how well trained and experienced he or she is. That is why, to produce a thoroughly researched book, *The Pregnancy Bible* was created with a team of experts in every related field including genetics, gynecology and obstetrics, midwifery, pregnancy nutrition and exercise, psychology, fetology, and pediatrics. Additionally, teachers in natural childbirth techniques, breastfeeding, and baby care were consulted. Ten years on from its initial publication, we've gone back to the experts and revisited the material to bring out a comprehensively revised edition.

This new edition of *The Pregnancy Bible* continues to cover every aspect of pregnancy, birth, and new parenthood but has been brought up-to-date with all currrent practices, particularly in regard to Cesarean deliveries, which about one-third of new mothers will experience. Although it cannot replace the care and attention that you'll receive from your healthcare providers, who will know you as an individual, it can supplement that advice, explain procedures, give handy hints, and answer any questions you may have.

Past readers have come to appreciate its special features such as the helpful illustrations and color photographs, including those that enable you to see how a baby develops week by week and the gatefold pages, which show at a glance what can be expected in each of the three trimesters. And this new edition is augmented by a comprehensive and useful glossary of pregnancy and neo-natal terminology.

Its definitive chapters on nutrition, exercise, maintaining good health, the essentials of prenatal care and managing emotions, will help you to achieve a healthy pregnancy, while those on childbirth choices, getting ready for birth, and the labor and birth experience, should prepare you for the birth that you want. Once your baby is born, further chapters will explain how to take care of yourself and your newborn. Two reference sections provide comprehensive coverage of all the prenatal tests and procedures that may be used as well as the medical complaints and problems that can affect you or your newborn.

Most importantly, *The Pregnancy Bible* has been designed to help you to achieve a positive attitude, which has been shown to be one of the most significant factors in a rewarding birth experience. With knowledge and understanding, you and your partner can take on pregnancy and parenthood with confidence.

Joanne Stone, MD and Keith A. Eddleman, MD

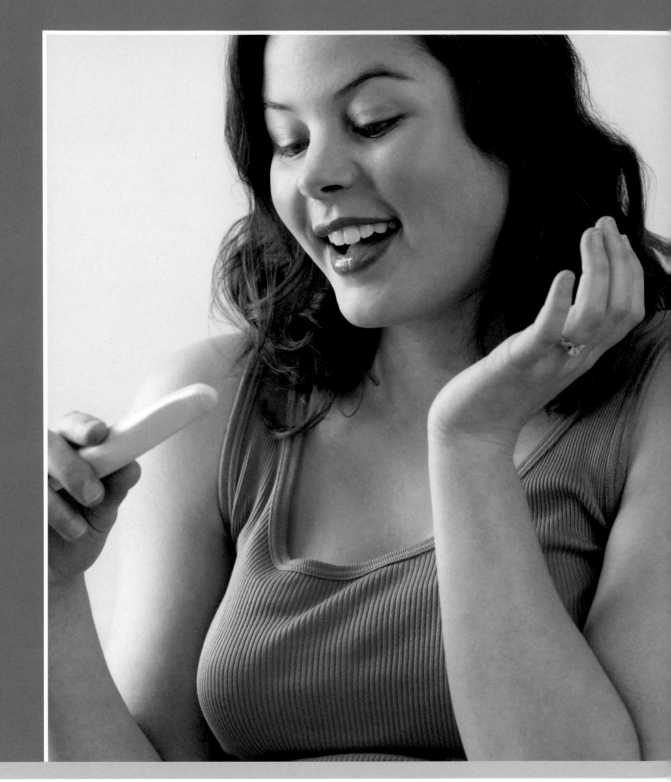

PART I MIRACULOUS BEGINNINGS

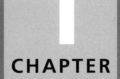

The story of pregnancy

When a woman conceives, it's just the beginning of an amazing process. This chapter tells the story of how the fertilised egg reaches the uterus, how your baby inherits your characteristics and how he or she develops week by week. It also outlines the major external changes to your body and the important milestones of the following nine months.

Sperm meets egg

An amazing process begins when an egg, no larger than a speck, unites with a single sperm, the sole winner of a race with several million competitors.

To meet, the egg and sperm undergo an arduous journey that is unlikely to work out. However, if they succeed, their meeting leads to the creation of a single cell containing genetic information from each partner. It's this unique blueprint that forms the basis of a new life.

Conception takes place in three basic stages: ovulation, fertilisation and the division of the fertilised egg, which then implants in the uterus – it's not until this is successful that pregnancy begins.

The egg comes first
A woman is born with approximately two million eggs (ova) in her ovaries but from the moment of birth, they begin to die off, so by the time she reaches puberty, only an estimated 40,000 eggs remain. Of these, some 400 to 500 will mature over her lifetime and be released during ovulation. By her menopause, however, less than 1,000 eggs are left

and natural pregnancy will no longer be possible. Most women ovulate every month in response to luteinising hormone (LH), which is released by the pituitary gland. Each month about 5 to 15 ova begin to ripen inside protective, fluid-filled sacs called follicles. Usually only one of these reaches maturity, and as this happens, oestrogen is released into the bloodstream, stopping the ripening of other eggs. This hormone also triggers the lining of the uterus to thicken, forming a blood-rich cushion in preparation for the development of an embryo.

How ovulation happens
At ovulation, which occurs about midway through the menstrual cycle, the follicle that has outgrown the others finally ruptures, and an egg bursts out. The ruptured follicle goes on to form the corpus luteum ('yellow body'), which produces a hormone, progesterone, that sustains the growing baby until the placenta takes over the role. At this stage, the egg is barely visible to the naked eye.

As the egg is released from the ovary it's moved along the Fallopian tube towards the uterus by tiny, hair-like projections called cilia. Conception (fertilisation) occurs when a sperm fuses with the egg, usually toward the outer end of the tube, near the ovary. The optimum time for conception is when a man and woman make love during the woman's fertile period – that is, when ovulation has just happened or is imminent.

If the egg isn't fertilised within 12 hours of being released, it dies, the follicle dries up and a menstrual period occurs 14 days after ovulation, when the lining of the uterus is shed. This is all due to a drop in the level of progesterone. However, if the egg is fertilised, progesterone levels will increase and the uterine lining will continue to thicken.

Signs of ovulation
Although most women are completely unaware of ovulation, around 25 per cent experience lower

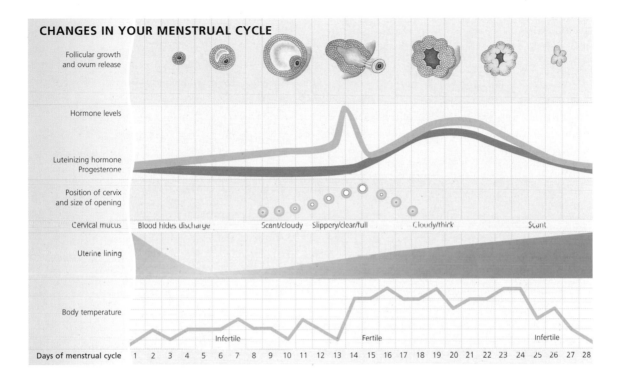

CHANGES IN YOUR MENSTRUAL CYCLE

Follicular growth and ovum release	
Hormone levels	
Luteinizing hormone Progesterone	
Position of cervix and size of opening	
Cervical mucus	Blood hides discharge · Scant/cloudy · Slippery/clear/full · Cloudy/thick · Scant
Uterine lining	
Body temperature	Infertile · Fertile · Infertile
Days of menstrual cycle	1 2 3 4 5 6 7 8 9 10 11 12 13 14 15 16 17 18 19 20 21 22 23 24 25 26 27 28

abdominal pain, usually on the side near the ovary that's ovulating. The pain is called *mittelschmerz* (literally, 'middle pain') and is thought to be caused by irritation from fluid or blood from the follicle when it ruptures. However, this pain is not always a reliable predictor of ovulation because as it doesn't occur with every cycle.

A more consistent sign of ovulation is a change in the cervical mucus. Just after menstruation, this is scanty, thick and sticky, making it impenetrable to sperm. As ovulation approaches, it becomes thinner and more liquid, allowing healthy sperm to travel through it at speed. After ovulation, the mucus reverts to its usual, more inhospitable consistency.

Another sign of ovulation is body temperature. Progesterone causes a small but measurable rise in body temperature from 36.4 to 36.7°C.

'Ferning' of your saliva, which occurs during the few days leading up to ovulation, can be checked for with special pocket-sized portable microscopes sold in salivary ferning kits – a type of ovulation predictor kit (see also page 12). As your oestrogen levels rise, the salt content of your saliva increases and when dried, crystallises into a fern-like pattern.

The great sperm race

When the man ejaculates into the vagina he releases hundreds of millions of sperm at a speed of around 16 km (10 miles) an hour. (Sperm are made from puberty onwards, although their quantity and quality begin to decrease from about the age of 40. The average healthy young man produces 2 to 6 ml of semen per ejaculation, with each millilitre containing 50 to 150 million sperm.) The sperm are mixed with a sugar-containing fluid that gives them energy for the testing journey ahead. The fastest will reach the egg in 45 minutes, the slowest take about 12 hours. However, most don't even make the journey – they either trickle out of the vagina or are lost or destroyed along the way. Only a few hundred of the strongest swimmers will eventually arrive at the Fallopian tubes where fertilisation can take place. Sperm have to traverse the vagina, cervix and uterus to reach the egg – a distance of some 15 to 18 cm, but equivalent to a human being swimming over 100 lengths of an Olympic-sized pool. Millions get lost in the numerous crevices of the vagina or arrive at the wrong Fallopian tube. Others, mainly weak or damaged sperm, are destroyed by the lethal acidic environment in the vagina. Interestingly, it seems that female sperm, which contain an X chromosome

(see page 18), are more comfortable with the acidic conditions in the vagina than male sperm, which contain a Y chromosome. Millions more sperm are pushed back by microscopic hairs inside the uterus.

However, other factors give the sperm a helping hand. If a woman orgasms during intercourse, it's thought that wavelike contractions in her vagina draw the sperm in towards the cervix – although you don't have to have an orgasm to become pregnant. During a woman's fertile period (see diagram, page 11), the mucus that usually forms a barrier to the cervix becomes slippery and thin, so helping the sperm's progression into the uterus. The opening of the cervix also becomes wider in readiness for receiving sperm, and it's estimated that some 40 million healthy sperm make this journey through the cervix and across the uterus, a journey

that takes around 45 minutes. The Fallopian tubes release an alkaline mucus, which nourishes the sperm as it waits for the egg to be released.

A matter of timing

The moment of conception is wholly dependent on timing. A woman must have a ripe egg ready as a healthy sperm arrives in the Fallopian tube. Sperm can survive for up to four days in the female body, but any longer than this and they'll die before the egg arrives. This means that if a woman has intercourse two to three days before ovulation, she can still conceive. If sperm arrive after ovulation they never have the chance to meet the egg in the Fallopian tube.

And the winner is...

Only around 200 sperm make it to the site of fertilisation, but the race isn't yet over. The egg is surrounded by thousands of cells that nourish it. The sperm fight their way through these cells, flipping them out of the way with their tails. When they reach the wall of the egg, a sticky substance on the surface helps them to attach. The objective now is to burrow through the outer layer of the egg, called the corona radiata, and through a further layer, the zona pellucida. Several sperm may break through the outer layer, but usually only one reaches the nucleus. When this happens, the head of the sperm fuses with the nucleus of the egg, and the egg immediately throws up a chemical barrier around it to stop other sperm from penetrating.

The beginning of life

As the egg and sperm fuse together, the sperm loses its tail and its head enlarges. The egg and sperm form a single cell containing 46 chromosomes of genetic information – 23 from each parent. The inside of the cell swirls around, forcing chromosomes to mingle. In a matter of hours this single cell will duplicate material known as deoxyribonucleic acid (DNA) and split into two. The building blocks of life are now forming.

Your chances of conceiving

Fertility varies widely, so it can take longer for some couples to conceive than others. On average, among couples having regular intercourse, 25 per cent of women will conceive within one month, 60 per cent within six months, 80 per cent within a year, and 90 per cent within 18 months.

However, certain factors on both the male and female side can mean that it may take longer to conceive. For example, smoking, drinking alcohol, certain medications, obesity and exposure to heat and chemicals can all affect sperm quantity and quality. Insufficient and poor quality sperm won't survive the journey to the egg. Even if they meet, damaged sperm or eggs may not be able to fuse successfully or they may produce a fertilised egg that can't survive the early stages of growth. The quality of a woman's eggs deteriorates with age, and, after the age of 35, she may not ovulate every month, even though she still has regular periods. Smoking and abusing drugs or alcohol also can damage eggs.

Some women may have a blocked or scarred Fallopian tube, which can hinder the movement of a ripe egg down the tube. If you're trying to conceive, you can improve your chances with the following:

- *Avoiding smoking* Smoking has a damaging effect on many aspects of health; it can reduce female fertility and affect the quality of sperm. If you smoke, quit before pregnancy.
- *Keep your weight healthy* Women with a BMI>30 (see page 64) can have problems with ovulation. A healthy diet containing plenty of iron, calcium and folic acid will be sensible, and the folic acid will benefit the baby by reducing the risk of neural tube defects.
- *Check with your doctor* Determine whether you are immune to Rubella, and if you feel you may be at risk, have a STD check-up.
- *Timing of sex* Make love at least every other day to improve the chance of conception.
- *Don't drink too much alcohol* A high alcohol intake is bad for a man's reproductive function as well as his general health. There is less convincing evidence linking alcohol with female fertility problems, but more than two units a week can harm the developing fetus.

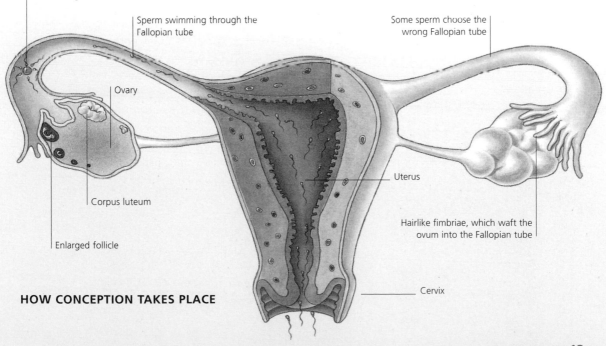

Ovum being fertilised

Sperm swimming through the Fallopian tube

Some sperm choose the wrong Fallopian tube

Ovary

Corpus luteum

Enlarged follicle

Uterus

Hairlike fimbriae, which waft the ovum into the Fallopian tube

Cervix

HOW CONCEPTION TAKES PLACE

The journey to the uterus

Between 12 and 20 hours after the egg is fertilised, the cell that is formed begins to divide in two, replicating its DNA as it does so. This division continues rapidly, and all the while this bundle of cells is heading towards the uterus, where the fetus will eventually grow.

It takes the fertilised egg around five to seven days to reach the uterus after leaving the ovary. This journey along the Fallopian tube is helped along by the cilia (hair-like feelers) that line the tube. The Fallopian tube also nourishes the developing cells and removes waste products produced by the cells as they divide. During this time the fertilised egg goes through several stages of development.

From egg to blastocyst
The fertilised egg is called a zygote, and this divides and subdivides until it forms a solid ball the size of a pinhead. Consisting of 16 to 32 cells, this is now called a morula. The morula continues dividing at 15-hour intervals so that by the time it reaches the uterus, some 90 or so hours later, it has approximately 64 cells. Of these, only a few cells will actually develop into the embryo; the rest will go to form the placenta and the membranes that surround the baby in the uterus.

The morula gradually goes from being solid to being a fluid-filled ball of cells, and at this stage it is called a blastocyst. The surface of the blastocyst consists of a single layer of large, flat cells called trophoblast cells. These later develop into the placenta. Inside the ball is a small cluster of inner cells that will become the embryo.

In the early stages of development, when the zygote is no bigger than a few cells, each one of these has the potential to become a human being. If the zygote splits, identical twins are formed.

Implantation takes place
About five to seven days after ovulation occurs, progesterone production is at its height, stimulating the growth of the rich blood vessels that supply the endometrium (the lining of the uterus). This coincides with the arrival of the blastocyst in the uterus ready for implantation. At this stage, the blastocyst is less than 0.2 mm (1/100 inch) across. It floats freely in the uterus for a few days as it continues to develop and grow. Approximately nine days after fertilisation, the blastocyst attaches itself to the uterine wall by means of spongelike projections of trophoblast cells, which burrow into the endometrium. These cells grow into the chorionic villi (see page 140), which will later develop into the placenta. Occasionally, implantation causes a small amount of bleeding, known as spotting.

If the blastocyst doesn't implant, it will be swept out with the next menstrual period, and the woman won't even be aware that she had conceived.

THE DEVELOPING EMBRYO

Zygote

Morula

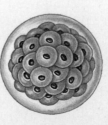

Blastocyst

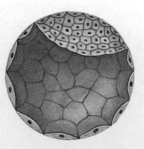

Cross-section of blastocyst

Finding nourishment

By the time it implants, the blastocyst is made up of hundreds of cells. It releases enzymes that penetrate the lining of the uterus and cause tissue to break down. This provides a nourishing mix of blood and cells on which it can feed. Occasionally, the lining of the uterus doesn't supply a rich enough source of food for the blastocyst. In this case, a miscarriage occurs, rather like a late, heavy period.

It's also after implantation that the placenta begins to develop and the embryo begins to produce the pregnancy hormone human chorionic gonadotrophin (HCG). It's this hormone that can be detected by pregnancy testing kits.

What happens next

It takes about 13 days for the embryo to implant firmly in the lining of the uterus. Miscarriage is still a possibility but is less likely after implantation. The embryo begins to produce progesterone of its own, encouraging the endometrium to develop. It's also at this stage that the embryo's first organs start to form, beginning with the nervous system and, later, the heart. Thirteen days is the latest date that an embryo can split into two to become twins. If the split occurs later, conjoined (Siamese) twins are formed.

Conceiving twins and more

Over the past 20 years, largely because of better nutrition and increased fertility treatments, the chances of conceiving twins – and more – have increased. In the United Kingdom there over 12,000 multiple births each year. Twins occur naturally in about 1 in 35 births, and triplets occur naturally in about 1 in 4500 births. However, most pregnancies with three or more fetuses result from treatments for infertility. During the process of IVF, drugs are used to stimulate the release of more than one egg and create several embryos. HEFA (Human Fertilisation and Embryology Authority), which oversees fertility treatment in the UK has advised that only one or

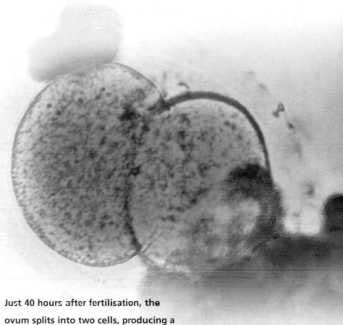

Just 40 hours after fertilisation, the ovum splits into two cells, producing a genetic copy of itself.

two embryos be used in order to reduce multiple births from occurring.

Many more twins are conceived than are actually born. Known as the 'vanishing twin' syndrome, this is when one of the fetuses spontaneously miscarries, usually during the first trimester, and the fetal tissue is absorbed by the other twin, the placenta or the mother, making it seem that the twin has vanished.

DID YOU KNOW...

IMPLANTATION CAN OFTEN FAIL Attaching to the endometrium is a risky business. It's estimated that around 40 per cent of blastocysts entering the uterus never implant. Instead they die and are swept out with the next period. It appears that timing plays a part, with an early or late arrival impacting negatively on the blastocyst's success in implanting.

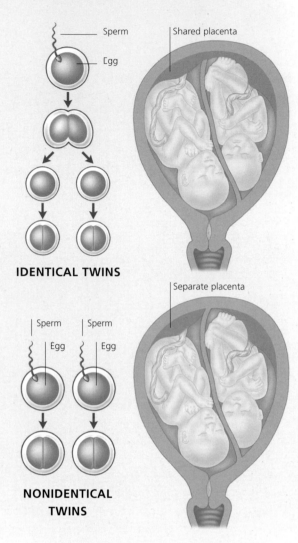

Sperm

Egg

Shared placenta

IDENTICAL TWINS

Sperm | Sperm

Egg | Egg

Separate placenta

NONIDENTICAL TWINS

not share a placenta and amniotic sac, but each twin has its own umbilical cord. These babies will have an identical genetic make-up and will be the same sex. They will also have the same hair, eye colour and blood type.

Nonidentical twins – also called fraternal twins – are produced when a woman releases more than one egg when she ovulates. This could be two eggs from one ovary, or one from each. Each egg is fertilised by a different sperm and two genetically different babies are conceived. They can be the same sex or boy and girl, and will look as much alike or different as any other siblings.

In the case of triplets, quads and more, there can be any combination of identical and nonidentical children. For example, three – or four or more – eggs can be fertilised, creating nonidentical triplets. Or, one fertilised egg can split into identical twins with another fertilised egg making it a triplet pregnancy with two identical babies and one non-identical. Or a single egg can divide into three, thereby creating identical triplets.

The hereditary factor

One factor influencing the conception of twins is the mother's age; after 35, the chances of conceiving identical twins rises. However, the chances of conceiving nonidentical twins rises until about the same age and then drops off. This may be due to the fact that as a woman ages she naturally produces more ovulation-stimulating hormones, which could trigger her ovaries to release more eggs each month.

Your chances of having twins also increase with each subsequent pregnancy, and it seems that larger, taller women are 25–30 per cent more likely to have them. Nonidentical twins also may run in families, on the mother's side. Finally, there seems to be an ethnic predisposition: twins are more common in women of African origin and occur least frequently in women of Asian origin.

An early ultrasound may show an empty sac in these circumstances.

Identical or nonidentical twins

About a third of twins are identical – technically monozygotic – and two-thirds are nonidentical – technically dizygotic – twins.

Identical twins develop when, as in a normal conception, an egg is fertilised by a single sperm. The fertilised egg then splits into two, causing two separate embryos to develop – if it splits into three, triplets result, and so on. Identical twins may or may

Your baby's inheritance

Your baby's genetic endowment is determined at the moment of conception. Half of it will come from the egg and half from the sperm. So both you and your partner have contributed equally to her inherited make-up.

The process whereby you pass on characteristics to your children is amazingly intricate, but the natural rules that govern it can be easily understood. To understand more about how you and your partner influence your baby's characteristics, you first have to be clear about some basic genetics.

Genes and chromosomes

Your body is made up of millions of cells, all of which are copies of the fertilised egg from which you developed, and the nucleus (centre) of each of these cells contains a copy of all your genes. Genes are the blueprints that instructed your body how to form when you were an embryo and determine how it functions now. These blueprints are encoded in miniscule units of deoxyribonucleic acid (DNA).

DNA influences how your baby will look. The colour and efficiency of her eyes, the texture of her hair, the shape of her nose, her blood type, her bone structure and many more of her characteristics are determined by her genes, which she inherits from you – and you inherited from your parents. There are about 30,000 genes in each of the body's millions of cells, so it takes little imagination to realise that they're extremely small – too small to be seen even under a very powerful microscope. All these genes combine to make a person unique.

Genes don't float around loose inside the body's cells; they're packaged systematically onto structures called chromosomes. Normally, in each cell, your baby has 46 chromosomes that exist in matching pairs. One chromosome in each pair came from you and the matching one from your partner. Each chromosome carries thousands of genes and is large enough to be seen under a powerful microscope.

Your genetic make-up

You have one pair of genes for each characteristic: one from your mother and one from your father. For some characteristics, both your parents may have given you the same version of a gene, and for others, they different versions. Sometimes, one version of a gene dominates over another; in other cases, both influence the outcome equally. It's the total effect of the combination of all your genes that determines your hereditary make-up.

Variety is the spice of life

Many genes exist in a variety of different forms, just as there are many possible recipes for chocolate cake. If this weren't the case, people would all look exactly alike and the world would be a very boring place. Since there are many versions of the thousands of genes you inherit from your parents, you are

Your child may resemble you more than your partner because of the way the genes you gave her have mixed.

genetically unique, unless, that is, you have an identical twin. Even your brothers and sisters will be genetically different, because their inheritance depends on the unique combination of genes in a particular egg and a particular sperm. This idea carries through for your baby and any children you have in the future.

Some genes do not form correctly. If one or both genes of the pair are abnormal, this can result in problems. Cystic fibrosis or sickle cell disease are disorders said to be inherited recessively (see below). Other abnormal genes, dominant ones, cause problems even if the other gene of a pair is normal, for example in Huntington's disease. Some abnormal genes that are carried on the X chromosome cause problems only for boys. These so-called X-linked disorders include Duchenne muscular dystrophy and haemophilia. For information on these diseases, see page 240. More information on genetic counselling, can be found in the Antenatal Directory.

Who will your baby look like?

If you and your partner both passed on your full complement of 46 chromosomes in the egg and sperm, your baby would have 92 chromosomes in her cells, and the numbers would continue to double with every generation. This system wouldn't work. Instead, in the formation of eggs and sperm, called meiosis or reduction division, the cells go through a specialised division, in which they halve the number of chromosomes within each – so each egg and sperm contains only 23 chromosomes. Therefore, for any given chromosome you will give your baby either the one you received from your mother or the one your received from your father; your partner does the same.

Your baby will receive some chromosomes that you inherited from both your parents, so she could have, for example, your father's build and hair colour but your mother's eye colour. If you plan to expand your family in the future, your next child will inherit a slightly different combination, so will be another unique addition to your family.

Silent genes

Your baby can inherit genes from you that you didn't know you had. This is because some genes are dominant and others are recessive and, in the pairs of chromosomes that are formed, the dominant genes override the information coded on the recessive genes. For example, you and your partner may carry both the gene for black hair, which is dominant, and the gene for red hair, which is recessive. In each of you, the black hair gene dominates. However, if you both pass on your red hair gene, your baby will have red hair as there is no dominant gene to override the recessive one.

Gender determination

Your baby's sex is also decided at the moment of conception. Of the 23 pairs of chromosomes, only one pair determines whether your baby is a boy or a girl. This crucial pair are the sex chromosomes: X and Y. Girls have two X chromosomes, boys have one X and one Y chromosome. Because of the way that eggs and sperm are produced, all eggs contain a single X chromosome. Sperm can contain an X or a Y chromosome. At fertilisation, when the sperm and egg pool their chromosomes, if the sperm carries an X, the baby will be a girl and if it carries a Y, the baby will be a boy; in other words, the sex of the baby is determined entirely by the father.

DID YOU KNOW...

IVF CAN PRODUCE BABIES FREE FROM GENETIC DISORDERS Couples who are carriers of lethal or severely crippling conditions such as muscular dystrophy can benefit from pre-implantation genetic diagnosis. Using IVF techniques, eggs are collected and fertilised in the laboratory. One or two cells are removed from the resulting embryos and screened for abnormal genes or to check whether the correct number of chromosomes are present. Healthy embryos are implanted (or frozen for later use).

The first signs of pregnancy

Some women just intuitively know when they're pregnant and are even able to pinpoint the exact moment that they conceived. For other women, it might not be so obvious.

You don't have to 'feel' pregnant to actually be pregnant and while there are certain telltale symptoms of pregnancy, you might not necessarily experience them all.

Early indications

You may experience one or two, or all, of the following symptoms of pregnancy. Morning sickness is the classic giveaway sign, but you may be one of the lucky ones and hardly have it at all. Likewise, while missing a period is another classic symptom, if your periods have always been irregular, it can be difficult to tell if you're late because you're pregnant or late because of the irregularities in your cycle.

Missing a period

This is one of the clearest indications of pregnancy. However, there are other reasons why menstruation may be delayed. Stress, illness, extreme fluctuations in weight – excessive gain or anorexia – or coming off the oral contraceptive pill can all stop periods for a while. Irregular periods are a common symptom with polycystic ovary syndrome, a condition in which periods can occur several months apart.

Breast tenderness

Changes in the size and feel of your breasts are one of the earliest signs of pregnancy. As early as a few days after conception your breasts will begin to enlarge in readiness for breastfeeding, and you'll probably experience heaviness and soreness. Many women report that their breasts are very sensitive and experience a sharp, tingling sensation, too, although this often disappears a few weeks later. These breast changes may be less dramatic with subsequent pregnancies.

Nausea and vomiting

Feeling sick is the most common complaint in early pregnancy and is experienced by most women from around 5 to 6 weeks of pregnancy, but it can also begin as early as two weeks after conception. Although termed 'morning sickness', the nausea can occur at any time of day and can vary from an occasional, faint sensation to an overwhelming feeling of nausea and vomiting (see page 67). By and large, these symptoms disappear by around 14 to 16 weeks of pregnancy.

Tiredness

Many women report feelings of extreme tiredness during pregnancy, especially at the beginning. Typically, after getting in from work in the evening all you want to do is go to bed, or you may be

Carried out correctly, home pregnancy testing kits are 98 to 99 per cent accurate, so you can trust the results.

desperate for a mid-afternoon nap. When you reach week 14 of your pregnancy, your energy levels should start to pick up.

Frequent urination

As early as two to three weeks after conception you will find yourself wanting to urinate more frequently. This is due to the pressure of the enlarging uterus on the bladder, literally reducing the capacity of your bladder. At about 14 weeks the uterus rises up into the abdomen, which often relieves this annoying symptom until the last few weeks of pregnancy when the baby's head engages (drops down in the uterus), again causing pressure on your bladder. Rising levels of the pregnancy hormone progesterone also relax the bladder muscle so that you feel your bladder is full even when there's not much urine in there. In addition to this, your kidneys are working harder in response to being pregnant, and an extra 6 to 7 litres (13 to 15 pints) will be added to your circulation to increase the blood flow around your body.

Changes in taste and smell

Don't be surprised if certain foods suddenly make you feel queasy or if you start to crave particular foods (see page 99) or are bothered by certain smells. You also may have a strange metallic taste in your mouth.

Constipation

A common early symptom of pregnancy, this is caused by high levels of progesterone, which relaxes the bowel and slows your digestion (see page 72).

Mood swings

High levels of pregnancy hormones flood your body in early pregnancy, making you extra emotional and sometimes weepy (see page 151).

Confirming your pregnancy

Two weeks after conception your baby is just a ball of cells, not much bigger than a pinhead, starting to develop in the lining of the uterus. Already the placenta is forming and starting to produce a hormone called human chorionic gonadotrophin (hCG), which passes into your bloodstream and urine from the day of your first missed period.

Home pregnancy tests

These tests, which you can buy from most chemists, confirm pregnancy by detecting hCG in the urine. They are very accurate, so don't be surprised if your midwife or other healthcare provider relies on your own home test for confirmation of your pregnancy. Normally, a test would only be repeated if complications arise, such as a concern about miscarriage. However, if you receive a positive result, you should make an appointment to see your midwife to get started with antenatal care.

Pregnancy blood tests

If urine tests are inconclusive, your doctor may use a blood test to detect and date a pregnancy. The test may simply give you a positive or negative result, or it may test levels of hCG (human chorionic gonadotropin), depending on your symptoms and medical history. The more sophisticated blood tests can detect a pregnancy from as early as two weeks after conception. If the levels of hCG are measured, these help to establish your dates, as the values of this hormone change as pregnancy progresses. However, ultrasound is still the best way to date pregnancy, and you may be offered one at your first antenatal visit (see page 87). Pregnancy blood tests are useful if there are any concerns about miscarriage

DID YOU KNOW...

YOU CAN HAVE 'A PERIOD' WHEN YOU'RE PREGNANT Some women experience light bleeding about nine days after the egg was fertilised. This bleeding is usually lighter than a proper period and is thought to be caused when implantation occurs as the ovum first attaches to the uterine wall.

or if your doctor or midwife suspects an ectopic pregnancy (see page 255). In these situations hCG blood levels don't usually rise as fast and may even fall, indicating that the pregnancy has failed.

Internal examination

Four to six weeks after conception, your doctor can receive definite proof of pregnancy by examining you internally, if necessary. He or she will be looking for telltale signs such as the uterus softening and an alteration in the texture of the cervix. The vaginal tissues thicken and produce more secretions, resulting in a heavier discharge. The uterus grows so quickly – it's already about the size of a small orange by eight weeks – that its size can help your doctor to date a pregnancy accurately. However, in practice, if you are sure of your dates and your

pregnancy test is positive, your doctor will not need to examine you internally.

HOW TO use a pregnancy testing kit

You can perform a home pregnancy test from the first day that you've missed your period and onwards. There are several different home kits on the market, so always read the manufacturer's instructions carefully.

It is best to use the first urine passed when you get up in the morning; this will be the most concentrated, so even tiny amounts of hCG can be picked up by the test. Later in the day your urine tends to get diluted from what you've been drinking and eating, so very early pregnancy hormone levels may be too low for a home kit to detect.

Some tests ask you to hold a stick in your urine flow **1**, others require that urine is passed first into a clean container and then a few drops squeezed from the dropper provided **2** onto a window on an oblong stick.

Usually the result appears within minutes and can be read by looking for

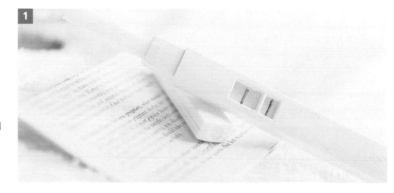

a coloured line in a window on the stick. Often there is also a line indicating that the test has been carried out correctly. If the test is negative, but you still feel that you may be pregnant, repeat the test in five to seven days. It may be that the pregnancy is too early to detect and you became pregnant later than you thought. This is most likely if you have irregular periods.

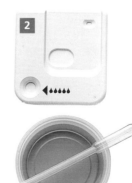

HOW TO CALCULATE YOUR DELIVERY DATE

Once your pregnancy's been confirmed, one of the first things you'll want to know is when your baby will be born. Your pregnancy, which is described as being 40 weeks long – according to Naegele's rule of dating (see box, right) – is dated from the first day of your last menstrual period (LMP).

If you have a regular 28-day cycle and know the date of the first day of your LMP, you can use Naegele's rule to work out your baby's due date by counting on nine months plus seven days – or 280 days – after the first day of your LMP. You can adjust the date according to the length of your cycle. If you have a 26-day cycle, count on nine months plus five days from your LMP – or 278 days. If you have a 32-day cycle, count on nine months plus 11 days from your LMP – or 284 days – and so on.

Alternatively, use the chart below to find out your estimated date of delivery (EDD). First, find the date of your last menstrual period by looking at the numbers in bold. Then look at the number in the line directly below it, which represents your EDD. If, for instance, your LMP was on 12 April, your baby will be due on 17 January the following year. Remember, however, that this is just a general guide and does not take into account women with cycles greater or less than 28 days. Only about 5 per cent of babies are born on their estimated birth date.

DATING PREGNANCY

In the 1800s, a German obstetrician called Naegele fixed the length of pregnancy at ten lunar months – nine calendar months or 280 days – and now all pregnancies are dated according to 'Naegele's Rule'. He based his calculations on the first day of the woman's LMP, but as conception usually occurs two weeks later, a pregnancy is actually 38 weeks long – or 266 days – not 40 weeks. So, two weeks after you conceived, you're described as being in week 4 of your pregnancy.

January	1	2	3	4	5	6	7	8	9	10	11	12	13	14	15	16	17	18	19	20	21	22	23	24	25	26	27	28	29	30	31
Oct/Nov	8	9	10	11	12	13	14	15	16	17	18	19	20	21	22	23	24	25	26	27	28	29	30	31	1	2	3	4	5	6	7
February	1	2	3	4	5	6	7	8	9	10	11	12	13	14	15	16	17	18	19	20	21	22	23	24	25	26	27	28			
Nov/Dec	8	9	10	11	12	13	14	15	16	17	18	19	20	21	22	23	24	25	26	27	28	29	30	1	2	3	4	5			
March	1	2	3	4	5	6	7	8	9	10	11	12	13	14	15	16	17	18	19	20	21	22	23	24	25	26	27	28	29	30	31
Dec/Jan	6	7	8	9	10	11	12	13	14	15	16	17	18	19	20	21	22	23	24	25	26	27	28	29	30	31	1	2	3	4	5
April	1	2	3	4	5	6	7	8	9	10	11	12	13	14	15	16	17	18	19	20	21	22	23	24	25	26	27	28	29	30	
Jan/Feb	6	7	8	9	10	11	12	13	14	15	16	17	18	19	20	21	22	23	24	25	26	27	28	29	30	31	1	2	3	4	
May	1	2	3	4	5	6	7	8	9	10	11	12	13	14	15	16	17	18	19	20	21	22	23	24	25	26	27	28	29	30	31
Feb/Mar	5	6	7	8	9	10	11	12	13	14	15	16	17	18	19	20	21	22	23	24	25	26	27	28	1	2	3	4	5	6	7
June	1	2	3	4	5	6	7	8	9	10	11	12	13	14	15	16	17	18	19	20	21	22	23	24	25	26	27	28	29	30	
Mar/Apr	8	9	10	11	12	13	14	15	16	17	18	19	20	21	22	23	24	25	26	27	28	29	30	31	1	2	3	4	5	6	
July	1	2	3	4	5	6	7	8	9	10	11	12	13	14	15	16	17	18	19	20	21	22	23	24	25	26	27	28	29	30	31
Apr/May	7	8	9	10	11	12	13	14	15	16	17	18	19	20	21	22	23	24	25	26	27	28	29	30	1	2	3	4	5	6	7
August	1	2	3	4	5	6	7	8	9	10	11	12	13	14	15	16	17	18	19	20	21	22	23	24	25	26	27	28	29	30	31
May/Jun	8	9	10	11	12	13	14	15	16	17	18	19	20	21	22	23	24	25	26	27	28	29	30	31	1	2	3	4	5	6	7
September	1	2	3	4	5	6	7	8	9	10	11	12	13	14	15	16	17	18	19	20	21	22	23	24	25	26	27	28	29	30	
Jun/Jul	8	9	10	11	12	13	14	15	16	17	18	19	20	21	22	23	24	25	26	27	28	29	30	1	2	3	4	5	6	7	
October	1	2	3	4	5	6	7	8	9	10	11	12	13	14	15	16	17	18	19	20	21	22	23	24	25	26	27	28	29	30	31
Jul/Aug	8	9	10	11	12	13	14	15	16	17	18	19	20	21	22	23	24	25	26	27	28	29	30	31	1	2	3	4	5	6	7
November	1	2	3	4	5	6	7	8	9	10	11	12	13	14	15	16	17	18	19	20	21	22	23	24	25	26	27	28	29	30	
Aug/Sept	8	9	10	11	12	13	14	15	16	17	18	19	20	21	22	23	24	25	26	27	28	29	30	31	1	2	3	4	5	6	
December	1	2	3	4	5	6	7	8	9	10	11	12	13	14	15	16	17	18	19	20	21	22	23	24	25	26	27	28	29	30	31
Sept/Oct	7	8	9	10	11	12	13	14	15	16	17	18	19	20	21	22	23	24	25	26	27	28	29	30	1	2	3	4	5	6	7

Letting people know

You may be so excited when you discover the good news that you want to tell everyone you know or you may decide to wait until you're sure that your pregnancy is progressing well. However, as well as telling your partner, your doctor is someone who needs to know at the outset.

Midwife

If you've found out that you're pregnant with a home testing kit, one of the first things you should do is contact your local surgery or health centre to arrange your first antenatal visit (normally around 8–10 weeks of pregnancy). This is particularly important if you are currently receiving medical care as pregnancy may affect the treatment of any illness, both current and future. Your doctor should be able to advise you about antenatal care in your area and put you in touch with a midwife, if you wish.

Your midwife will assess what type of antenatal care you are going to need, arrange for your first scan and give you all the information you need to make informed choices (see also page 86).

Friends and family

When to tell your friends and family is very much a personal decision. You might choose to tell only your nearest and dearest at first, such as your partner and close relatives and friends, and then start to spread the news as your pregnancy becomes more obvious. Alternatively, you might choose to postpone making your pregnancy common knowledge until after the third month, once the risk of miscarriage has reduced – women who have suffered a previous miscarriage often choose to do this.

Your employer and colleagues

The question of how to break the news at work sometimes causes concern for mums-to-be. But you can make it easier on yourself if you plan what you're going to say beforehand and if you have familiarised yourself with maternity legislation and relevant company policies before you meet with your employer.

One of the major issues is deciding when to tell your employers and work colleagues, and this depends on a number of factors. If you're putting on weight and suffering from morning sickness and tiredness, you may want to tell others soon, before they draw their own conclusions. However, if you have a review coming up, you may want to wait until you've heard that you're going to get that promotion or pay rise.

Consider carefully how you tell your colleagues. Although most people will probably be very happy for you, the prospect of you taking maternity leave may create uncertainty about if and when you're going to return and who's going to cover for you.

If you work in an environment that you think might be harmful for your unborn baby, such as with chemicals or in high or low temperatures, it's best to talk to your employer as soon as possible to find out about the possibility of changing duties. For more information about your safety in the workplace, see page 79.

MORE **ABOUT**   trimesters

The nine-and-a-bit months of pregnancy are divided into three trimesters, which mark the major milestones in your and your baby's progress. The trimesters are of slightly uneven length. The first trimester represents the first 13 weeks, and is the period during which your baby's major systems and organs are formed. The beginning of the second trimester, at 14 weeks, is a turning point for both you and your baby: you will probably feel some relief from early pregnancy symptoms and your pregnancy may start to show, while your baby is now fully formed and will start to grow. The third trimester, starting at week 28, is the home stretch, as your body prepares for birth and your baby continues to grow in weight and size.

Your pregnant body

Although you're unlikely to put on much weight or look significantly pregnant during the first 13 weeks of pregnancy, momentous changes are happening inside you. Emotionally, you're adjusting to the idea of being pregnant and beginning to take on board the incredible changes this will make to your life. Expect to put on 0.9 to 1.8 kg (2 to 4 lbs) this trimester, of which just 20 g (⅔ oz) will be due to your baby.

Your healthcare provider will date your pregnancy from the first day of your last menstrual period, which will be written as LMP in your antenatal records. Pregnancy usually lasts about 280 days or 40 weeks.

Your ovaries have begun to ripen an egg, which will be released into the Fallopian tube in a process known as ovulation. This usually happens 12 to 16 days before the start of your next period. You may notice that your vaginal secretions are wetter and more transparent at this time, and some women even feel slight pain with ovulation.

If you haven't already been taking a folic acid supplement, start as soon as possible and continue for the rest of the first trimester. It's also a good idea to take a 10 mcgs of vitamin D throughout pregnancy and whie breastfeeding.

Conception has taken place. Your egg has fused with a single sperm to create the unique cell destined to become your baby.

Your uterus is beginning to enlarge and soften, and the texture of your cervix is changing.

You may experience some breakthrough bleeding as the fertilised egg embeds in the lining of the uterus.

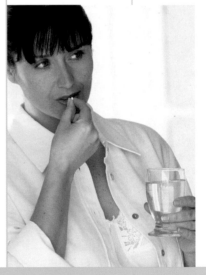

1-4

- You won't look any different, but your baby is starting to develop and his brain and spinal cord are beginning to form.
- Some women 'feel' they are pregnant soon after conception even before they have missed their next period.

You've missed your period. An over-the-counter test confirms that you're pregnant.

You should consult your healthcare provider about a booking appointment. If there's any confusion about how pregnant you are, you may be offered an early scan to confirm

Now is the time to make recommended changes that could affect your baby's health; eat more healthily and stop smoking and drinking.

You may notice a change in your breasts, due to hormonal stimulation of the milk-producing glands. Your breasts may feel full and tender, and your nipples may already be more prominent.

The areolae, the brownish circles of skin around the nipples, become darker, and blueish veins may be seen just under the skin as the blood supply to the breasts increases.

You may start to experience the nausea and vomiting of 'morning sickness', and you're likely to feel extremely tired.

Your heart rate rises steeply and your metabolic rate increases up to 25 per cent

Your 'booking appointment' will be scheduled between now and week 10 (see page 87). In addition to various tests, You will be offered a 'dating' scan (between 11 and 13 weeks) to confirm baby's due date and check on his health.

Your uterus has doubled in size since you conceived.

Although you won't look pregnant yet, you might notice that your waistband is starting to get tighter.

Your first antenatal visit will include routine blood tests to check things such as your blood count and Rhesus status (see page 89).

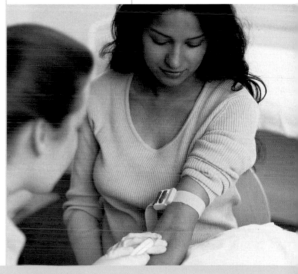

5-9

- A home pregnancy test can give you an accurate result from the first day of your missed period. If you subsequently start to bleed, you should be referred to an EPU (early pregnancy unit).
- The earliest physical signs of pregnancy, other than a missed period, include tiredness, changes in smell and taste and your breasts becoming fuller and more tender.
- It's very common to go off foods that you previously enjoyed.
- Mood swings are common, and you may feel emotionally vulnerable.

10　11　12　13

You may find yourself becoming upset or irritable over things that wouldn't normally bother you. This is due to hormonal changes, but can be exacerbated by natural anxieties about pregnancy and motherhood.

You may notice that your hands and feet feel warmer, due to the increase in blood volume. You may also find yourself feeling thirstier than usual, as your body signals that it needs extra fluids.

Your first ultrasound scan may be performed this week (or in the next two). It will give an EDD within five days, help screen for Down's syndrome and detect, if the present, whether you are carrying twins

It's normal to have gained around 1 kg (2¼ lbs) in weight by this stage, although some women actually lose weight in the first trimester if they suffer from nausea.

You may be offered a CVS test if there's a family history of cystic fibrosis, sickle cell disorder, thalassaemia or muscular dystrophy (see page 242).

If you suffered from morning sickness you should start to feel better now.

You can stop the folic acid supplement – your baby's nervous system is fully developed.

This marks the end of the first trimester, when the development of your baby's vital organs and structures is complete.

The risk of miscarriage is reduced by around 65 per cent.

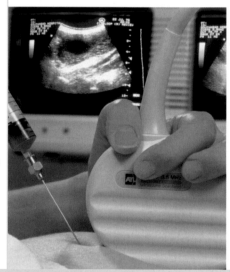

Chorionic villus sampling (CVS) can be carried out from around 11 weeks. It tests for chromosomal abnormalities and inherited disorders.

10-13

- ◆ You'll feel the urge to pass water more frequently.
- ◆ Changes in blood pressure make faintness or dizziness common, especially with changes in position, such as getting up from a chair quickly.
- ◆ Blood vessels may well be visible on your breasts and small nodules, called Montgomery's tubercles, may appear around your nipples.
- ◆ Hormonal changes may lead to a break out in spots.

23 24 25 26 27

23

As your abdomen grows, so does its impact on your digestive system. For some women this results in the discomforts of indigestion and heartburn.

To ease heartburn eat several small snacks, rather than two or three large meals, and, whenever possible, take a gentle walk after meals to aid digestion.

24

If you haven't already, start practising pelvic floor exercises now (see page 122) to strengthen your pelvic-floor muscles.

25

At your antenatal appointment, your healthcare provider sould check the size of your uterus, measure your blood pressure and check your urine for protein.

As your abdomen gets bigger and heavier, you may experience backache, pressure in the pelvis and cramps in the legs. Paying attention to your posture and getting plenty of rest will help.

Make sure you book your childbirth classes now. These will give you the opportunity to meet your healthcare providers and other mums-to-be.

26

From now until week 28, you may be offered a glucose screen for diabetes and blood test for anaemia.

If your are taking maternity leave, inform your employer in writing. Check the rights and benefits to which you are entitled.

27

This is the end of the second trimester. Your abdomen is now quite prominent, although its size depends on your height, weight and frame, whether or not you've been pregnant before, and the amount of amniotic fluid surrounding your baby.

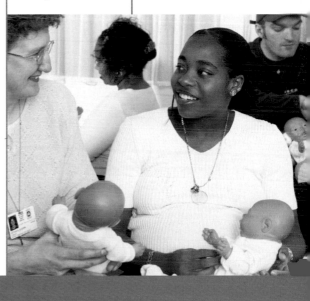

23-27

- ◆ With hormonal activity levelling out, you'll feel more relaxed and happy and less prone to mood swings.
- ◆ Pelvic-floor muscles are becoming stretched, which may result in stress incontinence (leaking urine when laughing or coughing).
- ◆ You'll be accumulating fat stores around your breasts and hips, and it's likely that your pre-pregnancy clothes won't fit anymore.
- ◆ Your heart and kidneys are working extra hard to maintain adequate blood circulation and process surplus fluids.

Your baby week by week

YOUR BABY'S SIZE

During the first trimester, babies follow a very predictable growth pattern, and measuring their body length, which can be done as early as 7 weeks, is the most accurate way of determining their age. It's easier to measure from crown to rump than from crown to heel, because the baby's legs are often bent. However, in later pregnancy, a baby's size can vary considerably, so measurements are less accurate at determining the baby's age.

The story of your unborn baby's development is an incredible one, beginning life as a fertilized egg and growing and maturing into a fully fledged human being, equipped with all the essential functions to survive in the outside world.

Conception usually occurs two weeks after a period. Most women, however, don't know exactly when they conceived, so it's easier for healthcare providers to date pregnancy from the first day of your last period. If, for example, your last period was ten weeks ago, you'll be considered in week 10 of your pregnancy, even though your baby will probably only be 8 weeks old. The descriptions below detail the development of your baby according to your weeks of pregnancy.

Pregnancy lasts for approximately 40 weeks. Babies born before 37 weeks are regarded as premature, while infants born after 40 weeks are regarded as postmature.

WEEK 4
...of your pregnancy.
Your baby is 2 weeks old.

Your baby measures between 0.36 and 1 mm (¹⁄₇₀ and ¹⁄₂₅ inch) from crown to rump.

This is a time of astounding development for your baby. At the end of the third week, the fertilized ovum (egg) is embedded in the lining of your uterus, where it continues to multiply and grow. What was originally a simple sperm and egg cell has become a blastocyst (fluid-filled ball) of several hundred cells. This blastocyst now divides into two, one half inside the other. The half attached to the wall of the uterus becomes the placenta. Its outer layer forms the umbilical cord, the amniotic and yolk sacs and the chorion (protective membranes in the uterus).

The inner half of the blastocyst will become your baby. This divides into three layers, known as germ layers, which grow to form different parts of your baby's body. The inner layer will form the liver, pancreas, bladder, thyroid gland and the lining of the gastrointestinal tract. The middle layer develops into muscle, bone, cartilage, blood vessels and kidneys, while the outer layer will become the brain and nervous system, skin and hair.

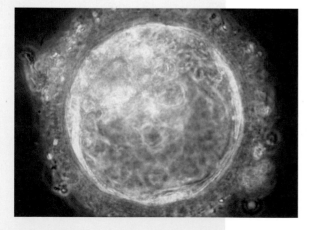

WEEK 5

...of your pregnancy.

Your baby is 3 weeks old.

Your baby measures about 1.25 mm (1/20 inch) from crown to rump.

What was a round mass of cells has begun to elongate and a head and tail are now distinguishable. The central nervous system begins to develop, and your baby's brain and spinal cord start to form.

Traces of the eyes and ears are discernible on the sides of her head, the liver and kidneys are beginning to develop, as are muscle and bone, although her bones will not ossify (harden) for a while yet. The walls of your baby's heart are now forming – it will begin to beat by the end of the week.

At this stage your baby derives most of her nourishment from the yolk sac and from nutrients stored in the uterine walls, but from as early as week 4 the placenta begins to provide nourishment.

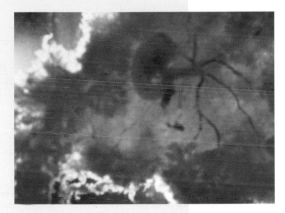

WEEK 6

...of your pregnancy.

Your baby is 4 weeks old.

Your baby measures about 2 to 4 mm (1/12 to 1/6 inch) from crown to rump.

Growth is very rapid this week. Your baby might look like a tadpole, with his curved back and tail, but he now has a brain. His tiny heart is no bigger than a poppy seed, but it is beating on its own. Other major organs, including the kidneys and liver, continue to develop, and the neural tube, which connects the brain and spinal cord, closes. Your baby's head now begins to take shape.

A rudimentary digestive tract begins to form, together with the abdominal and chest cavities and the backbone. What will eventually become the testes or ovaries appear as a cluster of cells. Rudimentary arms and legs appear as tiny buds on the body. Your baby now has his own bloodstream, which has started to circulate blood.

Your baby measures about 4 to 5 mm (⅙ to ⅕ inch) from crown to rump.

Your baby is beginning to look more human now, and her tail has almost vanished. However, her head is still bumpy and bent forwards. Dark spots on the sides of her head will be her eyes, two

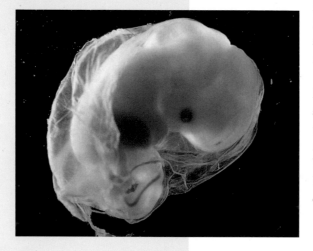

holes represent the beginning of nostrils, and her lips, tongue and first tooth buds are visible. Her arms and legs have lengthened, and she has rudimentary hands and feet.

This is a vulnerable stage for your baby when all her major organs are forming, so you need to avoid any potential hazards, which could adversely affect this development. Her heart has divided into the right and left chambers and is beating about 150 beats a minute – about twice the rate of an adult. Her liver, kidneys, lungs, intestines and internal sex organs are all nearing completion.

Your baby measures just over 14 to 20 mm (½ inch) from crown to rump.

Your baby's head is still larger than the rest of his body, and his facial features continue to develop. He now has a tongue and nostrils – you can even see the tip of his nose – while his jaw is fusing to shape his mouth. The next eight days are crucial for the development of his

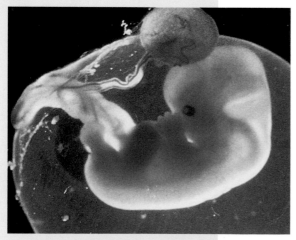

eyes and inner ears, responsible for balance and hearing.

Most of your baby's internal organs such as his heart, brain, liver, lungs and kidneys have developed in their basic forms. His intestines are starting to develop in the umbilical cord. His heartbeat has normalized and the pumping capacity has increased. Under his paper-thin skin, you can see a network of blood vessels.

Up to now, your baby's framework has been made up of cartilage. Now bone cells begin to replace this. His leg and arm bones are hardening and lengthening, and his joints start to form. He begins to move around, although you can't feel him yet.

WEEK 9

...of your pregnancy.

Your baby is 7 weeks old.

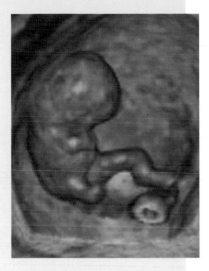

Your baby measures about 22 to 30 mm (1 inch) from crown to rump.

Your baby is now beginning to look like a proper baby. This three-dimensional (3D) ultrasound scan clearly shows her head bent forwards onto her chest, and her developing limbs. Her hands, feet and limbs are growing quite fast. Her fingers and toes are nearly complete, and touch pads form on the fingers. Her eyelids almost cover her eyes and her nose has taken shape.

During the next few days your baby's diaphragm will develop; this is the muscle that will enable her to breathe after birth. Her intestines now begin to move out of the umbilical cord, where they started to form, and into her abdominal cavity where the space is increasing as her body gets bigger.

WEEK 10

...of your pregnancy.

Your baby is 8 weeks old.

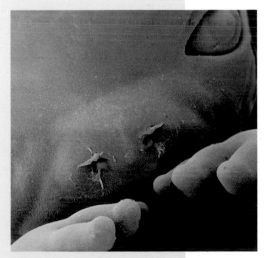

Your baby measures about 31 to 42 mm (1¼ to 1⅝ inches) from crown to rump and weighs about 5 g (⅕ oz).

Your baby switches from being an embryo to a fetus – meaning 'little one' – this week. His brain has grown so much that his head still looks too big for the rest of his body. His eyes and nose are clearly visible. Twenty tiny tooth buds are forming in his gums.

Your baby's wrists and ankles have formed by now, and you can make out fingers and toes. Most of his joints are formed. Genitals have begun to form, but still it's too early to distinguish the sex.

Your baby's nervous system is responsive and many of his internal organs begin to function. His lungs continue to develop, and his stomach and intestines are developing in his abdomen. His kidneys are moving into their final positions in the upper abdomen, and his heart is almost completely developed.

WEEK 11
...of your pregnancy.
Your baby is 9 weeks old.

Your baby measures about 44 to 60 mm (1¾ to 2¼ inches) from crown to rump, and weighs about 8 g (⅓ oz).

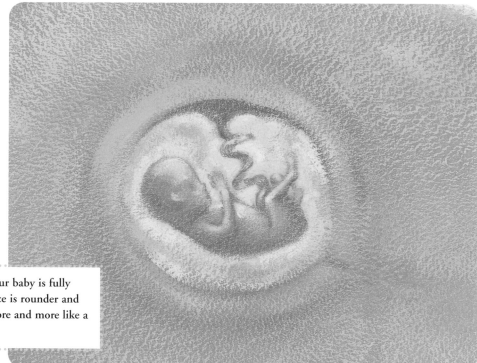

Your baby's development has passed its critical stage, and from now on she'll be at less risk of developing any sort of congenital abnormality or being affected by most infections and certain drugs.

By the end of the week her body will double in length, and her head will be almost half the length of her body. Underneath her fused eyelids, the irises start to develop, and these will later protect her eyes from too much light. However, her ears won't be fully developed for some time. Even this early on, your baby can yawn, suck and swallow.

Your baby's vital organs – liver, kidneys, intestines, brain and lungs – are fully formed and beginning to operate. For the rest of the pregnancy they just need to grow. Finishing touches, such as fingernails and downy hair, start to appear. Her heart carries on pumping blood to all her internal organs, including the umbilical cord, which transfers blood to the placenta.

At week 12, your baby is fully formed. His face is rounder and he's looking more and more like a human baby.

WEEK 12

...of your pregnancy.
Your baby is 10 weeks old.

Your baby measures about 61 mm (2½ inches) from crown to rump, and weighs between 8 to 14 g (⅓ to ½ oz).

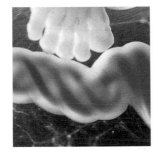

Your baby is fully formed from head to toe, although his organs continue to develop, particularly the brain. His fingers and toes have separated, and his hair and nails are growing. His bones continue to harden. The genitals begin to take on their gender characteristics. Your baby's vocal chords are forming, and the pituitary gland at the base of the brain is beginning to make hormones.

It's astonishing what your baby can do at this stage: he can move his arms, fingers and toes; he can smile, frown and suck his thumb.

His digestive system is now capable of absorbing glucose (sugar). However, the umbilical cord is busy circulating blood between the placenta and your baby to provide nourishment and get rid of waste products produced by his rapid growth.

WEEK 13

...of your pregnancy.
Your baby is 11 weeks old.

Your baby measures 65 to 78 mm (2⅗ to 3 inches) from crown to rump and weighs between 13 to 20 g (½ to ⅔ oz).

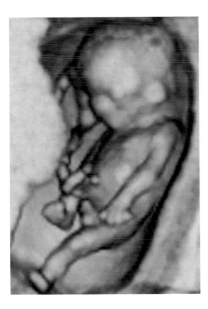

Although fully formed – as seen on this 3D ultrasound scan – your baby wouldn't be able to survive outside the uterus yet, as her internal organs, particularly her lungs, haven't matured sufficiently. The intestines have moved farther into her body, while her liver begins to secrete bile, and her pancreas starts to produce insulin. The external genital organs continue to grow.

Your baby's neck is fully formed and can support head movements. Her eyes are moving into position on the front of her head, and her ears move to their normal position. Research suggests that your baby starts to sense sounds now. The ears aren't fully formed until around 24 weeks, but it's thought that babies 'hear' sound through vibration receptors on their skin.

WEEK 14

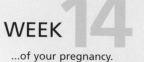

...of your pregnancy.

Your baby is 12 weeks old.

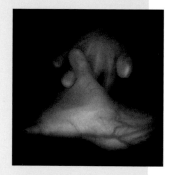

Your baby measures about 80 to 93 mm (3¼ to 4 inches) from crown to rump now and weighs almost 25 g (1 oz).

This week marks the beginning of the second trimester. Your baby's growth speeds up as his internal organs mature. The placenta is now his support system, producing hormones and supplying him with essential nutrients and oxygen.

Your baby's movements are now less jerky, and he can bend, flex and twist his fingers, hands, wrists, legs, knees and toes. His nervous system has begun to function. His eyelids, fingernails and toenails continue to develop, and he has a sprinkling of hair on his head.

Your baby now 'practises' the movements of breathing in and out, in readiness for life outside the uterus. He doesn't need to breathe in his watery world, as his oxygen comes straight from you, via the umbilical cord and the placenta.

WEEK 15

...of your pregnancy.

Your baby is 13 weeks old.

Your baby measures 104 to 114 mm (4 to 4½ inches) from crown to rump and weighs about 50 g (1¾ oz).

Your baby's ribs, blood vessels and retinas – which appear as dark spots on her head – are clearly visible through her wafer-thin skin, but her skin now starts to be covered with lanugo, extra-fine hair that helps to regulate her body temperature. This body hair follows the pattern of her skin, creating patterns that look like fingerprints all over her body. She also starts to develop eyebrows and the hair on her head continues to grow, but this hair may change its colour and texture after she's born.

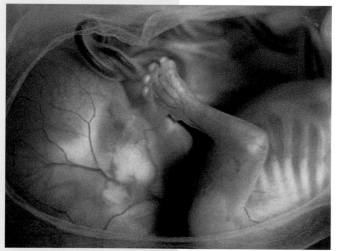

The mechanisms enabling your baby to hear are developing. Very small bones in her middle ear have begun to harden, but as her brain's auditory centres haven't developed yet, she won't be able to make sense of the sounds she hears. The amniotic fluid she swims in acts as a sound conductor, so over time she'll begin to hear your voice and your heartbeat.

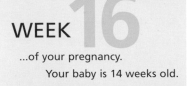

WEEK 16

...of your pregnancy.

Your baby is 14 weeks old.

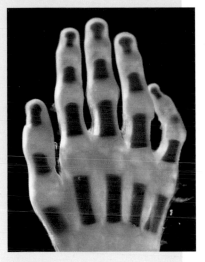

Your baby measures about 108 to 116 mm (4⅓ to 4⅗ inches) from crown to rump and weighs 80 g (2¾ oz).

Your baby's arms and legs are complete and his joints are working. Bones that have already formed are getting harder and retaining calcium – a process known as ossifying. On the picture, left, hardened bone shows up as dark red.

Your baby's nervous system is operating and his muscles are responding to stimulation from his brain, so he can coordinate his movements. He continues to be very active in his private space, rolling over, doing somersaults and kicking. However, you won't feel more than a fluttering sensation, as amniotic fluid cushions your baby's more vigorous movements. If this is your first baby, you won't usually recognize these movements for another few weeks.

You can now tell your baby's sex on an ultrasound scan. He also sheds cells and secretes chemicals into the amniotic fluid, and a sample taken via an amniocentesis (see page 243) can reveal important information about his health.

WEEK 17

...of your pregnancy.

Your baby is 15 weeks old.

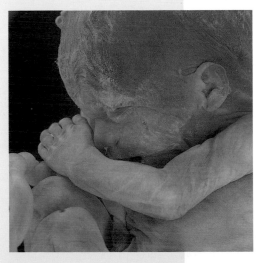

Your baby measures about 11 to 12 cm (4½ to 5 inches) from crown to rump and weighs about 100 g (3½ oz).

Your baby's head, while still big, is beginning to look in proportion with the rest of her body. Her eyes are still closed but are much larger, and her eyelashes and eyebrows have grown longer. This is a period of rapid growth, as fat starts to be laid down under your baby's skin, helping her to keep warm and giving her energy. She's getting more hair on her head, eyebrows and eyelashes, and she has fingernails and toenails in miniature. Her small heart is pumping as much as 24 litres (42 pints) of blood a day.

Your baby can now hear sounds outside your body, and some can even make her jump. As she practises breathing, her chest rises and falls. Her lungs are beginning to exhale amniotic fluid.

Your baby measures 12.5 to 14 cm (5 to 5¾ inches) from crown to rump and weighs about 150 g (5¼ oz).

There's no stopping your baby now as he begins his most active phase. He's twisting, turning, wriggling, punching and kicking, and generally giving his reflexes a good work-out.

Inside his fast-growing lungs, tiny air sacs called alveoli begin to develop. Pads have formed on his fingertips and toes, and the unique swirls and whorls that are your baby's fingerprints begin to appear. His eyes have moved to their correct position. Meconium, which forms your baby's first bowel movement, is accumulating in his bowels. If your baby is a boy, his prostate gland is forming.

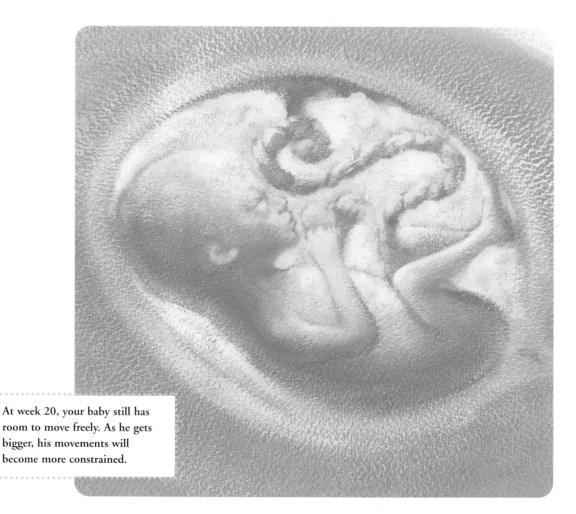

At week 20, your baby still has room to move freely. As he gets bigger, his movements will become more constrained.

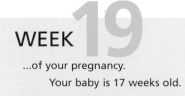

WEEK 19

...of your pregnancy.
Your baby is 17 weeks old.

Your baby measures about 13 to 15 cm (5¼ to 6 inches) from crown to rump and weighs about 200 g (7 oz).

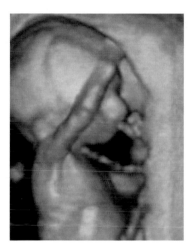

A thick, white greasy substance called vernix caseosa is being secreted by glands in your baby's skin. This acts as a waterproof barrier, to prevent her skin from getting waterlogged in the amniotic fluid.

Throughout your baby's body, nerves are being coated with a fatty substance called myelin, which insulates the nerves, allowing the smooth, rapid exchange of information necessary for coordinated, skilful movement. The poorly coordinated movements of newborns – and particularly premature infants – are for the most part due to their comparative lack of myelin.

Your baby's gut has begun to produce gastric juices that help to absorb amniotic fluid and pass it to her kidneys where it's filtered and excreted back into the amniotic sac.

WEEK 20

...of your pregnancy.
Your baby is 18 weeks old.

Your baby measures about 14 to 16 cm (5½ to 6½ inches) from crown to rump and weighs about 255 g (9 oz).

Your baby has reached the halfway mark. He's still tiny but growing rapidly. This is a crucial stage for the development of his senses – taste, smell, hearing, sight and touch. Now your baby can finally hear and recognize your voice. The nerve cells serving each of the

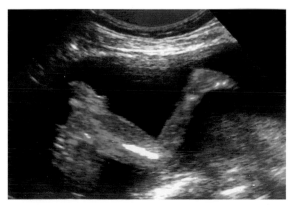

senses are now developing into their particular areas of the brain. The increase in the number of nerve cells is slowing, but the complex connections required for the development of memory and thinking functions are being formed.

If your baby is a girl, she already has roughly 2 million eggs in her ovaries. However, by the time she's born, this number will have reduced to a mere million.

She can also enjoy a good stretch of her limbs – a tiny leg is coloured blue on the ultrasound, left – as her nervous and muscular systems have developed enough to allow this.

WEEK 21

...of your pregnancy.

Your baby is 19 weeks old.

Your baby measures about 16 cm (7¼ inches) from crown to rump and weighs about 300 g (10½ oz).

Your baby's digestive system is developed enough to absorb water from the amniotic fluid she swallows. At full term, your baby can swallow as much as 500 ml (18 fl oz) of amniotic fluid in a 24-hour period. In the early stages, amniotic fluid is produced by the placenta. Once the baby's kidneys start functioning, from about the fourth month, they take over this production. Although your baby's kidneys remove some waste products from her blood and make urine, there isn't much urine in the amniotic fluid. Most waste products are conveyed through the placenta to your bloodstream and are then filtered by your kidneys.

The senses your baby will use to learn about the world are developing daily. Taste buds have formed on her tongue, and the development of her brain and nerve endings are advanced enough to let her sense touch. She can be seen on ultrasound sucking her thumb or stroking her face.

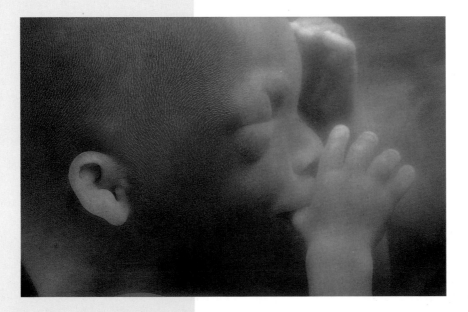

WEEK 22

...of your pregnancy.

Your baby is 20 weeks old.

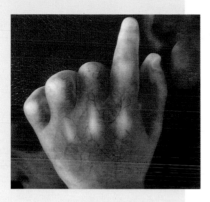

Your baby measures about 19 cm (7½ inches) from crown to rump and weighs about 350 g (12¼ oz).

Your baby now has sweat glands and his skin is less transparent, although blood vessels can still been seen. His fingernails are fully formed and continuing to grow. If your baby is a boy, his testes have begun their descent from the pelvis to the scrotum. Primitive sperm have already formed in the testes.

Your baby's brain has begun to grow very quickly now, especially in the germinal matrix, a structure in the centre of the brain that manufactures brain cells. This structure vanishes before birth but your baby's brain will keep on expanding until the age of 5.

WEEK 23

...of your pregnancy.

Your baby is 21 weeks old.

Your baby measures about 20 cm (8 inches) from crown to rump and weighs almost 455 g (1 lb).

Your baby's body is becoming better proportioned each day and looking like a full-term baby, but her bones and organs are still visible beneath her transparent skin.

Her hearing is much more acute now, as the bones of her inner ear have hardened. She can distinguish different noises from outside the uterus and from inside your body. You'd be surprised just how noisy your body is, with the gurgling of your stomach, the thump of your heartbeat and the rushing of your blood around your body.

At birth, your baby will recognize your voice by its pitch and cadences, so talk to her as much as possible now. Fathers should talk to their unborn babies as well. Research shows that deeper 'male' voices are easier for your baby to hear than high-pitched 'female' voices. Playing games such as patting your tummy and talking, may elicit a kick in response and help neurological stimulation.

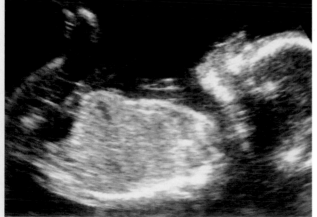

WEEK 24

...of your pregnancy.
Your baby is 22 weeks old.

Your baby measures 21 cm (8½ inches) from crown to rump and weighs about 540 g (1¼ lbs).

If your baby was born now, he'd have a one-in-four or five chance of survival. But he's still quite thin and covered in fine body hair. His body is starting to produce white blood cells to fight infection.

His lungs have developed just enough to give him a chance of surviving in a neonatal intensive care unit. But he continues to practise breathing by inhaling amniotic fluid into his developing

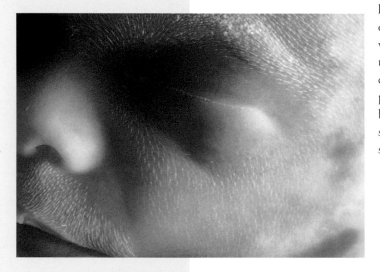

lungs. Airway passages form tubes in order to take in and expel air. Blood vessels and air sacs start to develop in the lungs – these will eventually exchange oxygen and circulate it to all parts of his body. The cells in your baby's lungs begin to produce surfactant, a substance that keeps the sacs from sticking together.

WEEK 25

...of your pregnancy.
Your baby is 23 weeks old.

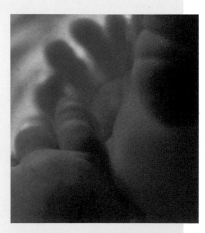

Your baby measures about 22 cm (8¾ inches) from crown to rump and weighs 700 g (1½ lbs).

Your baby can now hold her feet and curl her hand into a fist. Blood vessels continue to develop in her lungs, and her nostrils begin to open. High inside the gums, your baby's permanent teeth are developing in buds. These adult teeth won't descend until the baby teeth – also called primary teeth – start to fall out at about age 6. Meanwhile, nerves around the mouth and lip area are showing more sensitivity now, preparing your baby for the essential task of finding her mother's nipple once she is born.

That crucial lifeline, the umbilical cord, is thick and resilient now. A single vein and two arteries run through it, encased in a firm jelly-like substance that prevents kinking and knotting, protecting the blood flow between placenta and baby.

WEEK 26

...of your pregnancy.

Your baby is 24 weeks old.

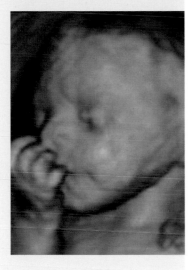

Your baby measures about 23 cm (9¼ inches) from crown to rump and weighs almost 910 g (2 lbs).

Your baby's lungs are still maturing and he still has some growing to do. His spine is getting stronger and more supple to support his growing body, and a friend may be able to hear his heartbeat just by putting an ear to your abdomen. Your baby can inhale and exhale. His eyes have completely formed. His pulse quickens as he reacts to sounds; he'll even move in rhythm to music. Studies of fetal brain activity show that your baby can now respond to touch.

WEEK 27

...of your pregnancy.

Your baby is 25 weeks old.

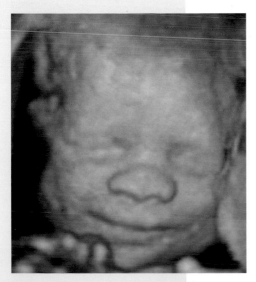

Your baby measures about 24 cm (9½ inches) from crown to rump and weighs a little over 1 kg (2 lbs).

Your baby is becoming plumper and rounder as the amount of fat under her skin increases. Thumb-sucking may now be one of your baby's favourite activities, strengthening her cheek and jaw muscles and possibly soothing her. Her lungs continue to grow. She now has fully functioning taste buds on her tongue and inside her cheeks, and her higher brain functions are becoming more sophisticated.

At about this time, your baby's eyelids begin to open, and the retinas begin to form. Babies now seem to be able to detect changes in light, and studies have shown that when a torch is shone against a mother's abdomen, the baby may move towards – or sometimes away from – its beam. Your baby's first visual impressions outside the uterus will be sorted into light and dark, too – that's why many toys designed for newborns are black and white. Her eyelashes are fully grown now, and will protect her delicate eyeballs from harmful matter once she's born.

WEEK 28

...of your pregnancy.
Your baby is 26 weeks old.

Your baby measures about 25 cm (10 inches) from crown to rump and weighs about 1.1 kg (2½ lbs).

Your busy baby is growing and developing at top speed. His lungs are capable of breathing air, but if he's born now he would find it hard to breathe properly. He will enjoy hearing your voice now so carry on talking to him. Next week you officially enter the third trimester, when your baby's main job will be to put on weight.

In baby boys, the testes are beginning their descent into the scrotum by this point. In baby girls, the labia are still small and don't yet cover the clitoris. The labia will grow closer together in the last few weeks of pregnancy.

> **At week 28, your baby's getting fatter and rounder and his muscle tone is getting better.**

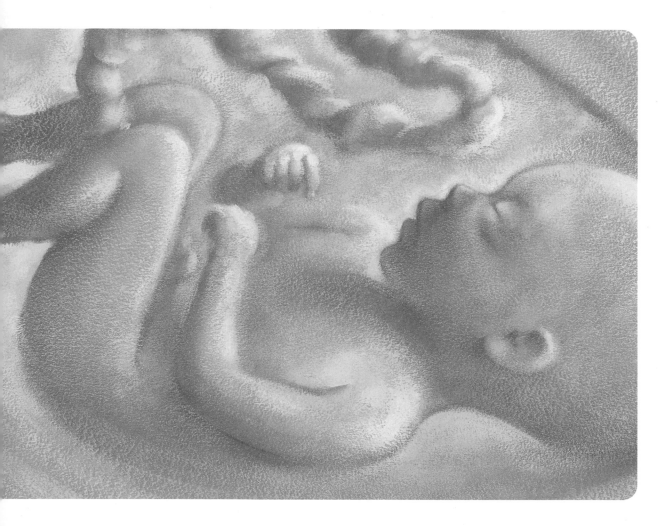

WEEK 29

...of your pregnancy.
Your baby is 27 weeks old.

Your baby measures about 26 cm (10½ inches) from crown to rump and weighs about 1.25 kg (2¾ lbs).

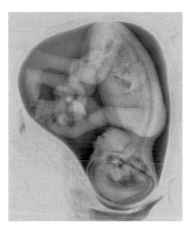

Your baby continues to fatten up as her brain and organs carry on growing. These soft tissues show up clearly on a magnetic resonance image (MRI) scan, which uses magnetic fields and radio waves. She doesn't have as much room now so she can't show off her acrobatic skills, but she's still managing to stretch and kick you from inside.

Your baby's brain is growing so quickly that the soft skull bones are being pressed outwards, and her head is now in proportion to the rest of her body. Her brain is looking more wrinkled as it gets faster and more powerful, building up connections between nerve cells. Her brain can control her breathing and body temperature. Her eyes can move in their sockets, and she's becoming more sensitive to light, sound, taste and smell. Through the wall of the uterus she can tell the difference between sunlight and artificial light.

WEEK 30

...of your pregnancy.
Your baby is 28 weeks old.

Your baby measures about 27 cm (10¾ inches) from crown to rump and weighs about 1.36 kg (3 lbs).

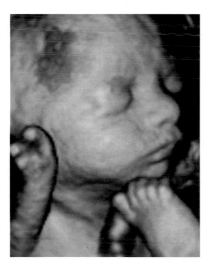

Your baby's lanugo (early body hair) is disappearing. The few fuzzy patches left at birth will rub off over the following weeks. The hair on his head is thicker, his eyelids open and close, and his toenails are growing. The bone marrow has taken over the task of red blood cell production from the liver. His skeleton is hardening (ossifying) even more and the brain, muscles and lungs continue to mature.

Many babies adopt the head-down position in the uterus now, the most common and most straightforward position for birth. Prepare to feel strong kicks under your ribcage and pressure on your pelvic floor when your baby presses down on it.

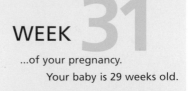

WEEK 31

...of your pregnancy.
Your baby is 29 weeks old.

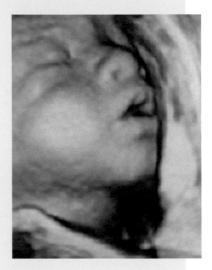

Your baby measures about 28 cm (11¼ inches) from crown to rump and weighs about 1.59 kg (3½ lbs).

While your baby's overall growth starts to slow, she will continue to put on weight. Her brain is continuing its growth spurt. Her lungs will be the last major organ to become fully mature.

Her eye colour begins to appear around now, but the real colour won't show for six to nine months after birth, as eye pigmentation needs light exposure to complete its formation. Dark-skinned babies usually have dark grey or brown eyes at birth, developing into a true brown or black after the first six months or year. Most Caucasian babies are born with dark blue eyes and their true eye colour may not be apparent for weeks or months. In the meantime, her eyes are being prepared for life after birth. Her pupils start to dilate in reaction to the reddish light that filters into the uterus. Her eyelids are frequently open during active times and closed during sleep.

WEEK 32

...of your pregnancy.
Your baby is 30 weeks old.

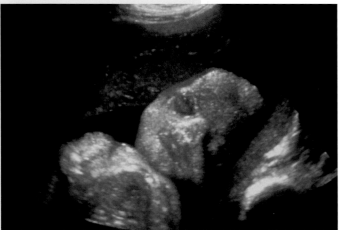

Your baby measures about 29 cm (11½ inches) from crown to rump and weighs 1.8 kg (4 lbs).

All of your baby's five senses are working and he can show off a new skill – turning his head from side to side. His organs are continuing to mature, his toenails are complete, and hair on his head is still growing. He continues to practise opening and closing his eyes, but he sleeps 90 to 95 per cent of the day.

Your baby's 'breathing lessons' continue to help his lungs to strengthen and mature. Recent studies have shown that this vital practice also encourages the lungs to produce more surfactant, the protein that's essential for the lungs' healthy development.

WEEK 33

...of your pregnancy.

Your baby is 31 weeks old.

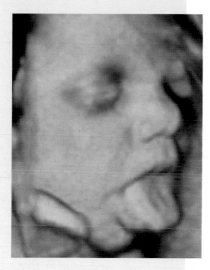

Your baby measures about 30 cm (12 inches) from crown to rump and weighs almost 2 kg (4½ lbs).

The amniotic fluid is at its highest level and will remain at this level until the birth. Rapid brain growth has increased the size of your baby's head by approximately 9.5 mm (⅜ inch) this week. Fat continues to accumulate, and this turns her skin from red to pink.

Your baby doesn't have much elbow room these days, as you can see from this 3D ultrasound scan, so her movements will feel more like rolls than kicks, and you'll be spared all those digs in the ribs. You may also notice that your actions affect her movements – how much and when you eat, what position you are in, and sounds from the world outside can all influence your baby's activity level.

Take some time each day to relax and check her movements. Your healthcare provider will be able to give you guidelines on how much movement you should feel – for example, you may be told to expect about six movements in one hour, but not every hour of the day.

WEEK 34

...of your pregnancy.

Your baby is 32 weeks old.

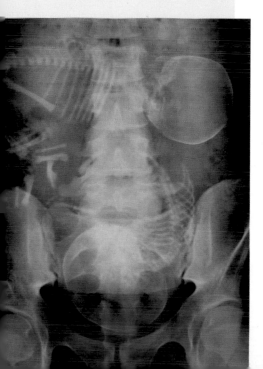

Your baby measures about 31 cm (12½ inches) from crown to rump and weighs almost 2.275 kg (5 lbs).

Your baby's developing his immune system to fight mild infection. The ends of his fingers are tiny, but he has sharp fingernails.

He's too big to float about in the amniotic fluid now and his movements are bigger and slower. He may have settled into the head-down position, although 3 to 4 per cent of all babies will be lying with their bottoms or legs towards the cervix in the 'breech presentation'. A doctor may sometimes encourage a baby to turn into the correct position with a procedure called 'external cephalic version'. This involves manipulating the baby through the abdomen manually, and is best carried out in a hospital so that mother and baby can be closely monitored.

With twins, as can be seen on the coloured X-ray, left, only one baby may be able to fit into the head-down position, while his twin fits around him as best he can.

WEEK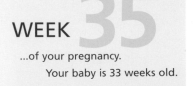

...of your pregnancy.

Your baby is 33 weeks old.

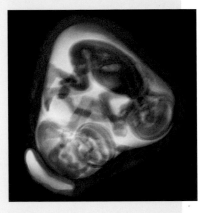

Your baby measures about 32 cm (12¾ inches) from crown to rump and weighs over 2.55 kg (5½ lbs).

Ninety-nine per cent of babies born now survive without any major problems. The central nervous system is maturing, the digestive system is almost complete, the lungs are usually fully mature, and respiratory problems are much less likely to occur if the baby is born prematurely at this stage.

   Your baby's arms and legs are plumping up nicely – in fact she's big enough to take up most of the uterus, and there's less room to move around. With twins, the conditions are even more cramped, as can be seen on this MRI scan – the pink area is the shared placenta.

WEEK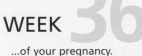

...of your pregnancy.

Your baby is 34 weeks old.

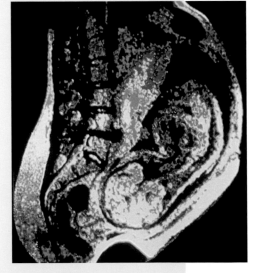

Your baby measures over 33 cm (13 inches) from crown to rump and weighs about 2.75 kg (6 lbs).

No doubt you've noticed a change in your baby's movements by now, as your uterus is getting very tight for space. He may wriggle about less because of this constriction, but his movements will generally be stronger and more defined. You may be able to see the outline of certain body parts such as an elbow or a heel appearing under your skin.

   By this stage, most babies will have assumed the head-down position ready for birth. This MRI scan shows the baby resting with its head in the lower part of the uterus.

WEEK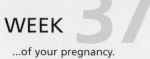

...of your pregnancy.

Your baby is 35 weeks old.

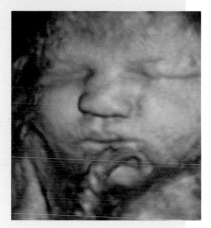

Your baby measures about 34 cm (13½ inches) from crown to rump and weighs almost 2.95 kg (6½ lbs).

Your baby is now considered full term, meaning that she can be born any day. As shown by a 3D ultrasound scan, she looks like a newborn. If your baby is lying in the breech position, your healthcare provider may offer external cephalic version now (see page 205). If labour starts now, no effort will be made to delay it. Research suggests that it's actually your baby who triggers labour, producing hormones as a reaction to her cramped surroundings.

Through most of the pregnancy, your baby has relied on you for protection against infections, but gradually her own immune system has begun to develop. It will carry on developing after birth, and breastfeeding will boost your baby's immunity. At first, your breasts produce colostrum, a substance rich in nutrients and antibodies. The breast milk that follows is nutritionally balanced and will help to protect your baby against infections and build her immunity.

WEEK 38

...of your pregnancy.

Your baby is 36 weeks old.

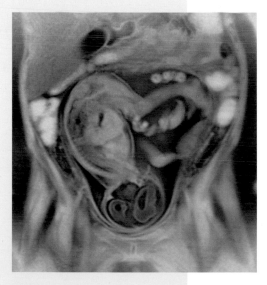

Your baby measures about 35 cm (14 inches) from crown to rump and weighs about 3.1 kg (6¾ lbs).

Your baby is clinically mature, and he's ready to be born any time now. All his body systems have developed, and it may be possible to see them on an MRI scan. His intestines have been accumulating waste material, a greenish-black, sticky substance called meconium, which he may pass before or after birth. His head and abdomen have about the same circumference.

Your healthcare provider will probably be able to give you an idea of your baby's size at this point, but be aware that this will just be an estimate – no one knows just how big a baby will be until birth.

The placenta starts aging now, as its role of sustaining your baby comes to an end. It becomes less efficient at transferring nutrients, and blood clots and calcified patches begin to show.

Your baby measures about 36 cm (14½ inches) from crown to rump and weighs just over 3.25 kg (7 lbs).

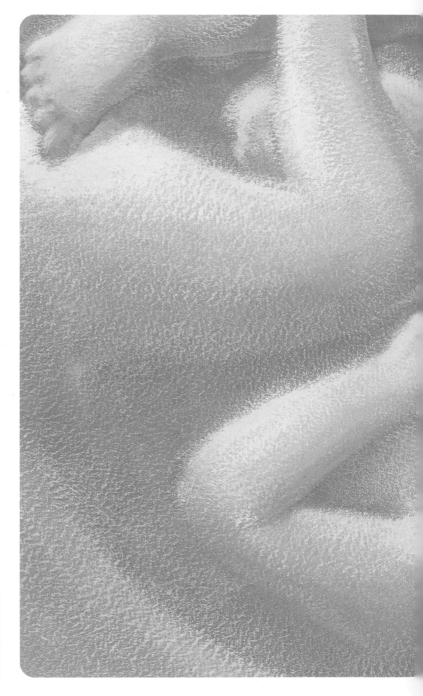

Most of your baby's lanugo is gone now as she prepares for birth. Your baby will swallow her lanugo, along with other secretions, and store them in her bowels. These will add to your infant's first bowel movement, a blackish waste called meconium. Her lungs are maturing and surfactant production is increasing. You may not feel all her movements at this stage. At 51 cm (20 inches) long, the umbilical cord is about as long as your baby from head to toe.

Pregnancy hormones produced by your body may cause the breasts in both newborn boys and girls to be swollen at birth and even produce tiny quantities of milk. The genitalia – the labia in girls and the scrotum in boys – may appear enlarged as well. All these side effects should disappear shortly after birth when your baby's detached from your blood supply. At the time of birth, your baby has no fewer than 300 bones, which is more than adults, who possess 206. Some of these bones fuse together as your baby grows.

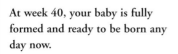

At week 40, your baby is fully formed and ready to be born any day now.

WEEK 40

...of your pregnancy.

Your baby is 38 weeks old.

Your baby measures about 37 to 38 cm (14¾ to 15¼ inches) from crown to rump, with a total length of about 48 cm (21½ inches).

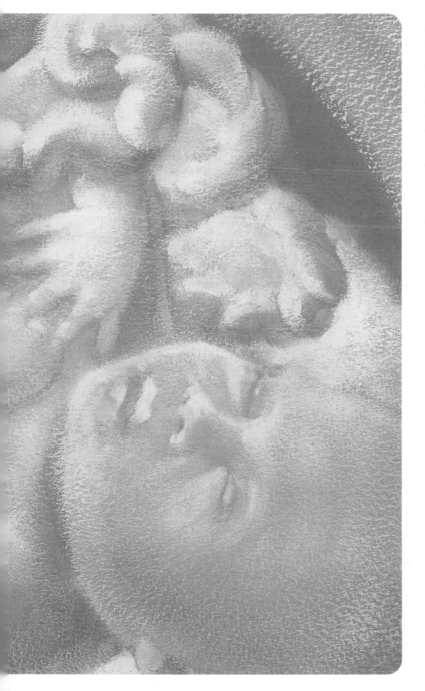

Equipped with over 70 different reflexes, your baby's ready to start his new life outside the uterus. At this point, most of the vernix is gone, 15 per cent of his body is fat, and his chest sticks out. At birth the placenta will peel away from the side of the uterus, and the umbilical cord will stop working as your baby takes his very first breaths of air. His breathing will trigger changes in the structure of his heart and arteries, which will divert blood to his lungs.

Weeks

28 | 29 | 30 | 31

Mentally and physically this is an exciting but demanding time, as you enter the last three months of your pregnancy. Some women feel great during this last trimester, others feel exhausted. Anxiety about the impending birth is very common, too. Expect to put on between 4.5 and 5.4 kg (10 and 12 lbs) during this last trimester, 3 to 3.6 kg (7 to 8 lbs) of which is due to your baby.

28

At your antenatal vist, your blood pressure and urine will be checked and the size and position of your uterus measured.

If you are rhesus (Rh) negative, you will be given anti-D treatment.

Between now and week 38, you will be offered the whooping cough vaccine.

Stretch marks may appear around now, usually on your tummy and breasts.

29

Sometimes pressure on the veins that take blood from the legs to the heart can cause varicose veins.

Your uterus has grown around 4 cm (1½) inches and will now be pushing up against the bottom of your ribcage, making the lower ribs spread out, which may cause mild discomfort.

If you want to have a birth plan, now is the time to start writing it, including issues such as the kind of birth you want and your views on pain relief.

30

The weight of your growing baby and changes to your centre of gravity can put increasing strain on your back.

31

At your antenatal vist, your blood pressure and urine will be checked and the size of your uterus measured. The results of any screening tests will be discussed.

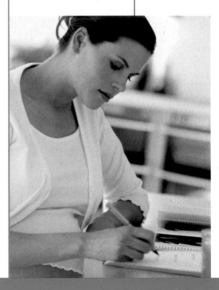

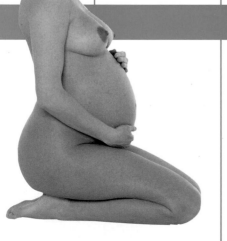

28-31

- Your belly button may be stretched and elongated, and may start to protrude, but it will return to normal after the birth.
- Your legs can feel heavy and tired in late pregnancy, and you will need to rest more often.
- Breathlessness is common, due to the increased effort needed to move around. Your lungs also have to absorb about 20 per cent more oxygen and expel more carbon dioxide with each breath as you breathe for your baby.

32

As your pregnancy progresses you continue to put on weight and may be doing so faster than at any other time in your pregnancy. Your uterus is approaching the highest position it will reach, with the top sitting about 12 cm (5 inches) above your belly button.

You may find that you are becoming unusually forgetful. Your baby takes up more and more of your concentration as you approach the birth.

33

If this is your first baby, he may have moved into the head-down position as he gets ready to be born. Once this happens, your breathing will become easier and any indigestion should start to improve.

You may notice that the rings on your hand feel tight, or that your feet and hands are swollen. This is due to fluid retention, but it can be made worse if tight clothing restricts your blood flow

34

At your antenatal visit, your blood pressure and urine will be checked and the size of your uterus measured. The results of any screening tests will be discussed. You will be given advice on recognising and coping with labour and about creating a birth plan.

You will be putting on weight faster than at any other time in your pregnancy and you may be surprised at how big your tummy is growing.

35

The pregnancy hormone relaxin, coupled with the weight of your baby, causes your pelvic joints to expand in readiness for the birth resulting in some aches and pains.

A Group B strep test (see page 363) may be done.

36

At your antenatal vist, your blood pressure and urine will be checked and the size of your uterus measured. Baby's position will be checked. You will be given advice on tests for and how to care for your newborn and safeguard your own health post birth.

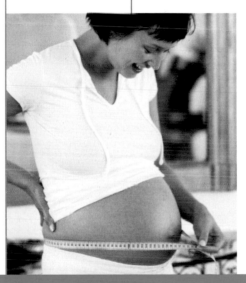

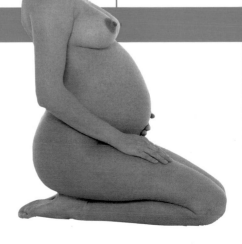

32-36

- The placenta reaches maturity at around 34 weeks and from then on it starts to age.
- The amount of blood in your body has increased by 50 per cent during the first two trimesters. After 34 weeks, it remains constant until you give birth.
- A common symptom at this stage is a tingling sensation or pressure in the pelvic area, due to your baby moving down the uterus.
- Your nipples enlarge and your breasts become heavier.

37

You are likely to experience 'practice contractions' known as Braxton Hicks contractions from now on. This is when your uterus hardens for around 30 seconds, then relaxes. These contractions should not be painful.

You may find that you dream a lot and that your dreams are extremely vivid.

38

At your antenatal vist, your blood pressure and urine will be checked and the position of your uterus measured. The options should you go overdue will be discussed.

Some women experience depression in late pregnancy, the result of a mixture of emotions – anxiety about the forthcoming birth, fatigue due to lack of sleep and a desire for the pregnancy to end. If you feel this way, talk through your feelings with your healthcare provider and try to take time out for yourself.

39

Your uterus is taking up all the space in your pelvis and a great deal of room in your abdomen so you may be feeling very uncomfortable.

The baby usually gets into the birth position at around 33 to 36 weeks. Your healthcare provider will examine you at each visit to check how your baby is lying.

40

If you haven't given birth (only 5% of babies are born exactly on their EDD), your blood pressure and urine will be checked and the position of your uterus measured.

41-2

You will continue to be seen for two weeks for regular checks. At 41 weeks, you may be offered a membrane sweep and at 42 weeks, options for inducing delivery will be discussed.

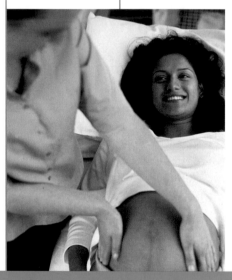

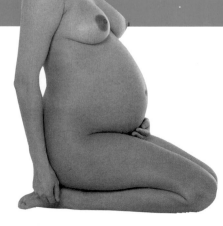

37-40

- ◆ Your feelings of excitement or nervousness may increase.
- ◆ Your weight is likely to plateau, and a few women actually lose weight in the last week or so before the birth.
- ◆ As the uterus presses against the ribcage you may experience some discomfort. Skin stretching tightly over the abdomen can become itchy.
- ◆ You may look a little flushed as your circulation works harder than ever before.

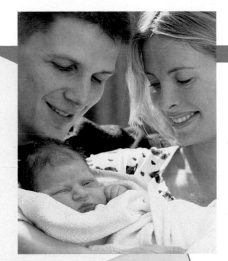

the moment of birth

Once his head is born, *your baby turns to straighten his neck, so he's facing your side* again. With the next contraction his shoulders are born, one before the other, with his arms held close to his body. Once his shoulders are through, the rest of his body slips out quickly – your baby has arrived at last.

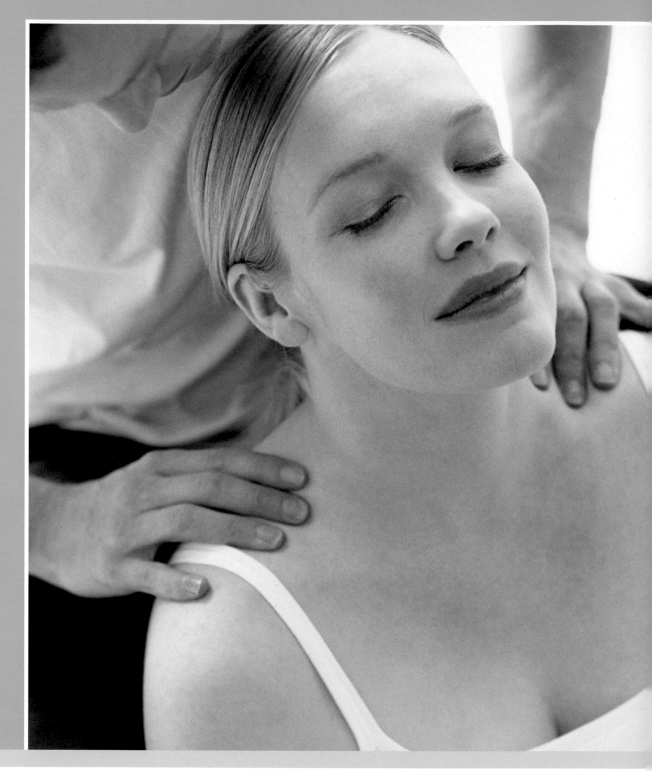

PART II ENJOYING YOUR PREGNANCY

Your pregnant body

Your body will be going through incredible changes

over the nine months of pregnancy, but your busy

lifestyle may continue at much the same pace. With

a little guidance and some minor adjustments, you

can carry on with most of your everyday activities,

safe in the knowledge that you're protecting your

baby's well-being.

Inner changes

From the moment you conceive, your body begins to make adjustments to nourish and nurture your growing baby. While some of these changes can be discerned, others are subtler and may not be noticeable right away.

Around the time of your first missed period early pregnancy symptoms usually start to occur. You may notice tenderness in your breasts, fatigue and feelings of nausea. These, and other changes that you may experience during pregnancy (see page 67), can be an irritation and may even cause you some discomfort, but in many cases they can be relieved. However, any unusual discomfort or pain should never be ignored.

Hormonal changes

Pregnancy is a time of great hormonal activity. Production of existing hormones is raised dramatically and new hormones are made specifically for pregnancy.

Human chorionic gonadotropin (hCG)

This hormone, released by the developing placenta as it begins to implant within the uterus, is widely known as the 'pregnancy hormone', because it's the one that is tested for in pregnancy tests. HCG is very important, because it triggers other hormonal activity needed to maintain your pregnancy and prevent menstruation from occurring. However, hCG does have some noticeable effects; in particular, it's thought to be partly responsible for the nausea and vomiting – morning sickness – that occurs in the first trimester.

Progesterone

This hormone is present in non-pregnant women, but at much lower levels. Produced first by the ovaries, and then by the placenta at around 8 to 9 weeks, progesterone plays an important role in sustaining your pregnancy, including preventing the uterus from contracting strongly and endangering

After a scan you may be offered a photograph that you can share with others, which will help to make your baby seem real.

your unborn baby. Some women who conceive after assisted conception techniques, such as IVF or GIFT, are put on progesterone supplements, in the form of pills, suppositories, vaginal gel or injections.

Progesterone maintains the functions of the placenta, strengthens the pelvic walls in preparation for labour and relaxes certain ligaments and muscles in your body. This relaxant effect can cause some unwelcome side effects.

Progesterone makes your bowel muscles sluggish, leading sometimes to constipation as well as a feeling of 'fullness' after eating. Progesterone also relaxes the sphincter (ring of muscle) between the oesophagus and the stomach, at times causing heartburn. It also causes veins to dilate, which can lead to varicose veins.

Another key role of progesterone is that of preparing your breasts for milk production. The hormone helps to stimulate and develop the duct system in your breasts, so that by the second trimester there is milk available. Early on you may feel its effects as breast tenderness.

Oestrogen

This is another hormone present in high levels during pregnancy. Very early on, oestrogen helps to prepare the lining of the uterus for the pregnancy, increasing the number of blood vessels and glands present within the uterus. Oestrogen also is responsible for some increase in blood volume, which can lead occasionally to bleeding gums or nosebleeds. Its most noticeable effect is an increased flushing, or redness of the skin, resulting in the familiar 'glow' of pregnancy.

Other significant hormones

Besides hCG, progesterone and oestrogen, a number of other hormones have specific roles to play throughout pregnancy:
- *Human chorionic somatomammotropin (HCS)* Also called human placental lactogen (HPL), this

hormone is regulated by oestrogen and is produced within the placenta in large amounts. It plays a part in the development of your baby and helps your breasts to develop the glands needed for breastfeeding. It also mobilizes fat for energy and may promote the growth of your baby.
- *Calcitonin* This conserves calcium and increases vitamin D synthesis, which enables your calcium and bone strength to remain stable despite an increased need for calcium for your baby.
- *Thyroxine (T4 and T3)* This hormone is needed for the development of your baby's central nervous system. It also increases your oxygen consumption, and helps your baby to process proteins and carbohydrates. Moreover, it interacts with growth hormones to regulate and stimulate your baby's growth.
- *Relaxin* This encourages your cervix, pelvic muscles and ligaments and joints to relax, in preparation for birth.
- *Insulin* This helps your baby to store food in his body and regulates glucose levels. If you are diabetic and your condition is not well controlled, your baby can grow too much and have problems balancing his own glucose levels.
- *Oxytocin* This hormone works in a kind of positive feedback loop. Released in response to the stretching of your cervix during labour it, in

turn, causes your uterus to contract further. Similarly, oxytocin is released in response to stimulation of your nipples during breastfeeding and causes your milk to flow in the let-down reflex (see page 297).

- *Erythropoietin* Produced in the kidneys, this hormone increases the total red blood cell mass and plasma volume by retaining salt and water.
- *Cortisol* This helps your baby to use various foods properly within his body.
- *Prolactin* This hormone helps to prepare your breasts for breastfeeding and promotes the growth of your baby.

Circulation changes

Shortly after conception, profound changes begin to occur in your body's circulatory system. One of the most significant of these is that your blood volume increases during pregnancy so that by week 30 you'll have 50 per cent more blood circulating within your bloodstream. This massive increase is necessary for your body to provide an adequate blood supply to your developing baby, your enlarging uterus and the growing placenta.

Despite this increase in blood volume, some women's blood counts decrease during pregnancy. This is because a blood count is a reading of the proportion of blood cells in relation to the amount of plasma – the fluid in which the blood cells are suspended – and the plasma tends to increase in volume more than the number of blood cells. Such a condition is called 'dilutional anaemia'. Anaemia can also be caused by iron deficiency, in which case your healthcare provider may recommend that you take an iron supplement.

You also may notice that your heartbeat is a little faster. This is perfectly normal and an indication that your body is adapting to pregnancy. No one knows for certain why a woman's heart rate increases during pregnancy. One theory is that it's nature's way of making sure that the extra blood volume gets circulated throughout the body.

Changes in blood pressure

Another change to your circulation, and one that you might notice, is a difference in your blood pressure. Some pregnant women's blood pressure begins to fall in the first trimester, reaching its lowest levels midway through pregnancy. A sudden drop in blood pressure – for example, when you stand up quickly – can give you a feeling of dizziness, or you might even faint. This is nothing to worry about, but you should mention it to your healthcare provider.

Although it is usually symptomless, some women experience an increase in blood pressure. Your doctor or midwife might pick this up at a routine check-up, and it is a condition that he or she will want to watch closely as it is one of the signs of pre-eclampsia, a medical condition unique to pregnancy that can affect both mother and fetus (see page 253).

Respiratory changes

You may find that you become short of breath toward the end of pregnancy. This is because your growing baby prevents your lungs from fully expanding. Some shortness of breath is completely normal but if you suddenly develop severe shortness of breath or get a sudden chest pain, seek medical attention at once.

Changes in metabolism

If you feel hungry all the time, or especially late at night, you'll be glad to know that there really is a physiological reason for this. During pregnancy your growing baby extracts glucose and other nutritional substances from your bloodstream throughout the day and night. So, in between your own meals, or at bedtime, your own blood sugar levels may well drop, leaving you feeling hungry. If you find yourself constantly foraging for food, try eating frequent, small healthy snacks, instead of fewer, large meals.

Outer changes

Of course, most women expect a burgeoning belly and enlarging breasts when they're pregnant, but you may not be aware that the texture of your skin may alter, and that your teeth, hands and feet might undergo changes.

Many of the physical changes you experience during pregnancy will be flattering: softer curves, a rosy complexion and thick, shiny hair can make you feel sexier than ever before. However, be prepared, too, for a few changes that aren't so attractive: swollen ankles, varicose veins and flaky skin are also common in pregnancy.

Fuller breasts

One of the earliest and most amazing changes in your body happens to your breasts. As soon as you find out that you're pregnant, you may begin to notice that your breasts are fuller and more tender. From about week 16, the nipples and areolae (the darkened areas surrounding the nipples) will be noticeably darker. Your nipples will become more prominent and the little glands on the areolae – known as Montgomery's tubercles – enlarge, resembling goose pimples.

These changes are caused by the large amounts of oestrogen and progesterone your body produces during pregnancy. These hormones cause the duct system inside your breasts to grow and branch out, in preparation for milk production and breastfeeding after your baby is born.

As your pregnancy advances, the veins on your breasts will become more prominent, stepping up the blood supply to your breasts. Your nipples may secrete a clear or golden-coloured liquid from time to time. This is known as colostrum, and is the liquid that your baby will ingest initially before your real milk is produced. Taking good care of your breasts throughout pregnancy will help prepare them for breastfeeding, and will also help ease any discomfort you may experience.

Hair and nail growth

While you're pregnant, your fingernails and toenails are likely to become stronger than they've ever been before and will grow at an unprecedented rate. This is due to the increase in metabolism and circulation caused by pregnancy hormones. For information about caring for your nails, see page 134.

Pregnancy also speeds up hair growth, usually causing the hair on your head to grow faster and look thicker. However, sometimes hair might grow in places where it hasn't done before, such as on your stomach or face. The best way to remove it is by plucking or waxing. It is probably best to avoid using depilatory creams or bleach, as your skin may not react well to the chemicals they contain. Electrolysis and laser hair removal are not recommended during pregnancy even though there are no documented risks.

You may be amazed at how large you have become towards the end of your pregnancy.

A HEALTHY WEIGHT GAIN

Starting pregnancy at a healthy weight and gaining weight at a moderate pace can help ensure that your baby grows and develops normally and that you stay healthy. Exactly how much weight you gain depends on several factors, including how many babies you're carrying.

Before you can work out your ideal weight gain during pregnancy (see chart opposite), you need to know your body mass index.

YOUR BODY MASS INDEX

Locate your pre-pregnancy weight on the vertical line of the chart and your height on the horizontal line. The place where the points intersect is your body mass index (BMI).

The cream-coloured area indicates the ideal BMI range at which a woman should start pregnancy.

- If your BMI is 19 or below, you're underweight.
- If your BMI is between 19 and 26, you're a healthy weight.
- If your BMI is between 27 and 30, you're overweight.
- If your BMI is over 30, you're clinically obese.

BODY MASS INDEX

KG	LBS																	
92	203	39	38	37	36	36	35	34	33	32	31	31	30	29	29	28	27	27
		39	38	37	36	35	34	33	33	32	31	30	30	29	28	28	27	27
		39	38	37	36	35	34	33	32	32	31	30	29	29	28	27	27	26
89	196	38	37	36	35	34	34	33	32	31	30	30	29	28	28	27	27	26
		38	37	36	35	34	33	32	32	31	30	29	29	28	27	27	26	26
		37	36	35	34	34	33	32	31	30	30	29	28	28	27	27	26	25
86	189	37	36	35	34	33	32	32	31	30	29	29	28	27	27	26	26	25
		36	35	35	34	33	32	31	30	30	29	28	28	27	27	26	25	25
		36	35	34	33	32	32	31	30	29	29	28	27	27	26	26	25	25
83	182	35	35	34	33	32	31	30	30	29	28	28	27	26	26	25	25	24
		35	34	33	32	32	31	30	29	29	28	27	27	26	26	25	24	24
		35	34	33	32	31	30	30	29	28	28	27	26	26	25	25	24	24
79	175	35	33	32	32	31	30	29	29	28	27	27	26	26	25	24	24	23
		34	33	32	31	30	30	29	28	28	27	26	26	25	25	24	24	23
		34	32	32	31	30	29	29	28	27	27	26	25	25	24	24	23	23
76	168	33	32	31	30	30	29	28	28	27	26	26	25	25	24	23	23	22
		33	32	31	30	29	29	28	27	27	26	25	25	24	24	23	23	22
		32	31	30	30	29	28	28	27	26	26	25	24	24	23	23	22	22
73	161	32	31	30	29	29	28	27	26	26	25	25	24	24	23	23	22	22
		32	30	30	29	28	27	27	26	26	25	24	24	23	23	22	22	21
		31	30	29	28	28	27	26	26	25	25	24	23	23	22	22	21	21
70	154	31	30	29	28	27	27	26	25	25	24	24	23	23	22	22	21	21
		30	29	28	28	27	26	26	25	24	24	23	23	22	22	21	21	20
		30	29	28	27	27	26	26	25	24	24	23	22	22	21	21	21	20
67	147	29	28	28	27	26	26	25	24	24	23	23	22	22	21	21	20	20
		29	28	27	26	26	25	25	24	23	23	22	22	21	21	20	20	19
		29	27	27	26	25	25	24	24	23	22	22	21	21	20	20	20	19
64	140	28	27	26	26	25	24	24	23	23	22	22	21	21	20	20	19	19
		28	27	26	25	25	24	23	23	22	22	21	21	20	20	19	19	19
		27	26	25	25	24	24	23	22	22	21	21	20	20	20	19	19	18
60	133	27	26	25	24	24	23	23	22	22	21	21	20	20	19	19	18	18
		26	25	25	24	23	23	22	22	21	21	20	20	19	19	19	18	18
		26	25	24	24	23	22	22	21	21	20	20	19	19	19	18	18	17
57	126	26	24	24	23	23	22	22	21	21	20	20	19	19	18	18	18	17
		25	24	23	23	22	22	21	21	20	20	19	19	18	18	18	17	17
		25	24	23	22	22	21	21	20	20	19	19	18	18	18	17	17	17
54	119	24	23	23	22	21	21	20	20	19	19	19	18	18	17	17	17	16
		24	23	22	22	21	21	20	20	19	19	18	18	17	17	17	16	16
		23	22	22	21	21	20	20	19	19	18	18	17	17	16	16	16	16
51	112	23	22	21	21	20	20	19	19	18	18	18	17	17	16	16	16	15
		23	22	21	20	20	19	19	19	18	18	17	17	16	16	16	15	15
		22	21	21	20	20	19	19	18	18	17	17	17	16	16	15	15	15
48	105	22	21	20	20	19	19	18	18	17	17	17	16	16	15	15	15	14
		21	20	20	19	19	18	18	17	17	17	16	16	15	15	15	14	14
		20	20	19	19	18	18	17	17	16	16	16	15	15	15	14	14	14
45	98	20	19	19	18	18	18	17	16	16	16	15	15	15	14	14	14	13
		19	19	18	18	18	17	17	16	16	16	15	15	15	14	14	14	13
		19	19	18	18	17	17	16	16	16	15	15	15	14	14	14	13	13
41	91	19	18	18	17	17	16	16	16	15	15	15	14	14	14	13	13	13
		18	18	17	17	16	16	16	15	15	15	14	14	14	13	13	13	12
		18	17	17	16	16	16	15	15	15	14	14	14	13	13	13	12	12
		17	17	16	16	16	15	15	15	14	14	14	13	13	13	12	12	12

METRES	1.52	1.56	1.6	1.64	1.68	1.72	1.76	1.80	1.84

FEET	5'0	5'1	5'2	5'3	5'4	5'5	5'6	5'7	5'8	5'9	5'10	5'11	6'0

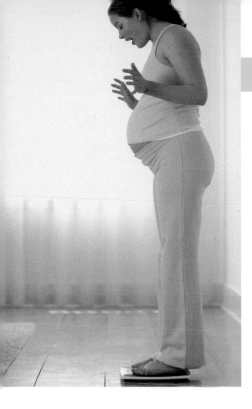

BODY MASS INDEX	RECOMMENDED TOTAL WEIGHT GAIN
Less than 19 (underweight)	12.5 to 18 kg (28 to 40 lbs)
19 to 26 (normal weight)	11.5 to 16 kg (25 to 35 lbs)
27 to 30 (overweight)	7 to 11.5 kg (15 to 25 lbs)
30 or more (obese)	7 kg (15 lbs) or less

These numbers refer to total weight gain during the entire pregnancy, so you won't know whether you hit the target until delivery day. These recommendations are for women expecting one baby. If you're expecting twins or triplets you may gain considerably more. An average total gain of 15.5 to 20.5 kg (34 to 45 lbs) for twins and 20.5 to 23 kg (45 to 50 lbs) for triplets is likely depending on the length of your pregnancy.

YOUR WEIGHT GAIN

The chart above gives the recommended weight gain for your body mass index. Bear in mind, however, that the figures refer to a singleton pregnancy. The rate at which you gain weight may vary from week to week. And, unfortunately, little is known about the best time to put on weight in pregnancy. Some research suggests that gaining very little weight early on – when you may be suffering from morning sickness – has less effect on fetal growth than poor weight gain late in the second or third trimester. Some women gain weight very inconsistently, piling on the pounds early and then much less later on. Nothing is necessarily unhealthy about this pattern.

Remember, too, that these weight gains are only a guide: women who gain very little or more than average can still have healthy babies. However, if you are underweight or very overweight, you may be advised to see a nutritionist or dietitian for specific advice on what and how much you should eat. See Chapter 4 to find out more about healthy eating during pregnancy.

It's important not to become fanatical about how much you weigh. In the United Kingdom doctors and midwives have stopped routinely weighing women at every antenatal check-up, because it is more effective to check your baby's growth by measuring the fundal height (see page 91) or, if there's cause for concern, by scheduling you for a series of ultrasounds (see page 236).

HOW WEIGHT GAIN IS MADE UP IN PREGNANCY

- BABY 39%
- BLOOD 22%
- AMNIOTIC FLUID 11%
- UTERUS 11%
- PLACENTA 9%
- BREASTS 8%

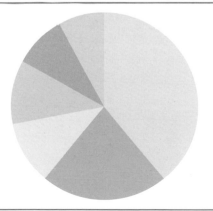

Skin changes

Overall, you may find that your skin becomes softer, due to its increased ability to retain moisture, and that you have the characteristic 'glow' of pregnancy, which is partly due to an increase in hormone levels. However, you may notice other changes to your skin. Pregnant women, for example, often perspire more as a result of the action of pregnancy hormones on sweat glands all over the body; for this reason, heat rashes are more common. Most skin changes go away in the first six months after the birth, but some may remain permanently.

Linea nigra

You may notice a dark line running from your pubic bone up to your navel. Called the linea nigra, this is usually more prominent in darker-skinned women.

Chloasma

The skin around your cheeks, nose and eyes may also darken. This is called chloasma or 'the mask of pregnancy' and appears dark in fair-skinned women and light in dark-skinned women. Chloasma is due to hormonal influences on skin pigment cells. Exposure to the sun can make these changes darker.

Spider angiomas

Tiny red spots, called spider angiomas or spider naevi, may suddenly appear anywhere on your body. These spots, which turn white when you press on them, are concentrations of blood vessels caused by the high level of oestrogen in your body.

Acne

Some women who suffer from acne find that their skin improves during pregnancy. Others find that the condition becomes worse, and women who do not normally have acne may develop it or be subject to spots. You may be able to help to control spots by cutting down on fats in your diet and exercising regularly. Always consult your doctor before taking any acne medication, as it may contain chemicals that could affect your baby. Acne and spots usually clear up in the second trimester.

Itchy hands and feet

Your palms and sometimes the soles of your feet may become red and itchy. Known as palmar erythema, this is caused by increased levels of oestrogen. If your skin is itching, make sure you see your doctor, as this could be a symptom of cholestasis (see page 255).

Skin tags, moles and freckles

Minuscule tags of skin are a common occurrence in high-friction areas, although it isn't totally clear why they occur. It's not a good idea to rush to have them removed. Existing moles, freckles or skin blemishes may become darker. If a new mole appears or an existing one changes appreciably in size or appearance, see your doctor.

MORE **ABOUT**   stretch marks

Stretch marks occur when fibres of the skin protein collagen are broken due to the rapid stretching or to hormonal changes that disrupt the fibres. They affect half of all pregnant women. They're most likely to appear on your stomach, the sides of your breasts and your thighs – areas where it's common to put on weight. Stretch marks initially appear as pinkish-red streaks, which fade to silvery grey or white several months after birth. You are more likely to get them if you've had more than one baby, gain an excessive amount of weight, or have a genetic disposition to getting them.

There's no surefire way of preventing stretch marks although two creams have been studied scientifically and showed a possible reduction in their formation. One study focused on using massage with a cream called Trofolastin, which contained Centella asiatica extract, alpha tocopherol, and collagen-elastin hydrolysates, while the other looked at massage with an ointment containing tocopherol, panthenol, hyaluronic acid, elastin, and menthol.

COMPLAINT	WHAT YOU CAN DO ABOUT IT

MORNING SICKNESS

Feelings of nausea and vomiting can occur at any time throughout the day, so the term 'morning sickness' is somewhat of a misnomer. Something like 75 per cent of women suffer from it from as early as week 5 or 6. Morning sickness usually goes away – or becomes much less severe – by the end of the first trimester. No one knows exactly what causes it, but most experts believe that it's related to hCG (see page 60).

Even when nausea doesn't actually cause you to vomit, it can be extremely unpleasant and truly debilitating. If your queasiness gets out of control – if you experience weight loss, if you can't keep down food or liquids or if you feel dizzy or faint – speak to your doctor, who will want to rule out hyperemesis gravidarum (see page 257). He or she may also be able to prescribe some helpful medication.

Above all, don't compound the problem by worrying about it – the nausea is harmless to you and your baby. Your optimal weight gain for the first three months is only 2 kg (4 lbs). Even losing weight probably isn't a big problem in early pregnancy – many women do.

- ◆ Eat small, frequent meals so that you never have an empty stomach. Avoid foods and smells you find off-putting; stick to bland, non-greasy foods such as baked potatoes and pasta.
- ◆ Wear comfortable clothes; avoid tight waistbands, which can make you feel worse.
- ◆ Get plenty of rest and sleep as often as you can; tiredness can make the nausea worse.
- ◆ Ginger – in the form of tea, tablets or biscuits – helps some women.
- ◆ Drink plenty of fluids.
- ◆ Keep cream crackers or dry toast by your bedside – eating them before getting out of bed can ease nausea.

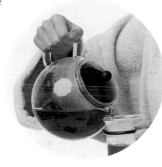

- ◆ Try acupressure wrist bands, sold in pharmacies and health food shops.
- ◆ If nausea gets worse when you brush your teeth, switching toothpaste brands may help.
- ◆ If your nausea is made worse by the accumulation of saliva in your mouth, suck lemon drops.

FATIGUE

Many women are astonished at how exhausted they feel in the first trimester; this is completely normal. Fatigue may be a side effect of all the physical changes taking place, including the dramatic rise in hormone levels. You'll probably find that your exhaustion goes away around weeks 12 to 14. As fatigue lessens, you'll begin to feel more energetic and almost normal, until about 30 to 34 weeks when you may feel tired again. At this point, part of the fatigue is due to carrying around extra weight. Try to rest when you can, and recognise that it's natural to reduce your physical activity and get more sleep at this time. Women often find their second or third pregnancies more tiring than their first, because they have to care for other children.

- ◆ Try to be realistic about what you can do, and don't feel guilty about what you can't get done. No one expects you to be Superwoman.
- ◆ Get as much rest as you can by sitting with your feet up during the evenings and going to bed earlier.
- ◆ Whenever possible, let other people help with household chores and other responsibilities. This is especially important if you already have children and can't just put your feet up when you feel like it.
- ◆ Make sure you are eating a healthy pregnancy diet (see page 101) and avoid caffeine and sweets, which will give you a quick energy lift and then leave your body feeling more fatigued as the blood-sugar level drops.
- ◆ Do some gentle exercise every day.

COMPLAINT	WHAT YOU CAN DO ABOUT IT

STRESS INCONTINENCE

During the last months of pregnancy, some women begin to leak a little urine when they cough, sneeze, laugh or move suddenly. Referred to as stress incontinence, this is perfectly normal and is caused by the growing uterus putting pressure on the bladder.

- Use the toilet before the urge to urinate gets too strong.
- Practise your pelvic-floor exercises (see page 122) regularly to help to strengthen pelvic-floor muscles and support the urinary sphincter.
- Urine loss can be a sign of a urinary tract infection (see page 260), so discuss it with your doctor.
- Continuous loss of fluid may also be a sign of ruptured membranes (see page 212). Your doctor can determine if this is the case.

DIZZINESS AND FAINTING

Feeling light-headed is common in pregnancy. In the early stages, it may occur as your blood flow strives to catch up with your increased circulation; later on, dizziness can be a result of the uterus pressing on large blood vessels. Low blood-sugar levels, low blood pressure, getting up too quickly or becoming overheated can all contribute to dizzy spells.

Fainting during pregnancy is rare, but if you do faint it's because the flow of blood to your brain is reduced temporarily. This will not harm your baby. Report fainting to your doctor right away as this may be a sign of severe anaemia (see page 252).

- Always get up slowly from sitting or lying down so that the blood has time to flow to your brain.
- When you're lying down, rest on one side or the other whenever possible; don't lie flat on your back.
- Drink plenty of liquids – dizziness can be a sign of dehydration – and don't avoid salt.
- Eat protein at every meal or try eating smaller, more frequent meals to maintain your blood-sugar levels.
- Carry raisins, a piece of fruit or some cream crackers in your bag for a quick blood-sugar lift while you are out.
- If you feel too warm, get some fresh air and loosen your clothes, especially around the neck and waist.
- Wear natural fibres, such as cotton, linen and wool, and refresh yourself with a cool, damp cloth as often as possible.
- If you feel faint, try to increase the circulation to your brain by sitting with your head between your knees or lying down with your feet higher than your head.

HAEMORRHOIDS (PILES)

Essentially varicose veins of the anal canal, haemorrhoids are caused by the uterus pressing on major blood vessels, making the veins enlarge and swell. Progesterone relaxes the veins, allowing the swelling to increase. Even if you manage to avoid getting haemorrhoids during pregnancy, it is possible to develop them during delivery.

Haemorrhoids sometimes bleed. While this bleeding isn't harmful, if it becomes frequent, talk to your midwife or doctor, who may refer you to a colorectal specialist. If your haemorrhoids become very painful, you may want to discuss further treatment.

◆ Avoid becoming constipated (see page 72). Straining during bowel movements puts added pressure on the blood vessels. Stool softeners are safe and effective.
◆ Exercise every day to help you to stay regular.
◆ Sit in a warm bath two or three times a day to help to relieve the muscle spasms that often cause the pain.
◆ Soothe the area with witch hazel, a cloth wrung out in ice water or special pads. If a pile protrudes, gently push it back inside using a lubricating jelly.
◆ Speak to your caregiver about medications.
◆ Take pressure off the area by sleeping on your side, and avoid standing for long periods.
◆ Do pelvic-floor exercises (see page 122) regularly, as these will help to improve circulation to the area.

ROUND LIGAMENT PAIN

Between 18 and 24 weeks, you may feel a sharp pain or a dull ache on one or both sides of your lower abdomen or near your groin. It's often stronger when you move quickly or stand, and it may fade if you lie down. This is called round ligament pain. The round ligaments are bands of fibrous tissue on each side of the uterus that attach the top of the uterus to the labia. As the uterus enlarges in the second trimester, the stretching of these ligaments may cause discomfort. While it can be quite uncomfortable, it's perfectly normal. The good news is that it usually goes away, or at least decreases considerably, after 24 weeks.

◆ Take breaks from standing or walking, and put your feet up when sitting.
◆ Always mention any abdominal pain when you have an antenatal check-up so that you can be reassured that there is nothing wrong.

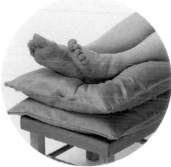

EXCESSIVE SALIVATION

Overproduction of saliva, which is sometimes called ptyalism, can be a problem but only in the first half of pregnancy. The symptoms include: producing double the amount of bitter-tasting saliva; a thickened tongue; and swollen cheeks, caused by enlarged salivary glands. Ptyalism appears to be more common in women who have morning sickness, and it can make the nausea worse temporarily.

◆ Cut down on starchy foods or dairy products, but still follow a healthy, balanced diet (see page 101).
◆ Eat fruit, as this can ease symptoms.
◆ Mints, chewing gum, frequent small meals and crackers can help to reduce the amount of saliva produced.
◆ Try brushing or rinsing your teeth with minty products to freshen your mouth.
◆ Suck on a piece of lemon or lemon drops.

COMPLAINT	WHAT YOU CAN DO ABOUT IT
NASAL STUFFINESS AND NOSEBLEEDS High levels of progesterone and oestrogen result in increased blood flow throughout your body, causing the lining of your nasal passages to become swollen. This can lead to congestion and overproduction of mucus. This increased blood flow also puts pressure on your nose's delicate veins, making you more prone to nosebleeds. Nasal stuffiness is likely to get worse before it gets better, after the birth. Don't use medication or medicated nasal sprays unless they are prescribed by your doctor.	◆ Increase your intake of fluids. ◆ Humidify your home, especially your bedroom, at night. ◆ Prop your head up when you sleep. ◆ With severe congestion, consider breathing steam from a bowl of hot water, or use a saline nasal spray. ◆ Blow your nose gently to avoid inducing bleeding. If your nose does bleed, sit with your head facing forward and using your thumb and forefinger, press the sides of your nose together just below the bony part for 10 minutes. Try not to swallow the blood. If the bleeding doesn't stop, repeat for a further 10 minutes, then seek medical advice.
WIND AND BLOATING Burping and passing wind at inopportune times can be highly embarrassing but are inescapable complaints in pregnancy. Even before the end of the first trimester, you may find that your belly looks bloated and distended – an unwelcome side effect of the hormone progesterone, which causes you to retain water. This hormone slows down the bowels also, causing them to enlarge. Oestrogen, the other key pregnancy hormone, causes your uterus to enlarge, which also makes your tummy feel bigger.	◆ There's very little you can do to prevent burping or passing wind, but try to avoid becoming constipated (see page 72), because that may make things worse. ◆ Avoid eating large meals, which may leave you feeling bloated and uncomfortable, or foods you know make the problem even worse. These vary from person to person, but some common offenders include onions, cabbage, fried foods, rich sauces and beans. ◆ Don't rush your meals. This can cause you to swallow air, which can form painful pockets of wind in your gut.
HEARTBURN A burning sensation, which occurs in the upper part of your abdomen, near the sternum (breastbone), is very common in the latter part of pregnancy. It's the result of acids produced in the stomach being pushed up into the lower oesophagus (the tube connecting your mouth to your stomach). Heartburn is more pronounced during pregnancy for two reasons. The high level of progesterone that your body is producing can slow digestion and relax the sphincter muscle between the oesophagus and the stomach, which normally prevents the upward movement of stomach acids.	◆ Eat small, frequent meals and sit up straight when eating; this takes pressure off your stomach. ◆ Munch on dry cream crackers when you feel heartburn. They may neutralise the wind. ◆ Avoid spicy, fatty and greasy foods. ◆ Avoid eating just before bedtime – heartburn occurs most readily when you lie down. ◆ Try sleeping with your head elevated on several pillows. ◆ If your heartburn is persistent, talk to your doctor or midwife about taking an antacid, which is safe during pregnancy. Apart from sodium bicarbonate, safe medications include alginates such as Gaviscon, ranitidine and omeprazole.

COMPLAINT	WHAT YOU CAN DO ABOUT IT

SHORTNESS OF BREATH

Two-thirds of all pregnant women occasionally experience breathlessness. This is caused by increased production of progesterone, which speeds up your breathing rate, and, in the last trimester, by your enlarged uterus, which presses against your diaphragm and lungs. Your breathing should improve as your baby descends into your pelvis in the final weeks.

- ◆ Relax and try to avoid stress. Try not to panic if you get breathless – it can make it worse.
- ◆ Don't slump. Stand tall and allow plenty of room for your chest to expand.
- ◆ If you experience wheezing, tingling lips or fingers, chest pain or blueness of your lips or fingers, get it checked out by your doctor as soon as possible. These could be signs of a problem such as anaemia, which may require treatment.

INSOMNIA

Many women complain of difficulty sleeping during the last few months of pregnancy. This may be due in part to normal anxiety about having a baby, but also may be due to the physical discomforts that can occur later in pregnancy such as heartburn, indigestion and having to urinate frequently. As your uterus grows, finding a comfortable sleeping position can sometimes be quite a challenge.

- ◆ Invest in a number of pillows. You may find that tucking one under your bump, and under and between your legs, makes it easier to find a comfortable position.
- ◆ Sleep lying on your left hand side. This prevents your unborn baby pressing on the inferior vena cava, the blood vessel that brings blood to your heart from the lower half of your body and will help to improve the function of your circulation and organs. Sleeping flat on your back in the last weeks of pregnancy can result in palpitations and other problems.
- ◆ Take a warm, relaxing bath before going to bed.
- ◆ Drink warm milk. Warming the milk releases tryptophan, a naturally occurring amino acid that makes you feel sleepy.
- ◆ Don't eat a heavy meal before bedtime; eat earlier in the evening and then have a light snack before bed.
- ◆ Get plenty of fresh air. Open a window so that you are not sleeping in a stuffy environment.
- ◆ Try to exercise on a regular basis.

COMPLAINT	WHAT YOU CAN DO ABOUT IT

BACK PAIN

Half to three-quarters of pregnant women experience back pain at some stage. Fortunately, only about a third of these will be significantly affected by it. There are two main reasons for back discomfort in pregnancy. In preparation for the birth, hormones cause your joints to become more relaxed than usual, and this, along with your growing bump, puts your body off balance.

If your backache becomes very painful, ask your healthcare provider to refer you to an obstetric physiotherapist who will give you advice and possibly some helpful exercises.

- ◆ Adjust your posture when standing to compensate for the shift in your centre of gravity (see page 116).
- ◆ Sit on chairs with good back support. Also, make sure your knees are elevated above your hips.
- ◆ Sleep on your side on a firm mattress. Keep a pillow between your legs and under your bump to support your back (see picture, page 71).
- ◆ Lift properly so that you don't strain your back: place your feet shoulder-width apart. Don't bend at the waist but at the knees. As you lift, push up with your thighs and keep your back straight.
- ◆ When carrying bags, make sure the weight is evenly distributed: if you're carrying groceries in your hands, divide the load into two bags and carry one in each hand; and if you're carrying a small backpack with straps, carry it on both shoulders.
- ◆ Wear low-heeled shoes.
- ◆ Apply a heated pad to painful areas for limited periods of time. Massage also can be very effective.

CONSTIPATION

Hard and difficult-to-pass stools may be the result of high levels of progesterone, which relax the bowel, meaning that waste matter passes through your system more sluggishly. At the same time, your expanding uterus squashes your intestine. Taking iron supplements can make the problem worse. If you have been prescribed a supplement, ask your caregiver if you can manage without or to change to another type.

- ◆ Eat plenty of high-fibre foods such as bran cereals, fruit and vegetables. Some women find it helpful to eat popcorn, but go for natural, air-popped versions, without added butter, oil or salt. Too much high-fibre food, however, can cause discomfort, bloating or wind so you may have to experiment to see which foods you tolerate best.
- ◆ Drink plenty of fluids – watered-down fruit juice, milk and water are fine.
- ◆ Eat prunes or drink a glass of prune juice every day.
- ◆ Your healthcare provider may recommend a bulking agent such as Fybogel or osmotic laxative, such as Lactulose, which can be bought over the counter. Stimulant laxatives, such as senna, may be prescribed on a short-term basis and usually not in the third trimester) as they can cause abdominal cramping and, occasionally, uterine contractions.
- ◆ Exercise regularly. It encourages the bowels to become more active and promotes daily bowel movements.

COMPLAINT	WHAT YOU CAN DO ABOUT IT

FLUID RETENTION AND SWELLING

Your body swells due to the accumulation of fluid in the tissues. The swelling is connected to the normal increase in body fluids in pregnancy, and three out of four pregnant women will develop oedema (swelling) at some time. Usually the swelling appears in feet and ankles, hands and fingers. It's most noticeable at the end of the day or after prolonged standing or sitting and in warm weather. Swelling could be a sign of pre-eclampsia, so you should mention it at your check-ups.

♦ Don't stand for long periods. Take regular breaks and sit with your legs elevated.
♦ If your hands are swollen, keep your hands elevated above your heart rather than down by your sides.
♦ Avoid wearing tight clothing or shoes.
♦ Wear support stockings or talk to your doctor or midwife about special prescription elastic stockings.
♦ Drink plenty of fluids to help to expel excess fluid.
♦ Don't restrict your salt intake unless your blood pressure is high (see page 265).

VARICOSE VEINS

Swollen veins often appear just under the surface of the skin of your legs and sometimes in the vulva and as haemorrhoids around the anus. They occur when the uterus puts pressure on the pelvic veins, increasing pressure on the veins in the legs and causing backflow. Blood pools in the veins in the legs causing them to distend. You may be more likely to get varicose veins if they run in the family, if you're overweight or stand or sit for long periods of time. They're usually painless, but occasionally they may be associated with discomfort, aches or pain. Varicose veins usually regress after delivery, but sometimes not completely. Swimming and walking, can help prevent them as can wearing elasticated stockings.

♦ Avoid standing still for long periods of time.
♦ Sit with your legs elevated as much as you can.
♦ Try to take several rest periods throughout the day so that you can get off your feet.
♦ Exercise your feet: rotate each foot 8 times in both directions and bend then stretch each one 30 times up and down.
♦ If you have to sit still for long periods, move your legs around from time to time to stimulate circulation. Flex your feet up and down to keep the blood from pooling.
♦ Wear support stockings or talk to your doctor or midwife about special prescription elastic stockings.
♦ Avoid wearing stockings or socks with tight elastic tops that grip around one part of your leg.

CRAMP IN YOUR LEGS AND FEET

Often worse when you've gone to bed, cramp occurs more frequently and painfully as pregnancy progresses. No one's sure exactly what causes cramp – one theory links it to low levels of magnesium or calcium. Fatigue and a build-up of fluid in the legs at the end of the day are also thought to be contributing factors. Some doctors believe that cramp in your legs may be related to a decrease in circulation, which gets worse when you're sitting down. Regular, gentle exercise, particularly moving your ankles and legs, will improve circulation and help prevent cramps occurring.

♦ Walking about in bare feet can help to ease the pain.
♦ Stretching and extending your legs or pulling your toes hard up towards your ankle should help to diminish the pain (see page 118).
♦ Leg massage may help to minimise the pain.

COMPLEMENTARY THERAPIES

Many women use complementary medicine to promote relaxation and help to cope with pregnancy complaints. Although generally safe, you should always consult a fully qualified practitioner before embarking on any treatment.

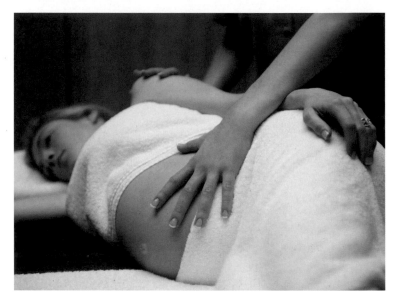

HERBAL REMEDIES

Pure fruit or mint teas are good alternatives to caffeine during pregnancy, and a slice of ginger in boiling water can ease morning sickness. However, teas and remedies containing herbs should be treated with caution, as herbs can be extremely potent, and in some cases, toxic. You should always consult your doctor before taking any herbal remedy and ask an expert to recommend a particular brand, as the quality of herbs can vary.

REFLEXOLOGY

This therapy operates under the premise that points on the feet and hands correspond to other parts of the body. It may help to relieve a number of pregnancy complaints including backache and circulatory problems, and reflexology has been used during labour to ease the pain of contractions. However, deep pressure should be avoided near the ankles, which correspond to the uterus and ovaries, as this may bring on premature labour. Some reflexologists also recommend it should be avoided during the first trimester if the woman has a history of miscarriage.

AROMATHERAPY

Essential oils derived from plants are often applied with massage in the practice of aromatherapy. They can be very effective in combating stress and promoting relaxation. However, a number of essential oils can be harmful to the extent that some experts advise against the use of all oils during pregnancy. The safest course is to consult a qualified aromatherapy practitioner.

ACUPUNCTURE

This ancient Eastern practice is usually perfectly safe during pregnancy as long as the treatment is carried out by a properly qualified acupuncturist. It may be especially useful for alleviating morning sickness, or reducing lower back pain during pregnancy. However, special precautions should be taken because certain acupuncture points may stimulate uterine contractions.

HOMEOPATHY

This therapy can be effective in combating minor pregnancy complaints such as heartburn, nausea and vomiting, and some women find it can help during labour. Homeopathic remedies are unlikely to cause side effects to either mother or baby, as only a very minute amount of the active ingredient is used in a specially prepared form. However, in pregnancy you should always consult a professional homeopath, as pinpointing the right remedy can be quite difficult.

Will it harm my baby?

Now that you're pregnant you'll probably want to take greater care of yourself in order to protect and nurture the little one inside you.

Your lifestyle can affect not only your body but your baby. The effects of alcohol and caffeine consumption are covered in Chapter 4, but here you'll discover the dangers in smoking, taking drugs or medications, or certain illnesses.

Smoking

Women who smoke run the risk of developing lung cancer, emphysema and heart disease, among other illnesses. Smoking when pregnant, however, means subjecting a baby to very serious health risks as well. The nicotine in the cigarette smoke will decrease blood flow to the baby, while carbon monoxide decreases the amount of oxygen this blood contains. As a result, women who smoke during pregnancy stand an increased chance of delivering babies with low birth weights. Babies weighing less than 2.5 kg (5½ lbs) at birth are 20 times more at risk of dying in their first year than babies of normal birth weight. They're also more likely to experience developmental problems. Babies born to smokers are expected to weigh an average of 0.25 kg (½ lb) less than those born to nonsmokers; the exact difference in birth weight depends on how much the mother smokes. Passive smoking (where an expectant mother inhales the smoke of others) also may be a cause of growth problems.

Smoking during pregnancy is also associated with a greater risk of complications like miscarriage, preterm delivery, placenta praevia, placental abruption and preterm rupture of the membranes. Research has suggested that smoking during pregnancy may even be linked to sudden infant death syndrome or SIDS (see page 383).

Fathers who smoke also affect the health of their babies, before and after birth. The risk of respiratory problems and SIDS is increased.

Your midwife will ask about smoking at your first antenatal appointment. She will refer you to the local NHS Stop Smoking Services to see a Stop Smoking counsellor. Alternatively you can get support from the NHS Smokefree Pregnancy Helpline. These experts can provide you with a carbon monoxide monitor. This hand-held device measures the level of carbon monoxide in your body when you blow into it. See the levels drop as you successfully cut down or quit.

Nicotine replacement therapy (available as gum, lozenges, patches, sprays or electric cigarettes) may help with inevitable cravings for a cigarette but doctors are not certain about how safe this is in pregnancy. Your baby is still exposed to nicotine but not the other thousands of harmful chemicals that are present in cigarette smoke.

Giving up smoking can be extremely difficult, but it's the very best thing you can do for your baby. If you stop smoking in the first trimester, the risk of low birth weight drops to a similar level as that for a nonsmoker. If you find that you can't give up completely, even cutting down on the number of cigarettes you smoke is of benefit to your baby.

Illegal drugs

You should avoid taking all illegal drugs during pregnancy. Many studies have shown that they put you at a higher risk of delivering a premature or low-birth-weight baby. Also, some drugs can cause developmental and behavioural problems.

- *Marijuana* The data on marijuana isn't clear-cut, but it does suggest that pregnant women who use it stand a higher-than-average risk of delivering their babies prematurely or at low birth weights. Heavy marijuana use can lead to an increased chance of miscarriage and ectopic pregnancy.
- *Cocaine and crack cocaine* These are highly addictive drugs. Using them during pregnancy, puts you at higher risk of premature delivery and placental abruption. Cocaine also has been found

to increase the chance of birth defects, neurological problems, seizures, developmental problems and SIDS. In addition to these adverse effects on the baby, a pregnant woman who uses cocaine is at greater risk of having a stroke, heart attack or very high blood pressure.

- *Narcotics and opiates* This group of drugs includes heroin, methadone, codeine and morphine. Taking narcotics to treat medical conditions and under medical supervision – for example, to provide pain relief after surgery – won't harm your baby; taking narcotics continually and in substantial amounts will. Narcotic addiction puts you and your baby at a very serious risk. It's associated with fetal growth problems, preterm delivery, fetal death and small head size. Perhaps even more importantly, narcotic addiction places the baby at a high risk of complications after the birth – even death – due to withdrawal from the drug. If you're addicted to narcotics or opiates, beginning a treatment programme during your pregnancy can minimise the effects of the drugs on your baby.
- *Amphetamines and 'uppers'* This group includes crystal methamphetamine, blue ice and ecstasy. Because these substances historically haven't been used as widely as narcotics and cocaine, there's less information available about their side effects during pregnancy. However, they do decrease the appetite, which in turn, could lead to poor fetal growth. Also, evidence shows that the drugs themselves can increase the risk of fetal growth problems, including small head size, placental abruption and fetal stroke or death. Ecstasy may cause a number of birth defects.

It is worth bearing in mind that there are additional risks associated with drug-taking. Women who abuse drugs are more likely to be malnourished than other women, and generally suffer a higher incidence of sexually transmitted diseases. All of these factors, independent of drug use, can cause problems for pregnancy and for the baby.

Prescribed medications

Some women are reluctant to take any sort of medication in pregnancy, for fear that it might harm their babies. Many medications (such as paracetamol; most antibiotics, local anaesthetics and antacids), steroid creams such as hydrocortisone [if not used on large areas of skin or for too long] and constipation treatments [see also Common Pregnancy Complaints for specifics) are safe during pregnancy, but it's always a good idea to discuss with your doctor, perhaps at your first antenatal visit, the type of drugs you are likely to take over the next nine months – both over-the-counter medications and prescriptions you might need. With antihistamines and decongestants, your doctor should be able to prescribe the safest versions. You should, however, avoid medications that contain phenylephrine or pseudoephedrine (especially in the first trimester) and fluconazole.

If you visit a different doctor, make sure you tell him or her that you're pregnant.

If you have an pre-existing medical condition such as asthma, diabetes, epilepsy, high blood pressure or a thyroid condition (see page 270), it's likely that you'll need to continue taking your medication throughout your pregnancy. Stopping medication for a chronic condition will, in many cases, pose a greater risk to your growing baby than any possible side effects of the medication itself. Make sure you discuss your dose with your doctor as soon as you find out that you're pregnant, as it may need to be adjusted. In the case of epilepsy or diabetes or any long-term illness needing tablets, it's best to see your GP before conception to discuss what treatment is best. Don't stop taking a prescription medication or change the dosage without talking to your doctor first.

Many medications are labelled 'Do not take during pregnancy', because their effects haven't been adequately studied in pregnant women. However, this doesn't necessarily mean that adverse effects have been reported, or that you can't use them. Whenever you have a question about a particular medication, it's best to ask the advice of your doctor or pharmacist. However, opinions can vary; there is not always only one right answer.

Illnesses

Serious illnesses that can affect your baby are covered in the Antenatal Directory, but even common problems may have repercussions. If you think you may have come in contact with any infectious disease, make sure you tell your doctor.

Colds

As miserable as it can make you feel, a cold won't harm your baby. Check with the pharmacist before taking any cold treatments, however, as some aren't recommended in pregnancy (see opposite). Rest as much as you can and take in plenty of fluids in the form of juices, soups and water.

If a cough develops, try drinking some honey and lemon in hot water. A stuffy or runny nose can be relieved safely by inhaling steam (fill a large bowl with hot water) or taking a hot shower.

If you have a respiratory infection that does not improve after a week, speak to your GP.

Fever

Fever can pose a threat to your baby, especially in the very early weeks when all the crucial development is going on. If you have a fever, you need to bring it down, by taking paracetamol, bathing in tepid water, wearing fewer clothes and having cold drinks. If you've got a temperature of 38.9°C (102°F) or over, call your GP for advice.

Stomach upsets

Gastroenteritis is unlikely to affect your baby and fortunately, it's normally short-lived, lasting only a day or two. Rest and plenty of fluids are the best treatments for most stomach bugs. You can carry on eating, but stick to bland, easily digestible foods.

If symptoms fail to settle after 48 hours, however, you may have food poisoning or an infection, both of which will need medical treatment. Symptoms such as high fever, blood in the stools, severe abdominal pain or dehydration need urgent medical treatment if you're pregnant.

HEALTH FIRST
VACCINATIONS Live vaccines, such as polio, yellow fever and typhoid, shouldn't be routinely administered to pregnant women, because of possible harm to the fetus. Tetanus, whooping cough and flu shots are safe. If you need a vaccination, perhaps to travel, tell your doctor that you're pregnant. Where there's significant risk of infection, the need may outweigh the risk.

Everyday hazards

You and your baby can be affected by a number of factors such as chemicals, pets, temperature extremes, pollution and childhood illnesses.

Maintaining a healthy environment also involves avoiding harmful activities and situations.

Household products

Everyday household cleaners won't harm your baby, but try and avoid using highly toxic products, such as oven cleaners. If you can't avoid using products with strong fumes, make sure the room is well aired and take frequent breaks to get some fresh air.

If you're seized with an irresistible urge to decorate your baby's room, try to resist it in the last weeks of pregnancy, or get someone else to do the painting. It's important to avoid exposure to paint that may contain lead, and some latex paints, which may contain mercury. Most water-based paints can be used, but always check the label for contents that could be harmful. Painting should always be done in a well-ventilated room.

Insecticides

Occasional contact with an insecticide shouldn't harm you or your baby but repeated exposure to a chemical over a period of time will be dangerous. High levels of exposure have been linked with birth defects. There are plenty of environmentally friendly products on the market that won't pose a risk to your unborn baby. If you have unwanted insects in the house, try to avoid spraying, if possible, and use non-chemical alternatives.

Household pets

Having a pet usually doesn't cause any problems. Even if your large golden retriever jumps up to your bump occasionally, it's unlikely to hurt you or your baby. The one pet that may carry some risk is a cat; some outdoor cats carry a rare infection known as toxoplasmosis (see pages 111 and 257) while indoor cats cats become infected by eating raw meat contaminated with the parasite. Infected cats have the organism present in their faeces, so you should avoid changing your cat's litter tray. If this is impossible, you should wear disposable gloves and wash your hands immediately after cleaning the tray. It's recommended that trays should be cleaned daily and filled with boiling water for five minutes.

Jacuzzis, saunas and steam rooms

Studies suggest that pregnant women whose core body temperature rises above 38.9°C for more than 10 minutes during the first seven weeks of pregnancy stand an increased risk of miscarriage or having babies with neural tube defects such as spina bifida. For this reason, it's vital to avoid overheating. However, after your first trimester, occasional use of Jacuzzis, saunas and steam rooms for less than 10 minutes is reasonable and safe.

Pollution

Air quality may become an issue for some pregnant women, especially those who live in a city. There's no evidence that city life is harmful to a developing baby, but what you can do for your baby is minimise the time you spend in highly polluted or dirty areas. Bear in mind, too, that air quality can be up to two to five times worse in the home than outdoors. For this reason, keep your use of toxic household products to a minimum (see above), check for any signs of mould or damp, and have heating appliances checked to ensure that they're not emitting carbon monoxide.

Common childhood diseases

A number of common illnesses – rubella (German measles), shingles, chickenpox and fifth disease or slapped cheek syndrome (caused by the parvovirus B19) – can be dangerous to your developing fetus. Notify your caregiver at once if you are in contact with an affected child.

Working safely

With the exception of a few physically demanding or high-risk jobs, it's perfectly safe for most women who have no complications to continue working throughout pregnancy. And there are ways to make your day even more comfortable.

Many women find that work is a good distraction from some of their uncomfortable pregnancy symptoms. And, if you plan to return to your job after the birth, balancing the demands of work and the physical challenges of pregnancy now will be great practice for managing your future career when you have your kids.

Adapting your routine

Speak to your employer as soon as you know that you're pregnant so you can discuss ways to make your day more comfortable. It may be possible to arrange more flexible working hours to help you to cope with times when you're suffering from fatigue or morning sickness. You also should be given time off to attend antenatal appointments.

If your job is physically very demanding, your doctor may advise you to make more drastic changes to your routine. If your job involves long hours, long periods on your feet or working with any hazardous materials, you are within your rights to ask your employers to get you some additional help or give you alternative duties.

Minimise stress

Rushing to get to work on time, meeting deadlines or working late can exaggerate pregnancy symptoms, making you feel tired or down. Although there may be little you can do to reduce stress that's inherent in your work – for example, you can't change deadlines or stop dealing with customer complaints – you can change your own attitude to work. Always bear in mind that your baby comes first, and for the sake of your baby's well-being, as well as your own, try to find ways to eliminate any extra stress. For example, delegate when possible and learn to say 'no' to overtime, excessive travelling or entertaining. Take plenty of breaks throughout the day, walking around

---

ways to make your workplace more comfortable

1   If there are smoking areas at your company's premises try to avoid them.

2   Keep your desk drawer topped up with healthy snacks such as dried fruit, nuts and cereal bars.

3   If you work in a place where there are extremes of heat, such as a kitchen, ask to work elsewhere – overheating may damage your baby.

4   If you work in front of a computer screen all day, take frequent breaks to get up and move around.

5   Make sure your work station is properly set up. Sit in a height-adjustable chair with a back rest, wrist support and a footstool.

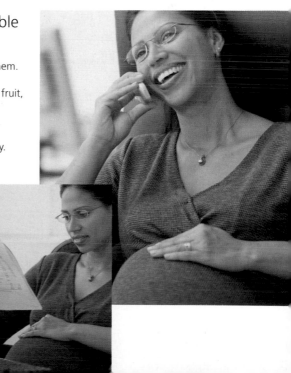

and stretching if you've been sitting at a desk, or sitting down and putting your feet up if you've been standing up all day.

Deciding when to stop

If your pregnancy proceeds without complications, there's no medical reason why you can't continue to work right up until your delivery date. Although most women find that they are too exhausted to carry on working past eight months, this is very personal. Some women are happy to carry on with their daily routine; others feel the need to stop earlier in the last trimester. If you want to stop work earlier than you'd planned, discuss it with your employer; you may be able to work part time for your last few weeks.

Occasionally, complications arise during pregnancy that make it advisable to reduce your workload or stop altogether. For example, if you develop high blood pressure or if there are problems with the baby's growth, your healthcare provider may advise you to stop working.

Avoiding hazards

As jobs are so diverse and individual pregnancies are so different, you may need to do a bit of research to find out if there are specific hazards in your workplace. Contact the Health and Safety Executive (HSE) for information and safety guidelines. At your first antenatal visit, talk to your doctor about the type of work you do.

Your daily tasks

Think about what you do each day. Do any of your tasks put you at risk of strain or injury? For example, if you work at a computer, incorrect seating can contribute to pregnancy backache, while prolonged typing or using a mouse may increase your risks of carpal tunnel syndrome (see page 260). Both of these hazards can be minimised with correct seating and positioning of equipment, and by the use of wrist supports. Speak to your employer to have your work station assessed. If your job involves lifting or carrying, check that you know how to lift correctly (see picture, page 72), and avoid carrying

heavy objects. If your job involves standing for long periods, take frequent breaks to reduce the chances of swelling and varicose veins (see page 73).

The equipment you use

In the office, there is little chance that any equipment you use will cause you any harm. Some women worry that computer monitors may emit harmful radiation. However, research has shown that the levels of radiation involved are well below international safety limits. Neither has there been shown to be a proven connection between mobile phone use and illness.

In other industries, risks are dependent on the type of work you do. Consider in particular any chemicals or biological agents you work with, such as drugs, laboratory specimens or pesticides. These are potentially harmful to pregnant women, so take all necessary steps to avoid contamination. If any machinery you use puts you at risk – such as the heavy metals present in semiconductor chip manufacturing, for example, ask about doing another job during pregnancy.

Your work environment

Smoking is no longer permitted in the workplace but there may be areas – outside the building, for example, where colleagues continue to smoke – so try to avoid them.

If you work in a place where there are extremes of heat, perhaps in a factory or kitchen, you may need to ask for work in a different area, as this can be damaging for your baby. The same is true if you work with potentially harmful chemicals, for example, in a dyeing, printing or photographic workshop; in a beauty salon; in a lab or on a dry cleaning machine or premises. Ask your employer for the safety data sheets for the products you work with and show them to your doctor.

Make sure your office chair, desk and immediate furnishings – window treatments, flooring and walling – are PVC-free and that you open windows frequently to ventilate your space.

Travelling safely

Being pregnant doesn't mean you have to stay at home and wrap yourself up in cotton wool. As long as your pregnancy is progressing normally and you follow a few precautions, you can still explore the world, if you want.

Bear in mind that going away will mean that you're away from the caregivers who know you. If you travel abroad the antenatal care may be very different and hard to access due to language difficulties. Importantly, care may not be free, so check that you have adequate medical insurance. Talk to your GP about which immunizations you might need and which medications you can take for common problems. It's also advisable to avoid travelling to areas at high altitudes – adjusting to the reduction in oxygen could be too taxing for you and your baby, especially during the last trimester.

When to go

One of the key questions is when is it safe to go away? In general, you're best off travelling during the mid-second trimester, between about 18 and 24 weeks, when the risk of miscarriage or premature labour is low. Obviously, you need to take into account your own particular circumstances – if you're expecting triplets, for instance, it wouldn't be advisable to travel at this time as you will require frequent medical check-ups.

Eating safely

Be careful of what you eat and drink in underdeveloped countries. Make sure that you stick to the healthy eating guidelines in Chapter 4, avoiding any potential hazards (see page 110). Choose restaurants that look hygienic, and make sure that you know what you're eating – if you're unsure of what a dish contains, don't eat it. Be wary of food bought from stalls and markets, where dishes, and meats in particular, may be only semi-cooked. Salads, fruits and vegetables can be problematical if you suspect the washing water isn't clean. Best to stick to fruit you can peel before eating. Before you travel, find out what the water supply is like. You'll need to keep up your water intake, so if you're at all unsure about the safety of the drinking water, drink still, bottled water. You should even use bottled water to brush your teeth. Avoid drinks containing ice.

Travellers' diarrhoea

It's very common to get diarrhoea when you're travelling. While not serious in itself, it can dehydrate you, which can lead to weakness, fainting, preterm labour, and reduced blood flow to your baby. If you develop serious diarrhoea, drink plenty of fluids and seek medical advice.

Looking after your health

It may be hard to find a pharmacy where you're travelling, so take along any medications that you feel you may need, provided that you have checked their safety with your GP. If you usually take prescription medications, for asthma or high blood pressure for example, make sure you carry enough to last you for your entire trip – and a little extra isn't a bad idea either. Again, discuss this with your doctor.

HEALTH FIRST

MALARIA   It's not recommended for pregnant women to travel to countries where malaria is common; malaria can pose a serious threat to a pregnant woman and her developing baby. While medications are available for the prevention of malaria, and some, such as Malarone, are safe in pregnancy, none is 100 per cent effective. If you cannot avoid the trip, ask your doctor for advice.

The basics of good care

After that first rush of excitement on finding out that you're pregnant, you need to start taking proper care of yourself and your baby and that means organising your antenatal care.

The ultimate goal of any antenatal care programme is a healthy pregnancy, for both mother and baby and the successful birth of a new life. It's never been safer to have a baby than today – if you're currently healthy, your chance of giving birth to a healthy baby is over 95 per cent. But this isn't a reason to miss your regular check-ups; in fact, the opposite is true – studies have shown a strong link between early involvement in antenatal care and healthy babies of a good birth weight.

The purpose of antenatal care

The tests and check-ups that make up antenatal care are designed to provide as much information as possible about your pregnancy. They will:

- *Assess your general health* Examinations and tests will uncover any existing medical problems, such as high blood pressure (see page 265). If a problem surfaces, it will be monitored at your subsequent visits and you'll be advised on how the condition may change as a result of your pregnancy and how it may affect your baby.
- *Check on your well-being* Professionals on your antenatal team can monitor your physical and emotional well-being when they see you.
- *Check on your baby's well-being* Your schedule of tests is designed to monitor the normal development and growth of your baby. If anything unusual is found, you'll be offered other tests to confirm the problem and determine the cause. Your midwife or doctor can then explain your options and help you to take whatever steps are necessary to safeguard your baby's health.
- *Detect complications* Common pregnancy complaints such as heartburn or haemorrhoids are minor, but a nuisance all the same. Your

healthcare provider can give you advice on how best to treat these and, if possible, prevent them from recurring. Antenatal check-ups are designed to detect any 'invisible' conditions, such as gestational diabetes or pre-eclampsia (see page 253), so that they can be treated successfully and therefore have minimal effects on your developing baby.

◆ *Educate and prepare you for parenthood* There's so much to learn about becoming a parent and your healthcare provider will give you advice on joining a parenting class.

◆ *Prepare you for the birth* It may seem a long way off now, but you'll be surprised how quickly your due date arrives. Your team is there not only to help you and your partner to make informed choices about the sort of birth you want but also to support you both throughout the miraculous birth experience.

Choosing your care

Most general practitioners (GPs) offer shared antenatal care with the local hospital if you are having a hospital birth. You will see your GP and community midwife for the majority of your checks and will usually only attend the hospital for one or two check-ups and your scans.

In some areas of the United Kingdom, women whose pregnancies are likely to be straightforward are looked after entirely by midwives. Midwives undertake all the antenatal care and the delivery – either in the hospital or at home – as well as providing postnatal care. This is called community midwife or 'low-risk' care. If any problems arise during your pregnancy, your midwife will refer you to the hospital.

If you have a pre-existing medical condition, have had a previously complicated pregnancy or delivery, or if there are factors that could make your pregnancy 'high-risk', your antenatal care will be under a consultant obstetrician at the hospital.

Private care is also available. You can be seen by a consultant obstetrician at a private hospital for all your antenatal care, delivery and postnatal care while private midwifery teams also are available to undertake all your care. With the latter, you will usually deliver your baby at home.

MORE **ABOUT**   your antenatal visits and notes

Most women use a store-bought pregnancy test to confirm a pregnancy (see page 21) and then ask their healthcare provider to recommend a midwife (community, independent or hospital-based). Once a recommendation is given, a booking appointment (see page 87) needs to be arranged between 8 and 10 weeks of pregnancy.

At your booking visit, you will be given a set of maternity notes, which you should carry with you to all your appointments and if you go on holiday. Each clinic has its own system, but the notes will include such information as the date of visits, the length of your pregnancy at the time, your weight, the results of urine and blood pressure tests, the height of fundus (see page 91), the baby's presentation, the presence of any swelling (oedema) and any other important observations.

After the booking visit, you will be seen according to your medical needs and those of your developing baby (see page 91). With a low-risk pregnancy, there will be around 10 visits.

Special tests are arranged at certain stages. For example, a dating scan will be performed between weeks 11 and 13 (which includes an early test for Down's syndrome, another scan at 18 to 20 weeks will check the baby's anatomy and growth, and your rhesus status (see page 90) will be assessed at the booking visit. Other scans or blood tests can be done to look for an increased risk of chromosome abnormality.

GENERAL PRACTITIONER

Most GPs provide antenatal care.

OBSTETRICIAN

This is a doctor who specialises in pregnancy, labour and birth. An obstetrician has special expertise in dealing with complications in any of these areas and you may be referred to one if your midwife has a particular concern.

MIDWIFE

All midwives have been specially trained to care for mothers and babies throughout normal pregnancy, labour and birth. Depending on their pre-training qualification, they may have a midwifery certificate or a degree. A supervisor of midwives has had extra training and education. He or she assists and supports midwives in providing the best quality maternity care. You should be given the contact details of the supervisor. All UK midwives are registered with the Nursing and Midwifery Council.

Midwives can work in hospitals, midwifery units or the community, attached to a GP's practice. One can deliver you at home. A community midwife continues to look after a mother and baby until their care is handed over to a health visitor at between 10 and 28 days after the birth. Independent midwives work outside the National Health Service, often in a group midwifery practice.

ANAESTHETIST

This specialist doctor is responsible for pain relief such as an epidural. He or she will provide appropriate anaesthesia for a caesarean or forceps or ventouse delivery.

PAEDIATRICIAN

This is a doctor specialising in the care of babies and children. One may check your baby to see that all is well after the birth and will be present if you have a difficult labour or if there is a suspected problem with your baby.

SONOGRAPHER

This individual is specially trained to carry out ultrasound scans. One will perform your dating and nuchal translucency and anomaly scans, and any additional ones you may require.

MEDICAL STUDENTS

Trainee midwives and medical students training in obstetrics and/or gynaecology may be present during antenatal visits. You can refuse to have them in the room and request that certain procedures are performed only by a fully-qualified doctor.

OTHER HEALTH PRACTITIONERS

An obstetric physiotherapist can give you advice and support about pregnancy-related aches and pains and also recommend exercises to speed your recovery after delivery (see page 334). Dieticians may advise you on healthy eating, particularly if you have a condition such as gestational diabetes.

HEALTH VISITOR

This is a specially trained nurse who will look after your baby from the early weeks.

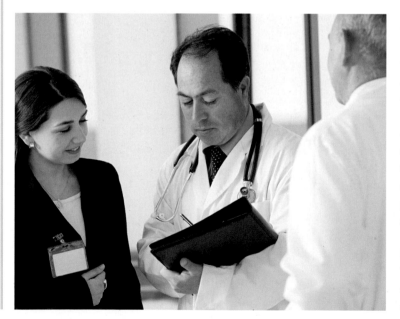

Your booking appointment

This should take place between weeks 8 and 10 and is one date you shouldn't miss. In addition to some base-line tests, your care options – shared care, hospital care, midwives alone, for example – will be discussed – and you will be given much information on different aspects of pregnancy and fetal development.

Your booking appointment can take up to two hours. This initial assessment may be done in hospital or at your GP's surgery or even at home (if you are using an independent midwife). If necessary, you will be sent to the hospital or clinic for tests.

Your midwife will probably start with a review of your past and current health and that of your partner. This is usually followed by a sequence of checks, such as your weight and blood pressure. You will be asked to give a urine sample and some blood will be taken from a vein in your arm for various laboratory tests (see page 89).

If you haven't had a recent cervical smear test (within three years), you will be advised to wait until your baby is born before you have one; pregnancy can make the result of a test harder to interpret.

Your midwife will give you information about nutrition, including taking folic acid and vitamin D supplements, and food hygiene; caution against smoking, drinking and recreational drug use, and inform you about and schedule, screening tests.

At the end of this visit, you'll be given the dates of future antenatal appointments, depending on your medical needs and be issued with hand-held notes to carry about with you for the rest of your pregnancy (see box, page 85).

Medical history

Gathering information about your health and that of your partner is one of the goals for your caregiver at your first visit. This questioning process is called taking your medical history. Your doctor or midwife will ask you various questions about all aspects of

your life (see the box on page 88) and it's important to be honest and accurate: all the details you give help to build a complete picture of your history so that any risk can be more easily spotted.

Don't be embarrassed about answering personal questions or become upset when revealing certain sorts of information, such as if you had a previous miscarriage; your caregiver is there to offer support and understanding. If you can't remember all the details of a previous episode, give as much information as you can and your midwife can try to expand on this information from records elsewhere.

Physical examination

Most women don't need a full physical examination but if you already have an existing medical problem, you may need extra checks such as tests of kidney function if you are diabetic.

A breast examination is not usually done unless you have concerns about the size of your breasts or the shape of your nipples.

Your caregiver will take your blood pressure at each check-up – high blood pressure is a common complication in late pregnancy.

A pelvic examination is not usually performed; there is no evidence that it predicts problems with delivering.

Measuring your weight

Your weight will be measured at your first visit and your BMI (see page 64) calculated. After that, you will only be weighed if you were over- or under-weight when you started your pregnancy or if you don't seem to be gaining weight at a reasonable rate.

Gaining too much weight can make it difficult for your healthcare provider to discern how your baby is growing and if you're overweight you're more likely to experience complications such as gestational diabetes (see page 253).

Being underweight isn't healthy either – your healthcare provider will want to monitor your baby's growth more closely if you're below average weight, because your baby may not be growing as well as expected (see page 261).

Blood pressure check

Your healthcare provider will check your blood pressure at every visit; it's an essential part of antenatal care because high blood pressure is an important – and common – complication, especially in late pregnancy. The reading taken at your first visit will form the baseline against which any fluctuations can be measured. You may become familiar with the numbers your healthcare provider

10 subjects that will be discussed at your booking appointment

Your first visit will be a successful and productive one if you prepare in advance. As well as considering the questions below, it's a good idea to talk to your mother to find out about her pregnancies – were they straightforward or were there complications and if so, what sort? Ask your partner to obtain similar information from his mother, too.

1 What is your medical history? Do you or your partner have any conditions that seem to run in the family? Have you had any operations – and therefore anaesthetic – or stayed in hospital for any length of time? Are you allergic to any medications?

2 Do you have any pre-existing medical conditions? Are you taking medication – and were you when you discovered your pregnancy – for a chronic condition, such as asthma or high blood pressure?

3 If this isn't your first pregnancy, how long ago was your last one? Was it a healthy, normal pregnancy or were there any complications? You should let your healthcare provider know about any previous terminations or miscarriages as well.

4 Do you exercise regularly? How healthy is your diet? Do you smoke? How much and how often do you drink alcohol? Do you use any recreational drugs?

5 What is your ethnic origin? Because certain medical conditions are more prevalent in particular ethnic

groups, your healthcare provider may want to know from where your family and that of your partner originate (see page 240).

6 What sort of job do you have? Could your job pose any risks or hazards to your unborn baby? Do you work with chemicals or X-rays? Do you work in a hot or cold environment? Do you travel extensively? Do you have a hectic work schedule?

7 Do you have a secure, permanent place to live? Is it clean and safe?

8 What date was the first day of your last period? Your due date is calculated from this date (see page 22). Typically, how regular were your periods and how far apart were they?

9 Were you using any form of contraception before you discovered that you were pregnant? If you have an intrauterine device (IUD) tell your healthcare provider, as there's a potential for it to cause complications. If you were on the Pill when you got pregnant, it shouldn't be harmful for your pregnancy or your baby, but your dates may not be accurate.

10 Do you have any problems with mental health, or are there problems in your relationship with your partner? You may be at increased risk of domestic violence or postnatal depressionl You may be referred for extra help and support if this is the case.

writes down for your blood pressure reading – a typical measurement is 120/70. Blood pressure is measured in millimetres of mercury – written as mmHg; the first number represents the systolic pressure (when the heart contracts), while the second number represents the diastolic pressure (when the heart relaxes). Your blood pressure will probably decrease during the first 24 weeks of pregnancy, with the systolic measurement dropping by about 5 to 10 mmHg and the diastolic by 10 to 15 mmHg. As you progress toward your third trimester, however, your blood pressure should return to your pre-pregnancy levels. If it starts to increase further, your healthcare provider will assess you for pre-eclampsia. Occasionally, blood pressure medication may be prescribed.

Urine tests

Changes within your body may mean that you're more prone to kidney and urinary tract infections during pregnancy – about 4 per cent of women are found to have bacteria in their urine samples. Recognising and then treating infection while you're expecting is important, because these types of infection can cause premature labour (see page 250).

To discount a bacterial infection, you'll be asked at your first visit to give a sample of urine, which will be sent off to a laboratory for testing. At your first and all subsequent visits, your urine is tested for the presence of protein, which could mean you have an infection or, more seriously, pre-eclampsia (see page 253) or kidney disease.

Normally, urine tests are done quickly on site using a specially impregnated dipstick; your healthcare provider may give you a supply of these dipsticks so that you can monitor your urine at

home on the day of your antenatal check and then report the result. It's imperative that you report any positive results of protein in your urine.

Your urine will also be tested for the presence of glucose. Pregnant women have sugar in their urine from time to time, but if it's found at consecutive visits or if your baby is very large for her dates, you'll be checked for gestational diabetes – a type of diabetes seen only in pregnant women, which disappears after their babies are born (see page 253).

Routine urine cultures aren't usually sent off, unless the dipstick indicates a possible infection, or the presence of white blood cells, blood or protein. Routine cultures may be done for women with a history of recurrent urinary tract infections, kidney infections, diabetes, or sickle cell disease.

Routine blood tests

You may have already received information from your healthcare provider explaining what blood tests are done and why, but if you're unsure about a specific test ask for clarification. At your first visit you'll be asked to give a blood sample and you might need to give further samples during your pregnancy depending on your health and if any complications occur. Fortunately, a whole host of tests can be performed on just one sample of blood.

Immunity to rubella (German measles)

It's likely that you have either had rubella or been vaccinated against it as a child, however, immunity can wear off over time. You will, in any event, be offered a rubella immunity test as part of your antenatal care. You are not able to have a rubella immunisation during pregnancy so if you are not immune, try to avoid anyone who has the virus but if you are unable to do so, inform your doctor. You can be vaccinated after your baby is born to protect any future pregnancies.

If you are pregnant less than three months after vaccination, don't feel concerned, as there have been no reports of adverse outcomes in children born under these circumstances.

Full blood count

As the name implies, this blood test checks the level of each type of blood cell: red blood cells (which carry oxygen), white blood cells (which fight infection) and platelets (which are involved in blood clotting). If you're anaemic (see page 252), for example, the level of red blood cells – and therefore haemoglobin, of which iron is an essential component – is low and your doctor will prescribe an iron supplement to remedy the problem. You may also be advised to include more iron-rich foods in your diet such as: dark green, leafy vegetables; red meat; cooked shellfish, particularly clams; dried fruit; fortified cereals; enriched pastas; and breads;

and eggs. Because iron-deficiency anaemia develops most often after 20 weeks – and especially in the third trimester – this check for low iron levels is normally repeated as your pregnancy progresses.

Blood group and rhesus status

This blood test, carried out at the beginning of pregnancy and again in the third trimester, identifies your blood group – A, B, AB or O – tests your rhesus status – positive or negative – and tests for blood antibodies, including rhesus. Knowing your blood group is important in case you need a blood transfusion during labour. Your rhesus status is vitally important, because if your baby is rhesus positive and you're rhesus negative, it's possible for you to form antibodies to your baby's red blood cells. If you become pregnant again and your next baby is rhesus positive, the antibodies you have formed can destroy his blood cells. This puts the baby at risk of developing a serious form of anaemia, called haemolytic disease. However, thanks to modern treatment this disease is now quite rare. Rhesus-negative mothers are given injections of Rh immuno-globulin (anti-D) during pregnancy and after delivery, which are completely safe and prevent the formation of the antibodies that attack your baby's blood cells. See also page 239.

Hepatitis B

Although this viral infection affecting the liver is more common among mothers who are born outside of the UK, all mothers are offered testing for hepatitis B at their booking appointments (see page 240). If you are a carrier, your baby needs to be vaccinated after birth and for extra protection, may be given an immunoglobulin injection to prevent him from developing hepatitis.

MORE **ABOUT**   testing for HIV

Although you cannot be tested for HIV without your consent, all pregnant women in the United Kingdom are offered an HIV test, as it's possible to be infected and not know that you have it. It's important to find out this information, as immediate treatment can reduce the risk of transmission of the virus to the baby, as well as keep the mother healthy. If you think you could have been exposed to any risk factors in the past – unprotected sex or sharing needles – opt for a test for your baby's sake.

If you are found to be HIV positive, you will be offered counselling and referred to a specialist for your care during pregnancy. The chances of your baby being infected can be drastically reduced – from about one-in-four to about one-in-fifty – with the antiretroviral treatments currently available and by considering an elective Caesarean. After the birth, you'll also be advised not to breastfeed your baby, because the virus can be transferred to your baby in your breast milk.

Subsequent visits

In sharp contrast to the detailed and lengthy first antenatal visit, later appointments are shorter and involve fewer checks.

If, for any reason, you can't make an appointment, make sure you reschedule; don't be tempted to skip it because you feel alright – regular checks are in place because they're the best way to keep an eye on you and your developing baby.

At each visit your doctor or midwife will ask you how you're coping and give you the opportunity to discuss any pregnancy-related complaints (see page 67) or concerns you may have. As with the first visit, a series of checks are performed – some every time and others at key stages – to keep a close eye on your baby's health and development.

Screening tests

Doctors can now detect a disease or problem before obvious signs or symptoms indicate that there's something wrong. A whole range of screening tests exist, including ultrasound scanning, nuchal translucency screening, amniocentesis, chorionic villus sampling, alpha-fetoprotein testing and cord blood sampling. These tests are covered in detail in the Antenatal Directory.

Blood pressure and urine protein

At every visit your blood pressure will be measured and your urine tested for protein – or you will be asked for your home result — to detect signs of pre-eclampsia (see page 253). Pre-eclampsia doesn't usually develop until the third trimester.

If your blood pressure rises or your urine test is positive for the presence of protein, your healthcare provider will refer you for further tests, and you may need to be admitted to hospital.

You may have certain blood tests to check for blood abnormalities that can occur with pre-eclampsia, such as low platelets and abnormal liver function tests.

Growth and fetal position

To follow the growth of your baby, your healthcare provider will palpate your abdomen at each visit and will measure your fundal height — the distance from the top of your uterus to your pelvic bone. This lengthens as your baby grows and so gives an estimate of his size for his age. If your baby is felt to be too big or too small, you'll be referred for an ultrasound scan for a more accurate measurement. If your baby isn't growing well or is growing too fast – for example, if you've developed gestational diabetes – you may need to deliver him early. With twins or triplets, your babies' growth will be assessed with ultrasound about every four weeks.

At each of your visits after 35 weeks, your abdomen may be checked to ascertain your baby's position. Because of natural constraints – such as the shape of a woman's pelvis and the shape of a baby's

An ultrasound scan not only enables your baby's development to be monitored, it also gives you a first glimpse of him or her.

head – over 95 per cent of babies are born head first. It's common for babies not to be in the head-down position before 36 weeks; however, after this time, it's more unusual, and your healthcare provider may advise you to take steps to try to turn your baby around into the correct position (see page 204) so that you can have a normal delivery.

Fetal heartbeat and movements
At each visit after 16 weeks, your caregiver will listen to your baby's heartbeat with a handheld Doppler device. At any time, if he or she has any concerns, ultrasound scanning and cardiotocography (CTG) may be used to check on your baby's progress.

From around 20–22 weeks' of pregnancy, you should feel your baby move – flutters, kicks and rolls – and such movements will rapidly acquire a regular pattern. During your antenatal visits, you may be asked about your baby's movements, how often you feel them and how strong they are. They become especially important after 30 weeks (see page 207).

Whooping cough vaccination
Following a rise in the number of cases of whooping cough in young babies, pregnant women who are between 28 and 38 weeks of pregnancy, will be offered vaccinations to protect their newborn babies. The temporary vaccination programme aims to boost the short-term immunity passed on by pregnant women to their newborn babies who normally cannot be vaccinated themselves until they are two months old. Even if you have previously been immunised, you are advised to be vaccinated again to boost your immunity.

YOUR FIRST SCAN

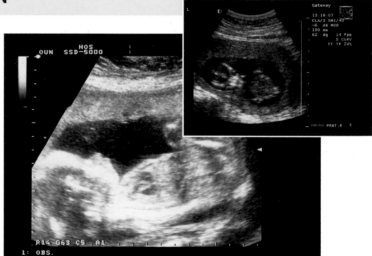

That first momentous ultrasound is carried out in a hospital and is done by an ultrasound technician. Watching your baby moving around inside and seeing his tiny heart beating is truly mesmerising and breathtaking. It may be the first time your pregnancy feels 'real', especially if you've been lucky enough not to have morning sickness and don't have any other obvious signs.

As wonderful as it may be to see your baby, the purpose of the scan is to make sure that your baby is developing properly and that there aren't any problems. Several measurements will be taken to check that he's growing well. Depending on the stage of the pregnancy, the baby's anatomy may be checked for problems such as neural tube defects (see page 375).

You can be given an idea of the sex of your baby at around 16 weeks – but it is only an idea and shouldn't be relied on for decorating your baby's room.

By the end of the appointment, your healthcare provider should be able to confirm your due date (within 5 days) or give a more accurate estimation based on your baby's size. As with all your antenatal visits, taking your partner, or a close friend or relative, is enormously important, both for support and for sharing the joyous experience. You'll almost always be offered a printout of your scan.

Special pregnancies

Every pregnancy is special, but there may be circumstances that necessitate you needing closer monitoring to ensure continued well-being. These include being older, carrying twins and having a pre-existing medical condition.

The questions you're asked as part of your medical history (see page 87) will identify whether you're more likely to need extra care. If, for instance, you're an older mother, have an existing medical condition such as asthma or diabetes, or have had a previously complicated pregnancy, you may be offered more screening tests and be asked to attend extra visits. If you're carrying twins or more, your team will want to keep an especially close eye on you all.

Being an older mother

If you're over 35, your prospects of a smooth and trouble-free pregnancy and birth have never been better. If you hear your caregivers referring to you as an 'elderly' or 'mature primip,' don't be insulted; this is simply a medical term that describes the fact that you're over 35 and having your first baby. 'Primip' is the shorthand form of primiparous; if you're having your second or third baby you will be referred to as "multip," which is short for multiparous.

Research shows that if you've waited to have children, you're more likely to be in good health and will make more of a conscious effort to promote your baby's well-being by eating healthily, exercising regularly, and avoiding hazards. If you are fit and healthy, you're likely to have a good pregnancy.

It's also been shown that children born to older mothers (no matter their social standing) are healthier and less likely to be admitted to hospital or to have accidents.

Age	Risk of Down's syndrome
25	1:1500
30	1:900
35	1:350
40	1:100
44	1:30

Health risks

The main risk for older mothers is the increased chance of chromosomal abnormalities. Chorionic villus sampling (CVS) or amniocentesis are the diagnostic tests used to identify such abnormalities. The good news is that many studies looking at neonatal outcome indicate that as long as the chromosomes are normal, the outcome for the babies is the same as it is for women under 35.

Older women also have a slightly increased risk of developing gestational diabetes (see page 253), pregnancy-induced hypertension (see page 253) and pre-eclampsia (see page 254). Because of this, you may be offered more antenatal visits and ultrasound scans to monitor your baby's development closely and to detect any problem as early as possible.

Down's syndrome

Any woman can have a baby affected by a chromosomal disorder, such as Down's syndrome, although this is more common as you get older. If you're 35, the chance of having a child with Down's syndrome is about 1 in 300. From a positive point of view, though, that means you have a 99.7 percent chance of having a normal, healthy baby.

Certain non-invasive tests, such as nuchal translucency screening (see page 237) and blood tests (see page 241), which can indicate the probability of your baby having the disorder, are routinely offered as part of prenatal care. But further tests will be needed to confirm the diagnosis. With these more invasive tests – CVS (see page 242) and amniocentesis (see page 244), a small sample of chorionic tissue or amniotic fluid is removed for analysis – your healthcare provider will offer you counselling to discuss the full implications should results come back positive. Your antenatal team is there to support you throughout your pregnancy, so don't hesitate to contact them between visits if you need more information, reassurance and/or advice.

An older father

'Advanced paternal age' (APA) is used to indicate older dads (generally 40+) fathering kids. It has recently been discovered that older dads have a higher risk of passing on chromosomal mutations in their genes, which are linked to a rise in autism and possibly schizophrenia in their offspring. Scientists now believe that older fathers account for 15–30 per cent of cases of autism and perhaps schizophrenia.

Older dads also have a slightly higher risk of passing on an autosomal dominant mutation – a disorder inherited from only one mutated copy of a gene. Compared to chromosomal abnormalities like Down's syndrome, autosomal dominant disorders (such as Huntington's disease) are much rarer, so since there is no test that will diagnose every autosomal dominant disorder (and there are thousands known), routine testing is not recommended for men.

Expecting twins or more

Discovering that you're going to have more than one baby can come as a shock and may seem overwhelming. Some women, especially if they're a

ways to take double care of yourself

Whether you're expecting twins – and triplets or more – you need to be extra careful. The tips below are designed to avoid or alleviate common complaints that are part and parcel of a multiple pregnancy and so make your pregnancy as safe and as comfortable as possible.

1   Eat little and often. Don't be surprised if you start feeling full even after a glass of fruit juice and an oatmeal bar – your stomach will have less space as your babies fill out and jostle for room. Nibble food on a little-and-often basis to keep up energy levels and obtain your essential nutrients.

2   Take a nap. Physically you'll need more rest as you may find daily life more tiring, so it's vital to build in some rest periods every day – especially in later months – in which you can sleep or practise some relaxation techniques. If you don't do this, you'll be exhausted before you know it and may even have to be admitted to hospital for the last month or so.

3   Beat backache. Be super-conscious of your posture – remember to stand and sit tall – as carrying the extra weight of your babies can exaggerate the curve of your spine and exacerbate backache, especially in your lower back. Ask your partner or a friend to try his or her hands at a back massage.

4   Swim for support. Being in water reduces the effect of gravity on your babies and offers some much-needed support. Swimming, especially crawl and

backstroke – which don't cause you to arch your back as breaststroke does – is great exercise and can soothe pressure on your pubic bone and help to alleviate any backache.

5   Make your pillow a friend. To relieve and prevent the extreme backache common in multiple pregnancies, buy or borrow a specially designed pillow to support your lower back. Carry it with you wherever you go.

6   Enlist your partner, friends and family in helping out around the house and in doing strenuous chores. In addition, try not to lift anything heavy, including bags of shopping and small children.

7   Take things slowly. You may feel dizzy or faint as your blood vessels are more dilated (open) than usual and blood rushes to your feet when you stand up – so don't leap up, get up slowly and learn how to get up from a lying-down position by rolling over onto your side first.

8   Sleep easy. When sleeping or resting, you may want to keep yourself propped up with pillows or a beanbag to avoid putting pressure on the major blood vessels, which could restrict the blood supply to the placenta. You'll probably have to try out a few positions until you find the one that is right for you.

You may be a little apprehensive about giving birth to twins, but your healthcare provider will be able to give you lots of advice and support.

twin themselves or if they've already had one baby, have an inkling that 'something's up' but can't quite believe it until they see conclusive proof on the ultrasound scan. Occasionally, if you're expecting twins, or more, you'll experience exaggerated pregnancy symptoms – compared with carrying a singleton – so severe morning sickness and extreme tiredness in the early days could be clues that something is different.

Multiple pregnancies are diagnosed by an early ultrasound scan; this early 'warning' enables you and your antenatal team to plan a specially tailored schedule of tests and check-ups. An ultrasound scan at 12 to 14 weeks will identify how many babies are present, and it is usually possible to determine if the twins are identical or not (see page 16).

How you feel

The unexpected news of a multiple pregnancy may make you feel extremely 'special': one of the few parents of twins, triplets or more. But after this exciting start, fears and ambivalence about the idea of having more than one baby may emerge. If you and your partner are first-time parents, your natural apprehension about approaching parenthood may be intensified further when you consider the reality of how you're going to cope with two babies at once. There's no denying it will be hard work initially but you'll soon find your feet and establish routines to nurture and love the new budding personalities in your life. For parents who had planned to have more than one child, finding out that twins are on the way is fantastic news – everything they wanted in one pregnancy and delivery.

Finding out that you're carrying twins early on in pregnancy allows time for you and your partner to adjust emotionally, so that you can get on with the practicalities that preparation for two babies requires. Of course, you'll need extra equipment – cots, clothes, car seats, nappies and so on – so double the number when making a list of everything you need (see page 199). This preparation also helps to reduce extra anxiety about the approaching births, because you feel more in control and ready to respond as necessary.

You may want to contact the Twins and Multiple Births Association (TAMBA) for specific advice and information. You'll discover all sorts of handy hints and tips from chatting to other parents of twins and listening to their stories.

What can you expect?

Carrying twins can be much more complicated than carrying a singleton, so your medical team will want to keep a close eye on how everything is progressing. You can expect:

◆ *More frequent check-ups* Your blood pressure and urine protein will be checked more regularly for signs of pre-eclampsia (see page 253), a common complication of a multiple pregnancy. If your initial blood test showed that your haemoglobin has dropped – not only because twins need more nutrients but also because your blood becomes more diluted – your healthcare provider may recommend a daily iron supplement – 60 to 100 mg – and folic acid – 4 mg – to normalise your levels and prevent further anaemia.

- *More ultrasound scans* Because it's difficult to monitor the growth and development of twins with a simple examination, your healthcare provider will want accurate and regular updates on how your babies are getting on in their uterine world. If your twins are nonidentical you'll probably have a scan every four weeks, or every two weeks if they're identical twins, as complications are more common.

- *Premature labour and early delivery* Babies are born early – by week 37 – in 50 per cent of twin pregnancies. Contact your healthcare provider immediately if you have any signs of pain, bleeding or watery vaginal discharge.

- *A hospital delivery* If you were planning to have your baby at home before you discovered that you're carrying two, you may be disappointed that you'll require a hospital delivery, but keep focused on the fact that your healthcare providers are thinking of your best interests. Although you can have twins normally, if the first baby is head first, keep in mind that it's not unusual for women carrying twins to require delivery by Caesarean (see page 188) so be flexible in your approach to birth. For more on twin positions and vaginal delivery see page 226.

- *Extra maternity leave* If you work, both your tiredness and your increased need for rest may mean you have to stop working earlier on in your pregnancy and take more time off.

Complicated pregnancies

If you suffered complications in any previous pregnancies, there's a risk that the same problem could recur and you should alert your healthcare provider to your history at your first antenatal visit. Of particular importance is severe pre-eclampsia (see page 253) and premature delivery. Having one previous miscarriage doesn't affect your chances for a normal and healthy pregnancy this time around; even after three miscarriages, you still stand a good chance of getting pregnant again and carrying your baby the full nine months. Talk through any

concerns with your healthcare provider, who may arrange more intensive antenatal care.
Pre-eclampsia recurs in up to 30 per cent of pregnancies, although it's likely to be less severe and occur later on in the pregnancy. If there is concern about you, you'll be offered more frequent antenatal clinic visits to check that your blood pressure is normal and to look for signs of oedema, such as swollen ankles and hands. Your healthcare provider may prescribe a small dose of aspirin – 75 mg daily – to be taken throughout pregnancy. Some studies suggest that this may help to reduce the risk of developing pre-eclampsia, or at least delay its onset.

If your last baby was born more than three weeks early, the same could happen again, although it depends on the cause of the previous premature delivery. Your healthcare provider may want to see you more often, especially in your last trimester and may also recommend that you take plenty of rest to lessen the chance of going into labour too far ahead of your due date. Ask what signs or symptoms could indicate a premature labour so that you can alert your healthcare provider as soon as possible, if the problem recurs.

Chronic conditions

Even though you may manage a long-term condition such as diabetes or high blood pressure excellently, you may be worried initially about how it will affect your baby. What's also important is how your pregnancy will affect your condition. It's imperative to discuss your condition with your healthcare provider, as you may need to visit another specialist for more frequent check-ups.

Depending on your condition, you may be offered more frequent visits for regular checks of your blood pressure, urine protein and your baby's growth. With diabetes, it's worth discussing your plans with your healthcare provider before getting pregnant next time, so your body can be in the best possible shape health-wise for conception. For information on how your condition could affect your pregnancy, see the Antenatal Directory.

Nine months of healthy eating

Eating a varied and balanced diet will give you the

energy and nutrients you need for a healthy

pregnancy. It also will be one of the biggest gifts you

can ever give your baby, providing him with a firm

foundation for his future health and well-being.

Making healthy adjustments

There's probably no other time at which you'll feel better motivated to adopt healthy eating habits than in pregnancy – and with good reason. Eating a varied and nutritious diet provides the best start for your baby and benefits you at the same time.

There's no great mystery to eating well in pregnancy; you simply need to eat a diet that's balanced in terms of the different food groups and that contains sufficient nutrients. Analyse what you eat each day using the food groups chart on page 102 and you'll probably discover that you're already following a fairly healthy diet. You may have to make some minor adjustments to this – for example, if you're not eating enough iron-containing foods, or eating too many sugary foods – and there are a few foods that you should avoid (see page 112), but there's no need to set yourself impossible targets.

Small changes for great rewards

Food is for enjoying, and this doesn't change even though you're pregnant. However, you will want to consider whether there are any improvements you could make to your eating habits. Maybe, for example, you usually skip breakfast, don't eat much fruit, or are often too busy to cook a meal when you finish work. While it's perfectly all right to have the occasional take away or ready-meal, these should be the exception rather than the rule, since they may not contain as many nutrients as fresh foods. When you find out how eating a good breakfast and sufficient fruit will benefit you and your baby, you'll want to make sure you get your fill.

Providing a nourishing diet for you and your baby doesn't mean you have to spend the whole day in the kitchen: cook meals in batches to store in the freezer; experiment with quick and healthy cooking methods, such as stir-frying, grilling and steaming; and if you're tired or feel sick, it'll be particularly helpful if your partner or a friend takes over some of the cooking or brings round the occasional meal.

Avoid drastic changes

Bear in mind that pregnancy isn't a time for radical change, so don't switch from being a meat-eater to a vegetarian or vice versa; it can take your body months to adjust to such a drastic difference in diet. It's much better to adapt your current eating habits so your baby receives the best nourishment possible. If you're concerned that you're not eating enough from a particular food group, speak to your healthcare provider or a dietician, who will be able to advise you on your individual requirements.

Your new eating patterns

During pregnancy, your taste buds, appetite and digestive system can be a little erratic, so prepare yourself for some weird and wonderful eating patterns. Initially, particularly if you're suffering from morning sickness, you may not feel like eating at all. Also, you might find yourself craving the strangest foodstuffs while shunning your favourite foods. Later on, in your second and third trimesters, you may feel like you're eating constantly as you move onto a little-and-often regime. Eventually, as your baby grows to take up most of your abdominal space, you may feel full even after a glass of milk and a banana.

Food cravings and aversions

Don't be surprised if you suddenly develop a passion or violent dislike for foods you felt differently about before you got pregnant. This is very common, particularly in early pregnancy. If you find you suddenly can't live without spicy or pickled items, sweets and chocolate, milk, fruit and fruit juices and very cold foods like ice cream, you're in good company, as these are the most common cravings. On the other hand, you may develop a sudden aversion to some things, such as tea, coffee, even some meats, too.

Some people believe that food cravings are a sign that your body is lacking in a particular nutrient, but this theory has yet to be proved. The exact reasons for pregnancy food fads aren't known, but changes in hormone levels, such as of oestrogen, are often thought to be responsible.

In general, as long as your cravings or aversions don't prevent you from following a sensible diet most of the time, indulge yourself and don't worry. Sometimes these feelings can work in your favour, for example, if you develop an aversion to coffee or alcohol, which aren't very good for your baby

---

MORE ABOUT strange cravings

Some pregnant women develop a very rare condition called pica, which is a compulsion to eat substances such as ice, clay, chalk, coal, toothpaste or burnt matches. Many theories have been put forward to explain this strange habit, but none has been widely accepted. One theory is that some pregnant women eat non-food substances because they are subconsciously trying to correct a deficiency in certain nutrients – some studies have linked pica to iron deficiency, even though the craved items don't contain significant amounts of iron. What is known, however, is that pica can interfere with the absorption of essential minerals, and if you fill up on pica substances, your intake of nutritious foods is reduced. If you're having any extreme cravings, discuss them with your healthcare provider.

---

anyway (see page 111). However, if you find that you're missing out on a food that's a valuable source of nutrients, try to make up for any lack by substituting it for a food of similar nutritional value from the same food group (see page 102).

Eating for two?

You'd assume that with a baby on the way, you'd need to eat twice as much food. In fact, you only need to eat more during your last trimester, and then you should aim for about 200 calories a day over your pre-pregnancy needs, which makes a total of 2150 to 2300 calories a day. These extra calories could be met easily with:

◆ A bowl of cereal and low-fat milk.
◆ Two slices of toast and butter or margarine.
◆ A glass of milk and a banana.
◆ A glass of fruit juice and a boiled egg.

However, requirements do vary with individual circumstances, and if you're concerned about your weight, speak to your healthcare provider. If you were underweight when you started your pregnancy, are expecting twins or triplets, or are a teenager, you'll need more calories. If you're overweight, you'll probably be advised to keep your weight gain to a minimum until the last trimester.

Pregnancy isn't a time to diet and you should never restrict your calorie intake to lose weight – sufficient calories are essential both to give you energy and to help your baby to grow. If you find that you're putting on too much weight, it will help to exercise regularly, limit your fat intake, and base your diet on fruit and vegetables and unrefined carbohydrates (see page 101). If you have an eating disorder, talk to your doctor or a dietician, who'll be able to help you to plan a good pregnancy diet.

200-CALORIE SNACKS: A COMPARISON		
	5 semi-sweet biscuits	Branflakes with low-fat milk
energy (kcal)	200	200
protein (g)	2.9	8.4
fibre (g)	0.7	6.5
vitamin B_1 (mg)	0.06	0.5
vitamin B_2 (mg)	0.04	0.8
vitamin B_3 (mg)	0.7	7.6
vitamin B_6 (mg)	0	1.3
folic acid/folate (mcg)	5.7	130
calcium (mg)	53	145
iron (mg)	0.9	10.1
zinc (mg)	0.3	2.1

Healthy choices

As well as making sure that you get enough calories, you need also to make sure they're from a healthy source. Eating nutritionally 'empty' foods, such as high-sugar or high-fat snacks, may satisfy your energy requirements but it won't meet your nutritional needs. There's no need to worry about every mouthful, but wherever possible, aim to eat a variety of fresh food. When choosing foods, study the nutritional information to find out what – apart from calories – you're gaining. The chart above shows how the values of two 200-calorie snacks can vary.

Managing meal times

If you have a busy life you may have got into the habit of skipping breakfast or lunch. But, just as pregnancy isn't a time to diet, it isn't a time to miss meals either, so make a conscious effort to eat properly at least three times a day.

At times, you may find that you can't manage to eat much at meals, so snack to make up your daily calories. Rather than eating nutritionally empty snacks like biscuits and sweets, go for fresh or dried fruit, raw vegetables, muesli bars, yogurts and fruit smoothies. If you're working, keep a supply of healthy snacks in your desk drawer or your bag so you've always got something to nibble on.

How to eat a balanced diet

Eating for optimal health doesn't depend on some magic formula or a definitive list of dos and don'ts – it's about balancing your intake from the different food groups and choosing the foods you want from within that framework.

An easy way to choose foods and plan your meals is to make use of the chart on page 102. This shows you the contribution that each of the five food groups should make to your daily diet.

What are the essential foods?

Most nutritionists divide food into five groups: complex carbohydrates; fruit and vegetables; dairy foods; meat, fish and protein foods; and oils, fats and sugars. Complex carbohydrates and fruit and vegetables are the two most important food groups and they should constitute the bulk of all your meals and snacks, together with smaller amounts of dairy and protein foods. Oils, fats and sugars do contain

Keep your refrigerator stocked with a variety of fresh foods, so you always have a selection from within the five food groups.

some valuable nutrients, but should be eaten only in moderation. Within each food group, eat a wide variety of foods in order to take in all the nutrients you and your baby need.

Complex carbohydrates

Breads, breakfast cereals, pasta, rice and potatoes should comprise roughly a third of your diet. Choose unrefined cereals, such as brown rice and wholemeal breads and pastas, as they're extremely nutritious. They contain both the bran, which is the outer protective coat of grain, and the germ, which is the small area at the base of each grain. When cereals are refined – to make white flour or rice, for example – most of the B vitamins, vitamin E and essential fatty acids are removed. In addition, about 20 per cent of the protein content and a high proportion of fibre is lost. Adequate fibre intake is important for your digestion and can help to prevent common pregnancy complaints such as constipation (see page 72).

Contrary to popular opinion, carbohydrates in themselves aren't particularly high in calories, but they are often served with or accompanied by high-fat, high-calorie toppings such as butter and creamy or oily sauces. If your healthcare providers are concerned that you are gaining too much weight during your pregnancy, cut down on the toppings and sauces but not on the carbohydrates, which help you to feel full and energised for longer, as they take longer for the body to break down.

Fruit and vegetables

A variety of fresh fruit and vegetables should form a major part of your diet, too. As well as providing water and fibre, fruit and vegetables contain many important vitamins and minerals (see page 106). Frozen produce is a great standby – it often has more nutritional value than fresh produce that has been been displayed in the supermarket for a day or two, because it will have been picked at its prime

A HEALTHY BALANCE OF FOOD

OILS, FATS AND SUGARS Limit your intake to less than 30% of your daily calories.

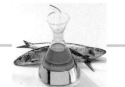

PROTEINS Eat 2 to 3 portions a day. A portion = 85 g (3 oz) meat, 115 g (4 oz) fish or 140 g (5 oz) cooked lentils.

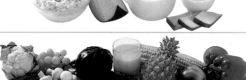

DAIRY PRODUCTS Have 3 portions a day. A portion = 200 ml (⅓ pint) of milk, 140 g (5 oz) yogurt or 40 g (1½ oz) cheese.

FRUIT AND VEGETABLES Aim to eat at least 5 portions every day. A portion = 1 glass of orange juice, 1 piece of fruit (e.g. an apple) or 3 tablespoons of cooked vegetables.

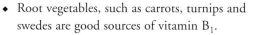

COMPLEX CARBOHYDRATES These should form the largest part of your diet. Eat 6 to 7 portions daily. A portion = 2 slices of bread, 140 g (5 oz) potatoes, 4 tablespoons cooked rice or 6 tablespoons cooked pasta.

and preserved within hours. To maximise your nutrient intake, eat a wide variety of fruits and vegetables, including, for example:

- Citrus fruit, strawberries, kiwi fruit and guavas, are rich in vitamin C, which boosts your body's absorption of iron.
- Yellow fruit, such as mangoes, peaches and apricots are good sources of betacarotene, the plant-based form of vitamin A.
- Oranges, tangerines, blackberries, raspberries and bananas contain moderate amounts of folic acid. This is important throughout your pregnancy but particularly in your first trimester.
- Dried fruit can be a good source of iron and other trace elements.
- Green leafy vegetables, especially dark green varieties such as spring greens, purple sprouting broccoli, brussels sprouts and spinach contain significant quantities of folic acid, vitamin C and betacarotene, as well as iron and other important trace elements.

- Root vegetables, such as carrots, turnips and swedes are good sources of vitamin B_1.
- Dried peas and beans, including lentils contain protein, fibre, B vitamins and minerals.
- Fruit and vegetable juices, such as apple, cranberry, orange, tomato and carrot contain lots of water, as well as being packed with vitamins and minerals.

Dairy products

Milk, cheeses and yogurt are rich in calcium, which is one of the most important pregnancy minerals. Calcium helps your baby to grow strong bones and teeth and protects your bones, too. Reduced-fat dairy products retain all the minerals and water-soluble vitamins (see page 106) of full-fat versions, so choose these when you can. Unless you buy enriched milk, all that is removed, besides fat, are the fat-soluble vitamins A and D, but milk isn't a major source of these vitamins, so don't worry that you're missing out. A 225-ml (8-oz) glass of cow's milk contain about a third of your daily recommended calcium requirements – drink three glasses and you've reached 100 per cent. Dairy foods are rich also in some B vitamins and protein. However, some cheeses should be avoided during pregnancy (see page 111).

Protein foods

Meat, poultry, fish, eggs, cheese, cereals, pulses (peas, beans and lentils) and nuts contain protein, an essential constituent of all living organisms. Protein is needed to build your baby's cells, tissues and organs. Protein foods are rich also in vitamins and minerals, such as B vitamins, iron and zinc.

Some of the amino acids that make up protein can't be made by the body and are provided only by food. But not all protein foods are equal in the amount and quality of amino acids they contain. Animal proteins – found in meat, fish, milk and cheese – contain a good range of essential amino acids. Plant proteins – in dried peas and beans, nuts, seeds and bread and other cereal products – tend to be low in one or more essential amino acids, so if you're vegetarian or vegan you'll need to eat a combination of plant-based proteins to get your full complement of essential amino acids (see page 104).

Oils, fats and sugars

This group includes foods that are high in calories and low in essential nutrients – so-called 'empty calories' – and consequently should make up the smallest proportion of your daily intake. Eating too many fatty or sugary foods on a regular basis may mean you eat less from the four other nutrient-rich food groups. You don't have to exclude fried foods, crisps, fizzy drinks, sugar, sweets and biscuits completely – you can have them as an occasional treat. But overindulging in these foods can lead to other health problems, such as obesity and heart disease.

However, small amounts of sugars and fats are essential to your health and that of your baby. They provide energy, help to maintain healthy skin and hair and transport the fat-soluble vitamins (see page 106). More importantly, the fats in vegetables, seeds and nuts and their oils, lean meat and fish, and fish oils supply you with essential fatty acids, which are compounds that the body can't make and must get from foods (see box, below).

Where possible, choose fats that are high in mono- or polyunsaturated fatty acids and low in saturated fatty acids. Unsaturated fatty acids come mostly from plant and fish sources and are generally liquid at room temperature. They are a healthy source of fats in your diet. Highly saturated fatty acids generally come from animal sources and are solid at room temperature. Eating too much saturated fat can contribute to heart disease.

Don't forget your fluids

An adequate fluid intake is essential during pregnancy, to help your blood volume to increase and to supply your baby with nutrients. Also, pregnancy boosts your body temperature so it's easy to become dehydrated. Aim to drink at least eight 225-ml (8-oz) glasses of fluids every day. As much as possible of this should be water, but milk, herbal teas and fruit and vegetable juices are also good choices. Limit your intake of caffeinated drinks and alcohol, as they can dehydrate you and have an effect on your baby (see page 111).

DID YOU KNOW...

SOME FAT IS GOOD FOR YOU

Oily fish, such as herring, sardines, salmon and mackerel, are rich in omega-3 essential fatty acids, which are key to the development of your baby's eyes and brain. Sixty per cent of your baby's brain is, in fact, made up of essential fatty acids, so it's particularly important to eat such foods during your last trimester, when your baby's brain increases in weight by four or five times. Essential fatty acids are good for you, too, as they have been linked with a reduced risk of high blood pressure during pregnancy. Pregnant women are advised to eat two portions of fish a week, one of which should be oily.

Balancing a vegetarian diet

While you're probably eating a healthy diet already, during pregnancy you may have to top up your nutritional reserves and you should make doubly sure that you're getting enough protein, iron, calcium, vitamin D and vitamin B_{12}. If you're concerned that you're missing out on any nutrients, ask your healthcare provider or dietician for advice.

Boost your protein

If you eat cheese and eggs, they will be valuable sources of protein. However, if you don't eat these, make sure you eat protein-rich foods from a variety of plant sources to ensure that you obtain the full range of essential amino acids. For example, try combining legumes (peas, beans and lentils) with wholegrain cereals. Also, any foodstuffs made from soya beans, such as tofu, tempeh or miso, are great protein providers.

Pump up your iron

Iron is essential for nourishing you and your baby (see page 108), particularly for producing new blood cells, and you need about 14.8 mg of iron a day during pregnancy. As iron from plant sources is less well absorbed than from animal sources, aim to increase your intake of iron-rich foods by consuming a range of legumes, dark green leafy vegetables and soya products. Snack on dried fruit for an iron boost. Remember, too, that vitamin C enhances iron absorption, so drink orange juice with an iron-rich meal.

Go calcium-rich

If you don't eat dairy products, you'll need to boost your calcium intake by eating plenty of green vegetables, such as broccoli, soya products, dried figs and sesame seeds. Topping up on vitamin D will help you to absorb calcium more efficiently, so eat

---

PREGNANCY MEAL PLANNER

If you're tired, it can be easy to opt for a takeaway or ready-meal, which may not give you the best balance of nutrients. Planning your meals in advance may save you some time and effort. Here are some suggestions for a week's worth of all-around healthy menus.

If you work and there aren't many healthy lunch options available locally, take a packed lunch. Dinner will probably be your main meal, so try to cook your favourite wholesome recipes then, including lots of fresh produce.

Try also to balance out your meals. For example, follow a rich main course with a light dessert, or eat a vegetable-based main dish followed by a protein-based dessert, such as yogurt or cheese.

BREAKFASTS

- Muesli with chopped dates and low-fat milk.
- Boiled eggs with wholemeal toast.
- Fresh fruit in season sprinkled with wheat germ.
- Rashers of lean bacon grilled with tomatoes and mushrooms.

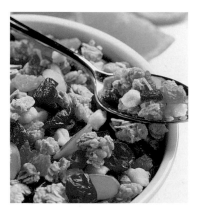

- Porridge served with low-fat yogurt and sprinkled with raisins or other dried fruit.
- Scrambled eggs on two slices of wholemeal toast.
- Fruit smoothie made with natural yogurt.

LUNCHES

- Bruschetta topped with roasted peppers and olives or tomato, basil and mozzarella.
- Pea or watercress soup and a slice of granary bread.
- A roast chicken and rocket sandwich on wholemeal bread.
- Fish goujons with an avocado dip.
- Roasted baby vegetables with tofu.
- Vegetable-topped pizza.

eggs, too. If you're a vegan, you can obtain vitamin D from fortified cereals, or speak to your doctor about taking a supplement.

Safeguard your vitamin B_{12}

This vitamin is primarily found in animal products such as eggs and dairy foods. However, fermented foods such as tempeh also contain vitamin B_{12}. Some yeast extracts, soya milk and vegetarian cheeses and spreads are fortified with vitamin B_{12}, so stock up on these, too. If you're a vegan, you may find it difficult to fulfil your vitamin B_{12} daily requirement, so speak to your healthcare provider about taking a supplement throughout pregnancy.

Other types of diet

If you are following a restrictive diet for medical or other reasons, seek specialised support and advice from a dietician or your doctor during pregnancy.

He or she will be able to tell you how you can maximise your nutrient intake so that your baby has access to all the essentials he needs. The following dietary tips are worth bearing in mind:

- If you're unable to tolerate lactose, boost your calcium levels by eating canned fish with bones, sesame seeds, tahini paste, dark green leafy vegetables, dried fruit and fortified soya milk.
- If you have a gluten intolerance you need to stock up on carbohydrates in the form of potatoes, gluten-free bread, rice and corn.
- If you're diabetic or develop gestational diabetes (see page 253), your healthcare provider will monitor you closely. As a rule, about half of your daily intake should come from carbohydrates, such as pasta, brown rice and whole grains.

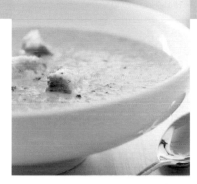

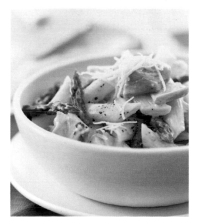

- Hummus with selection of crudités.
- Spinach and ricotta tart.

DINNERS

- Salmon and asparagus penne served with a green salad.
- Roasted Mediterranean vegetables (aubergine, tomato, courgette and yellow peppers) tossed with pasta.
- Lamb chops topped with tomato salsa and accompanied by couscous and broccoli.
- Baked cod, with green beans, boiled potatoes and salsa verde.
- Broccoli, leek and fennel gratin with a fresh green salad.
- Thai-style green chicken curry with baby corn and green beans, served on steamed brown rice.

- Stir-fry with lean pork, chicken, turkey or tofu and seasonal vegetables on boiled rice.
- Prawn and pea risotto or simple paella.
- Roasted sweet peppers filled with a rice and mince stuffing.
- Simple beef goulash, boiled potatoes, and peas and carrots.

DESSERTS

- Poached pear with chocolate sauce.
- Waffle with maple syrup and chopped strawberries.
- Flapjack or cranberry and oat biscuit.
- Lemon tart, with low-fat crème fraîche.
- Frozen fruit yogurt or passion fruit sorbet.

The essential nutrients

Nourishing your baby means more than eating the all-important body-building proteins and energy-providing carbohydrates; it means also giving him a range of vitamins and minerals.

Although your body can manufacture one or two vitamins, it relies mainly on the food you eat to provide it with nutrients. Refer to the chart on page 108 to find out the recommended daily intakes of vitamins and minerals during pregnancy and familiarise yourself with the good sources of each. Some foods are great providers of a range of nutrients, such as green vegetables (vitamins A, B_2, and C, and calcium) and whole grains (B vitamins, iron and zinc).

Essential pregnancy vitamins

There are 13 known vitamins, each with its own role to play in your and your baby's health. You can store some vitamins in your body and these are the fat-soluble vitamins A, D and E. However, your body cannot store the water-soluble variety – the B vitamins and vitamin C – so these have to be supplied on a regular basis.

If you were consuming ideal levels of all your vitamins before you were pregnant, then, theoretically, you could continue to eat the same diet throughout your pregnancy and still provide your baby with enough of each vitamin. This is because after 8 weeks, the placenta actively starts to concentrate most vitamins in your bloodstream. In reality, however, this can leave the mother with a deficiency – albeit a slight one. While it's important to take sufficient amounts of all vitamins during pregnancy, a few vitamins are especially important to the health of both you and your developing baby.

Vitamin A

This vitamin occurs naturally in two forms: retinol, which is a mature version found in animal products and betacarotene, which can be converted to vitamin A in the body and is found in plant foods. Vitamin A is involved in the development of your baby's cells, heart, circulatory system and nervous system. Consequently, when your baby's weight gain is at its greatest – in the last three months – the need for an adequate supply of vitamin A increases. Luckily, most women easily achieve their recommended daily intake of this vitamin.

Very large doses of retinol have, in fact, been associated with an increased risk of birth defects, but it is very unlikely that you will be consuming too much. Liver is the only food that provides high amounts of retinol, so pregnant women are advised to avoid liver and liver products such as pâté. Check that any supplements you take contain vitamin A in the form of beta-carotene rather than retinol.

B vitamins

This family of vitamins includes thiamin (B_1), riboflavin (B_2), niacin (B_3), pyridoxine (B_6) and cobalamin (B_{12}), as well as folates (see below). B vitamins, which help to convert food into energy, play a major part in new cell formation. They are particularly important in the early part of pregnancy when the rate of cell division is highest. At this stage, a good intake of B vitamins – notably thiamin and niacin – may be a strong predictor of a good birth weight. You need also to step up your intake of vitamin B_6, which is involved in the development of your baby's nervous system and vitamin B_{12}, which is vital for the manufacture of red blood cells. Foods rich in B vitamins include fortified breakfast cereals, vegetables, whole grains, meat, fish, eggs and milk.

Folates and folic acid

Belonging to the B vitamin family, folates and folic acid are particularly important during your first trimester. Studies have shown that women can reduce drastically the risk of giving birth to a baby with a neural tube defect such as spina bifida (see page 375), by taking a folic acid supplement before conception and during the first trimester. By 12 weeks, the baby's neural tube has formed completely and so the vulnerable period has passed.

Although folates are found naturally in foods such as green leafy vegetables, oranges and bananas, these alone are unlikely to provide adequate amounts. So it's essential to take a folic acid supplement (400 mcg) and to eat folic acid fortified bread and breakfast cereals. In contrast to other vitamins, folic acid (the synthetic version of the vitamin) is more readily absorbed than the natural version.

Vitamin C

Your need for this vitamin increases during pregnancy, as it helps you to manufacture new tissues. Your baby needs vitamin C for proper growth and development. Vitamin C also helps your body to absorb iron from food, so drink fruit juice with an iron-rich meal. Cranberries, citrus fruits and potatoes are all great vitamin-C providers.

Vitamin D

Vital for the absorption of calcium and for your baby's bone and tooth development, people whose skins are exposed to sunlight are usually able to synthesise enough vitamin D. However, there's recently been a rise in the number of young children suffering from rickets, a vitamin D deficiency, so current guidelines are that pregnant and breastfeeding women should take a daily supplement of 10 mcg, particularly if they have specific risk factors for a vitamin D deficiency. Your healthcare provider will advise.

Vitamin E

This is an antioxidant, so helps to counteract cell damage. Low levels of vitamin E have been linked to pre-eclampsia (see page 253), so make sure you eat plenty of avocados, seeds, nuts and vegetable oils.

Essential pregnancy minerals

Your body can't manufacture minerals; they have to be consumed within foods. Calcium, iron, and zinc are particularly important during pregnancy and they are discussed below. However, you should also make sure that you get an adequate intake of iodine, magnesium and selenium, which are involved in a range of functions, from the regulation of your metabolism to the development of genetic material.

Calcium

This is the most abundant mineral in the body with around 99 per cent of calcium being found in your bones and teeth. It is essential for blood clotting, muscle contraction and nerve signalling. It may also help to prevent high blood pressure, a major cause of pre-eclampsia (see page 253).

5 ways to get more nutrients

1   Much of the fruit we buy today is under ripe, so wait until fruit softens and the colour changes before you eat it – it will be at its tastiest and the vitamin content will be at its peak.

2   Fresh vegetables lose their nutrients quickly, so shop frequently and eat vegetables on the same day or soon after you bought them.

3   A high proportion of the nutrients in vegetables are stored just under the skin, so eat them with the skin on, if possible. Scrub root vegetables, such as carrots, rather than peeling them.

4   Fruit and vegetables lose vitamins wherever they're cut, so eat them whole or in large pieces.

5   Nutrients leach out into cooking liquid, so eat vegetables raw or cook them in a steamer. Cook meat and poultry using dry-heat methods, such as grilling and roasting, or use the liquid from braised or stewed dishes in sauces or gravies.

During pregnancy, your body adapts to absorb more calcium from your food and your own calcium stores are used to supply your baby. However, because many women have a lower intake than is recommended, it's vital to boost your levels throughout pregnancy, especially during the last trimester when the finishing touches are being put to your baby's bones and teeth. If you're under the age of 25, it's even more important that you get enough calcium, as peak bone health isn't reached until around this age.

Iron

This mineral is vital for new cell and hormone formation and constitutes a large part of haemoglobin, the oxygen-carrying protein in red blood cells. During pregnancy your blood volume may double, so iron is in great demand.

The recommended intake of iron is 14 mg a day for both menstruating and pregnant women. After conception, menstruation ceases and your body becomes more efficient at extracting iron from food, so in theory you shouldn't need extra iron during pregnancy. But because many women – particularly teenagers, those with heavy periods, or women who don't eat enough iron-rich foods – are already slightly deficient in iron, boosting iron levels can reduce your chances of developing iron-deficiency anaemia (see page 252).

Iron is present in both animal- and plant-based foods. Animal sources, such as red meat, poultry and fish, contain a form called haem iron, which is more readily absorbed than the non-haem iron from plant-based sources such as vegetables, pastas, fruit, grains, nuts, eggs and fortified breakfast cereals.

Vitamin C enhances iron absorption, so have citrus fruit juice or another source of vitamin C with meals containing iron. As tea and coffee are believed to inhibit iron absorption, wait for an hour or so after meals before drinking them.

Zinc

Essential for growth, wound healing and immune function, zinc is involved in cell replication. Low intakes during pregnancy have been associated also

HOW TO MEET YOUR DAILY VITAMIN NEEDS

VITAMIN	DAILY REQUIREMENT
A (retinol/betacarotene)	800 mcg
B$_1$ (thiamin)	1.1 mg
B$_2$ (riboflavin)	1.4 mg
B$_3$ (niacin)	16 mg
B$_6$ (pyridoxine)	1.4 mg
B$_{12}$ (cobalamin)	2.5 mcg
folic acid/folate	600 mcg (pre-pregnancy and first trimester) 300 mcg (last two trimesters)
C (ascorbic acid)	80 mg
D (calciferol)	10 mcg

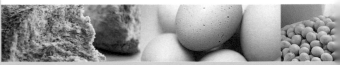

HOW TO MEET YOUR DAILY MINERAL NEEDS

MINERAL	DAILY REQUIREMENT
Calcium	800 mg
Iodine	150 mcg
Iron	14 mg
Magnesium	375 mg
Selenium	55 mcg
Zinc	10 mg

mg = milligrams
mcg = micrograms, sometimes written as μg

GOOD FOOD SOURCES

fish oils, kidney, dairy produce, egg yolk, yellow and red fruit and yellow, red and dark green vegetables

fortified breakfast cereals, wholemeal bread, dried peas and beans, pork, bacon, milk, yeast extract and eggs

milk, wholemeal bread and cereals, egg yolk, cheese and green leafy vegetables

wholemeal bread, fortified breakfast cereals, dried peas and beans, lean meats, fish and nuts

meat (especially pork), chicken, fish, eggs and wholegrain bread and cereals

lean meat, oily fish, milk, cheese and eggs

fortified breakfast cereals and bread, green leafy vegetables, bananas, orange juice, berries and dried peas and beans

citrus fruit and juices, rosehips, kiwi fruit, cranberries, strawberries, papaya, cauliflower, green vegetables, potatoes and peppers

oily fish, eggs, polyunsaturated margarine and butter

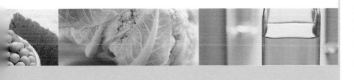

GOOD FOOD SOURCES

milk, cheese, yogurt, canned fish with bones (such as salmon and sardines), tofu and green leafy vegetables

saltwater fish, iodised salt, dairy products and eggs

lean red meat, fish, egg yolks, wholegrain cereals, spinach, legumes, fortified bread and breakfast cereals

legumes, nuts, wholegrains, spinach and peanut butter

oily fish, meats, wholemeal flour and brazil nuts

lean red meat, eggs, canned sardines, wholegrain cereals and dried peas and beans

---

with low birth weights. As with iron and calcium, your body becomes more efficient at processing this mineral, so if you were getting enough before, you probably won't need to increase your intake during pregnancy. However, if you're taking an iron supplement, this can interfere with zinc absorption. Generally speaking, zinc is associated with protein-rich foods such as meat and fish. Zinc from plant sources is less well absorbed.

Supplements: do you need them?

Generally, a healthy, well-balanced diet, precludes the necessity of taking vitamin and mineral supplements. However, supplementary folic acid prior to and during pregnancy is a necessity and nowadays, extra vitamin D (see page 107) is also recommended. Although you may be tempted to take other supplements to make up for what you think you lack in your diet, never do so without first checking them with your healthcare provider. He or she is your best source of advice about supplements.

You may be recommended a daily antenatal supplement containing a balance of vitamins and minerals. Recent research has shown that a supplement can produce babies with a larger birth weight, making them less susceptible to problems incurred by those who are small for dates. If your healthcare provider suspects that you're not getting enough iron from your diet, you also may be advised to take an iron supplement.

Taking supplements without your caregiver's knowledge is potentially dangerous and relying on them can create a false sense of security that you're meeting all your nutritional needs; an adequate intake of vitamins and minerals is only a part of what a healthy diet has to provide. You also need to have energy-rich carbohydrates, protein, essential fatty acids and fibre. Even if your healthcare provider recommends a vitamin or mineral supplement, this is no substitute for a healthy diet.

Some experts even question the effectiveness of supplements as nutrients in foods are absorbed alongside other constituents, which may have other health-promoting properties.

Avoiding food hazards

During pregnancy and particularly in your first trimester, you're susceptible to infections in food that can be transmitted to your baby. But, by following some simple rules, you can cook and eat meals that are nutritious and completely risk-free for you and your baby.

Bacterial toxins, contained in certain foods or caused by poor preparation techniques, can pass from your blood to your baby's via the placenta. Also, during pregnancy your natural immunity is slightly lower, because of metabolic and circulatory changes in your body. This is why it's paramount to minimise the risk of food-borne infections.

Buying wisely

Food safety starts in the supermarket. Always choose dairy products, meat, poultry and fish with the longest 'best before' date and try to select these products at the end of your shop, so they'll be out of a refrigerated environment for less time. Never eat

Select your foods carefully. Look for the freshest vegetables, avoiding those that look wilted or damaged.

foods past their 'sell by' date. When selecting other items during your shop, reject or discard any products with damaged packaging, such as a dented tin or torn plastic bag, so that the preservation of the food is guaranteed.

Should I choose organic?

Increasingly, you may have the choice between organic and regular foods. Organic foods are popular because many people believe they are healthier since they are grown without the use of chemical pesticides and herbicides. They believe that not only do such pollutants undermine the environment but that the cumulative effect of these chemicals and other pollutants – from the environment, smoking and drinking – can be damaging for your body.

However, this doesn't mean that conventionally produced food is unsafe: farmers' use of chemicals is strictly controlled and you can minimize your intake by thoroughly washing any fruit and vegetables you eat. Ultimately, the question of whether to 'go organic' is one of personal choice. You might consider, too, that organic food is more expensive and may not contain any more protein, nutrients or fibre than regular food.

Good food hygiene

You may already be aware of the safest ways to prepare food, but now that you're pregnant, you have a good reason to re-examine your hygiene around the kitchen. Check that you always:
- Unpack and store frozen and refrigerated food as soon as you return from shopping. Also, cover recently cooked leftovers, then refrigerate or freeze them once they've cooled.
- Store raw and cooked foods separately. Raw meats and poultry should be covered and kept on the bottom shelf of the refrigerator, to prevent their juices from dripping onto other foods.
- Avoid defrosting food outside of the refrigerator.

- Don't refreeze food once it has been defrosted.
- Wash your hands, cooking utensils and work surfaces before and after preparing food.
- Use one board for preparing raw meat and poultry and another for preparing other foods.
- Cook meat, poultry and eggs thoroughly.
- Make sure reheated food is piping hot all the way through, but don't reheat food more than once.
- Avoid eating honey and milk that is not pasteurised.

Avoiding infections

During pregnancy there are certain foods you should avoid to limit your chances of developing a food-borne infection. The most common infections caught from contaminated food are listeriosis and salmonellosis; less common is toxoplasmosis.

Listeriosis

The bacterium that causes listeriosis is *Listeria monocytogenes*, which is widespread in the environment, especially in soil. A third of all cases of listeriosis occur during pregnancy and severe cases, which are rare, can result in miscarriage (see page 278), stillbirth or premature labour and newborn infections such as meningitis (see page 363). Possible sources of listeria and therefore foods to avoid, include unpasteurised cow's milk and cheeses, mould-ripened cheeses (such as Brie), blue-veined cheeses (such as Stilton), unpasteurized sheep and goat's milk and their products, pâtés of all types, cooked foods chilled for reheating, ready-prepared coleslaw, hot dogs, undercooked poultry and raw fish and uncooked shellfish.

Salmonellosis

Because salmonella bacteria are hardy and can withstand light cooking, any potential source, such as eggs and poultry, should be thoroughly cooked to destroy all traces of infection. It's sensible during pregnancy to exclude raw and undercooked eggs and foods that may contain raw eggs, such as home-made mayonnaise, mousses or ice cream.

Toxoplasmosis

This infection, caused by the organism *Toxoplasma gondii,* can potentially lead to brain damage or blindness in your baby. It is a particular risk in your last trimester. The organism is carried in the faeces of animals, particularly cats, but is present also in soil and in raw and undercooked meat and poultry. Therefore, make sure that all the meat or poultry you eat is cooked thoroughly: only eat pork, for example, if it's 'well done'. In addition, wash all vegetables and fruit thoroughly; wash your hands after stroking pets; avoid dealing with cat litter trays; wear gloves when gardening and wash your hands before you prepare or eat food.

Common concerns

Besides the foods that are potential sources of infection, which all experts recommend you should avoid, there are several other foods and drinks that are subjects of debate. With changing notions of what is safe and potentially confusing advice from friends or the press, it can be difficult to know what you can or can't eat or drink. Here are some answers.

Can I drink alcohol?

When deciding whether you should drink alcohol during pregnancy, moderation and common sense must be your guidelines. There is much scientific data to show that daily drinking or heavy binge drinking can lead to serious complications. Moderate drinking – having one or two drinks a day or bingeing occasionally – has been associated with an increased risk of miscarriage, complications during labour and low birth weights. Pregnant women who heavily abuse alcohol – drinking five or more alcoholic drinks a day – put their babies at risk of a condition known as fetal alcohol syndrome (FAS), a term that covers a wide range of birth defects, including heart defects, learning difficulties, or structural abnormalities of the face and limbs, as well as the risk of growth problems or death.

Although there is little evidence that the occasional alcoholic drink will harm your baby, some experts say that the safest course is to avoid alcohol completely throughout pregnancy. Other healthcare providers agree that it is best to avoid alcohol at least while trying to conceive and during the first trimester, when the baby's major organs are forming. If you choose to have the occasional drink, bear in mind that it will pass to your baby through your bloodstream. Limit yourself to one to two alcoholic drinks once or twice a week at most, preferably taken with meals, as food reduces alcohol absorption. Within these guidelines, no type of alcohol is better than another: a small can or bottle of beer, a small glass of wine, or one measure of spirits all contain roughly the same amounts.

Is it okay to drink coffee and other caffeinated drinks?

Consuming over 200 mg caffeine a day reduces the absorption of some essential nutrients and increases the risk of low birth weight and miscarriage. An average cup of home-brewed coffee contains around 80 mg of caffeine so drinking one to two cups a day is usually okay during pregnancy. However, this is an average cup, not the larger coffees you get in many coffee shops. Caffeine is also found in other drinks and chocolate. New guidelines advise restricting daily intake to four cups of tea, or five cans of cola, or three energy drinks or five bars of chocolate.

Do I need to restrict salt?

Swelling (oedema) of the feet and ankles, which occurs in pregnancy is the result of water retention, caused by hormonal activity. Pregnancy hormones also increase the amount of sodium you lose in your urine. So don't over-use salt, but don't limit your intake either.

Are fish and shellfish safe?

Fish are good sources of nutrients, and you should aim to eat at least two portions of fish a week, one of which should be oily (see page 103). However, see box, left for restrictions. Some fish contain high levels of methyl mercury, a chemical harmful to a baby's nervous system.

Will eating nuts give my baby an allergy?

Peanut allergy in children is a growing problem but research has so far been inconclusive about the causes; further research is ongoing. Currently the advice is that if a pregnant or breastfeeding woman would like to eat peanuts, then she can do so, as long as it is part of a healthy balanced diet. Only women with food allergies or strong family histories (in particular the father of the baby or any siblings) of food allergies should avoid nuts and peanuts during pregnancy and while breastfeeding.

HEALTH FIRST

FOODS TO AVOID It can be confusing to keep track of everything you can and can't eat during pregnancy, so here's a list of what to avoid:

- All unpasteurised milk and cheese such as feta cheese, mould-ripened cheese such as Brie and Camembert, and blue-veined cheese such as Stilton and Danish Blue (even if pasteurised).
- Sheep and goats' milk and their products.
- All pâtés, whether meat, fish or vegetable.
- Unheated cooked-chilled meals and precooked poultry foods that can't be reheated safely.
- Raw or undercooked eggs or products containing them, including some desserts.
- Raw or undercooked meat and poultry dishes such as steak tartare or Parma ham. Take particular care with sausages and minced meat.
- Liver and liver sausage or pâté.
- Raw or undercooked fish and shellfish including sushi.
- Certain fish, including marlin, shark and swordfish. Limit fresh oily fish to 2 portions and week and canned tuna to 4 cans a week.

Keeping fit

Pregnancy makes demands on both your mind and

your body. Exercising and using relaxation

techniques can help you to maintain your health and

sense of well-being throughout pregnancy, during

labour and beyond.

Preparing for exercise

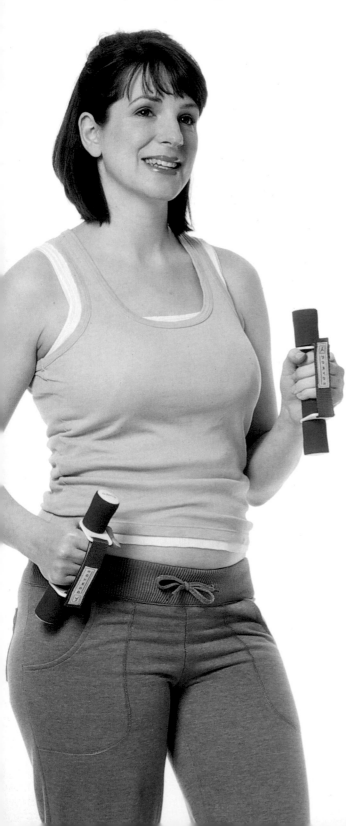

Regular exercise keeps your body in great shape for the physical challenges of pregnancy, but it's vital to learn how much or how little is best for you and the precious cargo you're carrying inside.

Exercising during your pregnancy will improve your heart and lung fitness, improve your posture, boost your circulation, help to control excessive weight gain, reduce digestive discomfort, relieve muscle aches and cramp and strengthen muscles.

Physical activity also causes the brain to release serotonin, dopamine and endorphins, chemicals which help to balance mood swings, reduce stress and promote a positive outlook. At a time when your body is changing dramatically, exercising can give you a much-needed sense of control over your body image. Studies show that a fitter body gives you more stamina to get through the lengthy hours of labour, and helps you to recover faster afterwards – you'll suffer less muscle soreness and will be up and about more quickly. Moreover, you'll be able to get back in shape sooner, and will have more energy to cope with the demands of your new baby.

Exercise safely

Whatever your fitness level, you need to take extra care when you exercise. Working out in pregnancy may carry certain risks, so check with your healthcare provider before you begin or continue with an existing exercise programme. Some women have, or develop, medical conditions that warrant caution in relation to exercise (see box, opposite). In some cases, you'll be able to exercise if the condition is controlled. However, some medical conditions prohibit exercise altogether.

Once you have the go-ahead, keep your caregiver updated with your progress. Learn to listen and respond to your body – pregnancy isn't a time to push yourself. Always err on the side of caution – if you're in doubt about an exercise, don't do it. Bear in mind, too, that pregnancy is a time to maintain, rather than improve, fitness, and you should never work out with the intention of losing weight. Regular exercise can, however, help you to keep weight gain within sensible limits.

Choose your exercise carefully

Pick an activity that you can do with your partner or a friend. You'll feel more motivated and are more likely to keep active if you are enjoying what you do. Do not perform activities in which you're in danger of falling, losing your balance or getting hit in the stomach, such as horseback riding, roller blading, downhill skiing or team sports such as basketball or volleyball. Avoid scuba diving throughout pregnancy, as it could cause gas bubbles to form in your baby's bloodstream. For recommended activities, see page 123.

Keep to a moderate level

Try to avoid or limit any strenuous activities, and always go at your own pace. Rest frequently, and take care not to overdo it, particularly in the first trimester. At altitudes greater than 2500m take particular care not to overexert yourself and spend four to five days acclimitising. Check your heart rate to gauge how hard you're working (see page 121).

In late pregnancy you may notice a shortness of breath, even when you're just sitting down. This is normal and may be because your resting heart rate is higher than normal – an average rise is about 15 to 20 beats per minute. When exercising, however, try to keep your breathing even and regular. Don't hold your breath at any point, as this increases pressure in your chest and can make you feel dizzy or faint.

Maintain a healthy body temperature

Your overall body temperature is raised by your baby's, and your body releases this extra heat through the skin, resulting in the healthy, 'rosy glow' of pregnancy. This rise in temperature means also that when you exercise, you're susceptible to overheating or hyperthermia. Getting too hot,

meaning a core temperature above 39.2°C, can be harmful to the baby – particularly in the first trimester. It's vital, therefore, to have adequate hydration and avoid exercising in very hot and humid conditions – particularly if you are not used to such conditions. Exercise at cool times of the day. Stop if you feel too hot and to drink plenty of water – you should drink around 2 litres (4 pints) of fluid a day (see page 103) and then take frequent sips of water before, during and after exercise.

Dress appropriately. Don't overdress on warm days and if it's cold, wear layers so that you can peel some off if you get too hot. Invest in a good sports bra and trainers that support your feet and ankles.

Stretch safely

During pregnancy your body produces the hormone relaxin, which is thought to soften the connective tissue around your joints, making them more flexible in preparation for the birth, but also more susceptible to injury. Stretching before and after exercise can help to prevent injuries, but stretch gently to protect your extra-supple body and take care not to overstretch. Also avoid exercises that jar your joints, such as jogging or high-impact aerobics.

Adapt your position

Don't exercise on your back past your fourth month, as the weight of your uterus presses on blood vessels and can restrict blood flow to your heart and baby. From the fourth month on, adapt any exercises that you would normally do lying flat so that you are sitting, standing or lying on one side. Also check that you maintain good posture during other activities. As your pregnancy progresses, you'll be carrying extra weight in front, so you may experience a shift in your centre of gravity, which can make you feel slightly unbalanced.

Eat right for exercise

Boost your energy by eating a light meal based on complex carbohydrates, such as wholemeal bread, pasta, rice or potatoes, at least 30 minutes to one hour before exercising.

Keep hydrated

Make sure you have water on hand while you exercise and that you take frequent small sips during your workout. Have a longer drink when you have finished exercising.

HOW TO maintain great posture

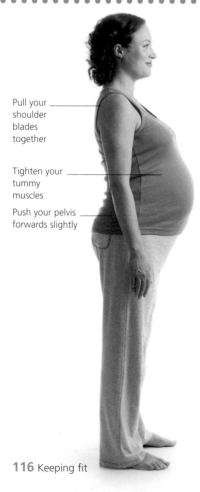

Pull your shoulder blades together

Tighten your tummy muscles

Push your pelvis forwards slightly

As your pregnancy progresses, the forward shift in your centre of gravity can result in bad posture, upper back and shoulder pain and lower back discomfort. Maintaining good posture in your everyday activities may help to eliminate these stresses and strains. Initially, you'll find that you have to make a conscious effort to correct and keep a balanced posture, but after a while you'll find it more natural.

To find a good posture, stand with your feet hip-width apart and your arms by your side. Check that your weight is evenly distributed between your feet. Stand tall and lengthen your neck – it can help to imagine a string pulling you up through the top of your head. Try to look straight ahead and keep your chin parallel to the floor.

Relax your shoulders. If you find that your shoulders are slumping forwards, push your shoulder blades together until you find a comfortable – but not rigid – position. This will help to open out your chest.

A common mistake many pregnant women make is to let the weight of their bump pull their spine forwards, which puts strain on the lower back. To keep your lower back strong and to support your baby, tighten your abdominals. Once you have found a comfortable position, try to maintain it. Never adopt the two extremes of pushing your pelvis all the way forwards or all the way backwards.

Core stability exercises such as Pilates can help greatly with posture and back pain in pregnancy.

Planning your programme

Find an exercise that you enjoy and try to build it into your schedule. You'll soon start to feel the benefits of your work-outs.

Your best source of information about exercise during pregnancy will be your healthcare provider.

If you were exercising regularly before you became pregnant and currently feel healthy, you'll probably be advised to simply carry on. However, you'll probably have to adapt your current level and the length of your sessions (see page 115).

If you haven't previously done much exercise, you may be advised against starting a new regime until your second trimester, when the risk of miscarriage and overheating has decreased, and you're likely to have more energy. Whatever your level of fitness, always be aware of warning signs while you are doing your work-outs (see box, right).

What makes a good work-out?

The ideal work-out components are: a warm-up; aerobic activity; muscle strengthening; and a cool-down. A good warm-up prepares you for your work-out. Doing some aerobic exercise works your heart and lungs. You can improve your muscular strength and endurance by performing conditioning exercises, in which groups of muscles are isolated and worked through repetitions. Careful stretching and breathing exercises are excellent ways of returning your body to normal at the finish.

Warming up and cooling down

These two stages are important before and after every activity – even gentle exercise, such as walking – as they prevent muscle soreness and stiffness. So make sure that you include short sessions – 5 to 15 minutes – of warming-up and cooling-down activities with any exercise routine.

The best warm-up consists of low-intensity, rhythmic activity, such as walking on the spot or stationary cycling, followed by slow, controlled stretches (see page 118). The initial gentle activity increases blood flow to your arms and legs. This warms your muscles, meaning that when you stretch them, they'll be less liable to damage.

Just as you should start slowly, a gentle cool-down is the best way to end your session. To cool down effectively, stretch each muscle group in turn. Gentle toning exercises are also safe if you want to include them here. Also consider including relaxation or deep-breathing exercises (see page 125) in your cool-down.

If you already go to a a gym or have a trainer, continuing your regular workout is safe but expect to modify it as you get further on in pregnancy. If you are new to the gym, start with 15 minutes of aerobic exercise three times a week and build up to 30 minutes four times a week or even daily. If you are too breathless to talk during your workout then you are probably exercising too strenuously.

SAFETY FIRST

SIGNS YOU SHOULD STOP If any of the following problems occur while you're exercising, stop immediately and seek medical advice:

- Bleeding from the vagina.
- Any gush of fluid from the vagina – a possible sign of rupture of the membranes.
- Unexplained pain in the abdomen.
- Persistent headache or changes in vision.
- Unexplained faintness or dizziness.
- Marked fatigue, heart palpitations, chest pain or excessive breathlessness.
- Sudden swelling of ankles, face or hands.
- Swelling, pain and redness in one calf.
- Reduced fetal movements.
- Painful uterine contractions.

STRETCHES FOR PREGNANCY

Stretching is an integral part of good warm-up and cool-down routines. These stretches also can help to relieve some common pregnancy complaints such as cramp in the legs and feet. However, always warm your muscles with gentle exercise before you stretch, and take care not to overstretch (see page 116).

CALF STRETCH Stand with your feet slightly apart. Take a step back with your right foot **1**. Bend your left knee until it's over your left ankle, and press your right heel into the floor. Lean slightly forwards **2**. Hold until you feel the stretch in your right calf, then release. If you can't feel it, move your right foot back. Repeat with the other leg.

FRONT-OF-THIGH STRETCH Stand with your feet hip-width apart and rest your hand on the back of a chair. Flex your left knee slightly. Lift your right knee in front of you and hold your shin **1**. Move your right knee back until it's directly under your hip and next to your left knee. Tilt your pelvis forwards slightly **2**. Hold until you feel the stretch, then release. Repeat with your left leg.

SIDE STRETCH Stand with your feet shoulder-width apart and your knees slightly bent. Place your hands on your hips. Stand tall and stretch your right arm up to the ceiling just in front of your head. Bend directly to the left, reaching your arm up and over to the side. Hold until you feel the stretch, then release. Repeat on the other side.

UPPER-ARM STRETCH Stand with your feet shoulder-width apart. Keeping your stomach pulled in, lift your right arm towards the ceiling **1**. Bend your right elbow and reach your fingers down between your shoulder blades. Place your left hand on your right elbow and gently pull the elbow behind your head **2**. Hold until you feel the stretch in the back of your right arm, then release. Repeat with your left arm.

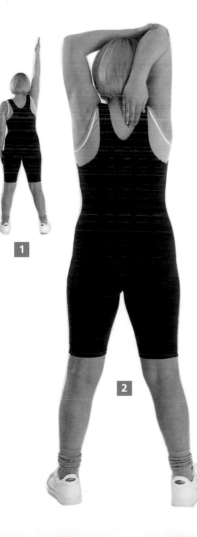

SEATED BUTTOCK AND THIGH STRETCH Sit on the floor with your legs in front of you. Place your right foot on your left thigh just above the knee **1**. Gently bend your left knee, sliding the foot towards you. Keep your tummy muscles tight **2**. Hold until you feel a stretch in your right thigh and buttock, then release. Repeat on the other side.

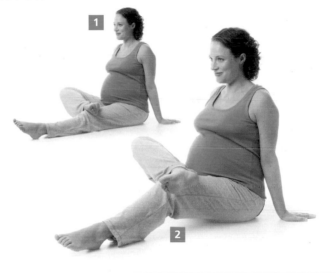

SEATED CHEST STRETCH

Sit on the floor with your legs loosely crossed. Rest your hands on your buttocks. Keeping your stomach muscles tight, lengthen your spine and draw your elbows back, squeezing your shoulder blades together. Hold until you feel the stretch across your chest. Repeat if required.

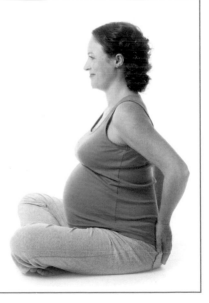

Swimming is ideal during pregnancy – your body weight is supported, so it's easy on your joints. Don't exercise in a pool that's too hot (over 32°C) or too cold – it should feel comfortable from the start.

Exercising your heart and lungs

Regular aerobic exercise boosts your circulation and improves the performance of your lungs. Also known as cardiovascular exercise, aerobic activities are those that involve moving large muscle groups – basically your arms and your legs – for a sustained period of around 15 to 30 minutes. To work effectively during this time, your muscles require a higher oxygen supply than when at rest, and to meet these extra demands, your heart rate and breathing rate have to increase. With repeated exercise, your heart and lungs begin to function more efficiently.

Whether you choose to walk briskly around your local park, swim or join a local antenatal fitness class, incorporating some form of aerobic exercise into your routine is essential to your all-round well-being – it will help you to get through the physical exertion of labour and delivery and will speed your recovery afterwards.

Muscle strengthening and conditioning

Pregnancy is almost a weightlifting exercise in itself, and because you're carrying those extra pounds, it's more important than ever to keep your muscles strong and toned. To promote muscular strength and endurance (your muscles' ability to perform an exercise repeatedly), you need to isolate groups of muscles and work them against a form of resistance, such as lifting weights at the gym or pushing against water in a water aerobics class. Before you begin this type of work-out, consider the following:

- *Use correct techniques* Make sure that you know how to perform exercises in a class or use free weights and weight machines correctly. If you're unsure, ask a qualified instructor to show you how – lifting a weight incorrectly is worse than not doing the exercise at all.

- *Never lift heavy weights during pregnancy* The general rule to follow is to use a weight that you can comfortably lift 12 to 15 times (one set). If you can't manage this many repetitions, use a lighter weight until you can. Aim to do two to three sets on each muscle. But don't get too tired.

- *Work within your limits* If you take part in a class using weights or resistance tools, don't push yourself above your target heart-rate zone (see opposite). Modify exercises that are normally performed on your back so you do them standing, sitting or on your side.

- *Keep breathing* When using weights or resistance tools, it's important not to hold your breath.

Learn to use your breathing to help you to carry out the exercise: exhale when you exert and inhale when you relax your muscles.

How much exercise should I do?

The FITT principle – frequency, intensity, time and type – will help you decide how often and how much aerobic (and other) exercise you should do.

Frequency

Unless there are medical reasons not to, experts advise that pregnant women should try to exercise moderately for at least 30 minutes on most, if not all, days. But with your enthusiasm at a peak, don't immediately start to run 5 miles or play tennis every day if you're not used to it – build up gradually. If you were already exercising regularly before you became pregnant, you can keep it up as long as there are no complications, but adjust the level of effort you put in. A good benchmark when starting to exercise is to work out three times a week – less than this and you won't see any improvement in your heart and lung fitness – then progressively increase the number of work-outs. If you get too tired at this level, cut down to three times a week.

Intensity

The amount of effort you use to perform an activity is called the intensity. Throughout your pregnancy, moderation is the key – too little effort isn't effective and too much can be exhausting or even dangerous. Intensity must be monitored carefully (see box, below) so that you don't overexert yourself. Because your heart is already pumping about 15 to 20 beats per minute faster than normal, it's essential that you don't push yourself too hard. Make sure that you exercise within your target heart-rate zone and that you know how to take your pulse.

HOW TO monitor your intensity levels

A good indication of whether you're working too hard or not hard enough is your heart rate, which is measured in beats per minute (bpm). Your ideal effort levels are indicated on the chart right. Look for your age along the bottom, then look at the highlighted band above it. When exercising, try to keep your heart rate within the minimum and maximum bpms. If you work out regularly, you can keep toward the higher limit of this zone; if you're unused to exercise, work at the lower limit. But always listen to your body: if you get too tired, slow down.

If you exercise at the gym, you may find it helpful to use cardiovascular machines, such as stationary bikes and cross trainers, that measure your heart rate through metallic pads or a clip on your thumb. Portable heart-rate monitors, which fit around your chest, are also available in fitness shops.

If you don't have access to these, you can take your pulse as you're exercising. To find your pulse on your wrist, place the index and middle fingers of one hand on the inside of the other wrist, just below the thumb. If you have trouble finding a pulse there, try the stronger pulse in your neck. To find this, place your index and middle fingers on the side of your neck about three finger-widths below your jaw.

When you have a pulse, count how many beats you feel in 10 seconds. Multiply this figure by six to get your heart rate in bpm.

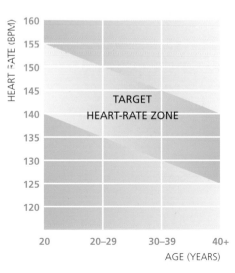

TARGET HEART-RATE ZONE

HEART RATE (BPM): 120, 125, 130, 135, 140, 145, 150, 155, 160

AGE (YEARS): 20, 20–29, 30–39, 40+

Another easy check is the 'talk test'. As you exercise, if you can continue a conversation without getting out of breath, then your intensity should be fine – as long as you stay within your target heart-rate zone. If you find that it's difficult to talk and that you're gasping for breath, reduce your effort levels, even if it means dropping below your target heart-rate zone.

Time

Start exercising in short sessions; pushing yourself too soon will only lead to exhaustion and sore muscles. For the first few weeks, do 15 minutes of aerobics at your target heart-rate zone. Once you're happy at this level, you should be able to increase your sessions in 2-minute steps, until you reach a maximum of 30 minutes. Experienced and regular exercisers can aim for a maximum of 30 minutes each session, again within their target zones.

However, even if you were exercising before pregnancy, it's not a good idea to increase the amount of exercise you do prior to week 14. The best time to start increasing the length of your sessions is in the second trimester, when you're likely to have lots of energy. In the third trimester, you may want to cut down again, if you tire easily. Listen to your body and reduce your number of sessions if you find that you're overly tired. Try to follow your aerobic sessions with muscle-strengthening exercises and always remember to include a good warm-up and an easy cool-down.

DAILY SUPER-STRENGTHENERS

As well as doing a good all-over work-out, strengthening your pelvic floor and your abdominal muscles can be helpful for a healthy pregnancy and delivery.

PERFECT PELVIC PRESS-UPS Your pelvic-floor muscles form a supportive 'hammock' within your pelvis, encircling the urethra, vagina and rectum. Pelvic-floor exercises –

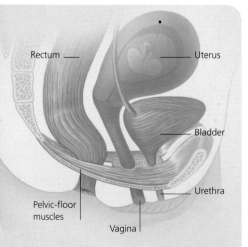

Rectum ———   ——— Uterus

——— Bladder

——— Urethra

Pelvic-floor muscles

Vagina

also called Kegels after Arnold Kegel, the doctor who introduced them – will help to tone these hard-working muscles, enabling them to support the weight of your growing baby and to help to push your baby out during delivery. Also, keeping these muscles toned will help them to recover more quickly after the birth, so helping to prevent problems such as stress incontinence (see page 68).

To practise Kegels you first have to identify the correct muscles. Next time you urinate, try to break the flow of urine briefly but without dribbling. Remember how this feels – the muscles that you use to stop the flow are your pelvic-floor muscles. Once you have identified these muscles, don't repeat this exercise during urination. If your bladder isn't emptied completely each time, you may get a urinary tract infection.

You can carry out your pelvic-floor exercises literally anywhere – sitting in the car, watching TV, even standing in the checkout queue. Simply tighten your pelvic-floor muscles, hold for a count of five, then slowly release them. It can help to imagine your pelvic floor as a lift. As the 'lift' ascends to each floor, try to pull up your muscles a little more until they're completely tight. Then, as the 'lift' descends floor by floor, gradually relax the muscles until it reaches the ground floor. Repeat this exercise five times.

Initially, it may seem like hard work even reaching a count of five because these muscles tire easily, but repeat the exercise several times a day and you'll soon be able to build up your repetitions.

Type

Activities that are excellent during pregnancy – for both aerobic exercise and muscle strengthening – include swimming, walking, stair-climbing, special antenatal aerobics and aquafit classes and stationary cycling. Walking and swimming are so safe that most women are able to carry them out until the day of their delivery. If you are an experienced runner or used to regular jogging, it is safe to continue during pregnancy but avoid running in the heat, especially in the first 12 weeks, as overheating could potentially harm your baby. Be aware that the pregnancy hormone, relaxin, loosens joints and ligaments so there is a greater chance of sustaining an injury. Always wear supportive shoes. Run on even ground, if possible, to avoid falling, particularly as your centre of gravity changes due to the enlarging pregnancy bump. Consider switching to walking or swimming in your last few weeks.

T'ai chi and yoga are other good choices, as they help you to relax and improve your body awareness. Some yoga poses, however, should be avoided during pregnancy, so always check with your instructor or choose a special antenatal class. If you find that your choice of exercise strains your weight-bearing joints, such as your hips, knees or ankles, try changing to one in which your weight is supported, such as cycling or a water-based activity.

SAFETY FIRST

DIASTASIS RECTI Before you start abdominal exercises, check that you aren't suffering from this condition, in which the vertical muscles of the abdomen begin to separate:

- Lie on your side with your knees bent.
- With your chin tucked in, reach for your knees with outstretched arms.
- If your abdominal muscles have parted, a bulge will appear down the central line of your stomach.

If you think you may have this condition consult your healthcare provider, as you may need to adapt your abdominal exercises.

TUMMY TIGHTENER Several groups of muscles run from your ribcage to your pelvis. Strong muscles here help you to maintain good posture and push your baby during delivery.

Although you would normally lie flat on your back to perform abdominal strengtheners, you should not do so after the fourth month of pregnancy (see page 116). Instead, perform this exercise when sitting, standing or lying on your side. You can have your hands on your lap, by your sides, or behind your head. Slowly curl your body towards your knees, contracting your abdominal muscles. Relax and repeat. Do as many times as you can without tiring yourself.

Support your lower back with a cushion

Pull your baby up and in towards you

Keep your feet flat

Using relaxation techniques

If you've never practised any relaxation techniques before, pregnancy is an ideal time to begin. Learning how to relax will help you to stay healthy while you are pregnant, cope well with labour and enjoy your baby after he is born.

Pregnancy is a wonderful time to learn how to make space in your day for relaxation. Get into the habit of prioritizing tasks you have to accomplish. What has to be done today? What can wait until tomorrow? And what doesn't really need to be done at all? Acquire the art of saying 'no' if people ask you to do something that's going to put you under strain. Plan a little time for yourself each day and time for you and your partner to spend together. Learn not to feel guilty because you're relaxing.

How to handle stress

A certain amount of stress is essential in life – it gives you the edge that helps you to rise to challenges and cope with any minor crises you encounter. Too little stress can mean that you function below your capacity, but too much can make you irritable, tired and ill. It is probably good for your baby to encounter stress hormones while he is developing in the uterus – it can prepare him for the stress he'll experience during the birth. But if your blood is continually flooded with these chemicals, your baby may be adversely affected. To handle stress well, it can help to raise your body awareness.

In this time of physical and emotional upheaval, every system in your body is affected: the respiratory, cardiovascular, nervous, excretory, endocrine and, of course, the reproductive. The prospect of being pregnant can be quite daunting and worrying, and you may suffer from unexpected headaches, stomachaches and muscular pains – messages that your body sends out to tell you that your muscles are tense. If you take some time to get to know your body better, you'll be able to reduce the daily wear and tear of stress and provide the best growing environment for the baby inside you. Set aside some time today to do the exercise *10 Steps to Stress-Relief* (see box, opposite). It will make you aware of how your muscles feel when they are tense and how they feel when you are really relaxed.

Learn how to breathe

You might not be aware of just how much space your lungs take up in your body. There is lung tissue above your collarbones, stretching right down to your diaphragm. If you use only part of your lungs'

Breathe deeply. Feel your tummy push against your hands as you breathe in and then fall back as you breathe out.

capacity for breathing, you're denying your body, and particularly your brain, the oxygen it needs to perform at its peak, and you'll find that your resources for coping with stress are reduced.

Take a few moments to find out whether you have a healthy breathing pattern. Sit down and put your hands on your bump. When you breathe in, you should feel your abdomen expanding to draw air into your lungs and when you breathe out, your abdomen should flatten again. Many people have an inverted breathing pattern and suck their abdomens in when inhaling.

Relaxed shoulders mean relaxed breathing. Try tensing your shoulders by pulling them up towards your ears. Notice how tight your breathing becomes; pulling your shoulders too far downwards or backwards has the same effect. When your shoulders are loose, your breathing is easy. Get in the habit of checking your shoulders regularly throughout the day, especially when you're feeling tense. Let your arms hang down and roll your shoulders backwards and forwards slowly, making sure that they're relaxed so that you can breathe well.

Instant stress relief

When you feel stressed, use this quick exercise for on-the-spot relaxation. Breathe in deeply. When your lungs are full, sigh out gently through your mouth and let the out-breath carry the tension away from the top of your body right down to your toes. When your lungs are ready, let them fill again. Then sigh out gently, relaxing your forehead, jaws, shoulders, hands, stomach and legs. The out-breath is the breath that cleanses your body of stress. If you feel tense at any time remember: sigh out slowly.

10 steps to stress-relief

Put aside 20 minutes in your day to find out the difference between muscles that are stressed and those that are relaxed.

1 Put the answerphone on, dim the lights and sit in a comfortable chair or lie down – don't lie on your back after your fourth month, try lying on your side with your bump supported by a cushion.

2 Spend a few moments settling down and trying to calm your thoughts.

3 Now stretch your toes and feel the tension. Let your toes gently relax, wiggling them a little.

4 Tighten your knees and your thigh muscles, feeling the effort. Hold for a few seconds and then relax, letting your thighs roll slightly apart.

5 Tighten your tummy muscles to give your baby a big hug. Relax, giving him as much room as possible.

6 Make fists with your hands, hold, and then let your fingers gently unfurl.

7 Pull your shoulders up towards your ears and let them drop. Shrug them a little and let them drop again. They should feel loose and easy.

8 Screw up every muscle in your face – don't worry, nobody's watching. Now relax so that there's no expression at all on your face. Your mouth should feel very soft; it may be slightly open.

9 Take a few minutes to become aware of how your body feels now that it's relaxed. Your baby will enjoy the extra oxygen he's receiving while your breathing is deep and your body is calm.

10 When you're ready, yawn, stretch, sit up gently, and prepare to get on with whatever it is you have to do.

Soothe with massage

In pregnancy, massage is an ideal way to help you to relax, as it stimulates the release of endorphins – nature's own opiates – which give you a sense of well-being. In addition, massage has beneficial effects on your circulation, digestion and excretory system, all of which come under particular stress when you're pregnant.

Although massage is largely risk-free, it's wise to check with your healthcare provider before you have any kind of massage, and always advise anyone giving you a massage that you're pregnant. Avoid massages of the abdomen and lower back during the first trimester. Also, if you find any techniques uncomfortable, immediately tell your masseur.

It's an excellent idea for the person who is going to be your companion during labour to practise massaging you throughout your pregnancy so that he or she understands which parts of your body are particularly prone to stress and what kinds of massage you find relaxing. The box below gives some simple techniques. Here, too, are some guidelines for the masseur:

◆ Try to relax.
◆ Tell your partner when you're going to start.
◆ Keep your strokes firm, rhythmical and slow.
◆ Always keep at least one of your hands in contact with the person you're massaging.
◆ Ask her if the pressure and the pace are right.
◆ Try to be aware of her body – what is it telling you? Can you feel where she's tense, and what helps her to relax?
◆ Tell her when you're going to stop.

The important thing is to experiment with different techniques and for your partner to build up a repertoire of strokes that enable you to relax. Bear in

STROKING AWAY YOUR ACHES

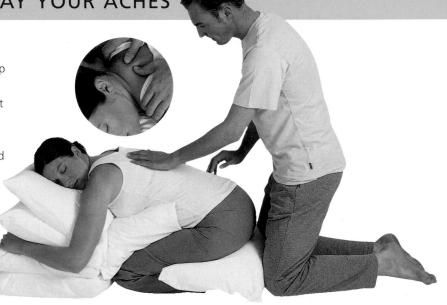

Massage can ease some of the discomforts of pregnancy and help your partner to get to know your body before labour. Spend at least 10 minutes on each technique.

BACK MASSAGE Kneel on a bed or the floor and relax into a large pile of pillows so that your bump and head are comfortably supported. Place a pillow between your calves and bottom to assist with your circulation.

Placing the flat of his left hand on your left shoulder, your massage partner strokes firmly and slowly down the side of your spine to your buttocks. Before removing his hand, he places his right hand on your right shoulder and strokes firmly down that side of your spine. He continues to alternate between each side. Tell him if the pressure is right.

Next, he uses his thumbs to make small circles in the grooves on either side of your spine, gradually working down, vertebra to vertebra. At the bottom of your back, he makes larger circles using his palms to circle down over your hips.

mind, however, that the kinds of massage you find enjoyable during pregnancy may not be the most effective in labour.

Which oils are safe?

Essential oils can provide wonderful aromas during massage and some are thought to have beneficial properties, such as relieving headaches and aiding sleep. However, you should use an essential oil for massage only if a qualified aromatherapist has recommended it to you. Some aromatherapists don't use any essential oils during pregnancy, and all experts agree that there are some – such as clary sage, rosemary, peppermint and pennyroyal – that should definitely be avoided.

A base oil, however, such as almond or olive oil, is always safe and will help the masseur's hands to glide smoothly over your skin. Your masseur should pour a little of the oil into his cupped hands and warm it there for a minute before spreading it lightly onto your body. He should position himself so that he can massage you without having to bend down or twist his back. It's important that he should be relaxed while he's massaging; otherwise, his hands will communicate tension to you and your baby.

Find peace with meditation

During pregnancy, you're in a state of heightened mental awareness. You may find yourself bursting into tears over something on the news that normally wouldn't have affected you. You may be very conscious of the changing seasons and of the different moods of nature. Certain objects in your home, perhaps from your childhood, may take on extra meaning and your thoughts may dwell on many memories as you make the transition

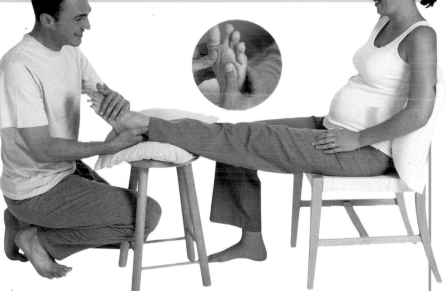

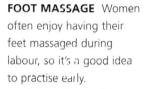

FOOT MASSAGE Women often enjoy having their feet massaged during labour, so it's a good idea to practise early.

Sit in a chair with one leg supported on a pillow placed on a stool. Your massage partner kneels in front of you. Gently resting your heel in his hand – without squeezing it – he uses his other hand to stroke firmly from your ankle to your toes. This movement is repeated slowly and regularly for several minutes.

Using his finger, your partner next strokes between each toe. He then flexes your toes upwards, supporting your heel on the pillow, and makes small circles with his thumbs across the sole. Provided that the pressure is firm, this shouldn't tickle you.

Gently lifting your foot by the ankle again, your partner then strokes you several more times from the ankle to the toes. The whole process is then repeated on your other foot.

to motherhood. You're very conscious of your body and of the changes it's going through. Meditation, which involves focusing on your thoughts and emotions, can help you to make maximum use of this self-awareness, while enabling you to achieve profound states of relaxation.

However, if you feel at all depressed, and certainly if you're being treated for depression, it's best to avoid meditation. The deep introspection it encourages may be distressing to you if your view of yourself and your life is unbalanced.

Meditation can't be learned in a single session, so it should be practised regularly. But there are two simple ways of focusing your mind: mantras and visualisation. Try alternating them day by day. As your mind learns how to still itself using the mantra, you'll find that visualisation stimulates an ever richer exploration of your thoughts and feelings.

Meditate with mantras

Find a peaceful room in which you won't be disturbed by harsh lights or sudden noises. Sit comfortably and start your meditation by focusing on your breathing. Breathe in deeply and, as you sigh out gently, let your whole body relax. Repeat until you feel fully relaxed.

Your mantra should be a word that you can match with your breathing, such as 'baby' or 'relax'. When you breathe in, say silently to yourself 'ba…' and as you breathe out, say 'by…'. Or you could think 're…' on the in-breath and 'lax…' on the out-breath. Or simply hold the word 'peace' in your mind as you breathe out.

Focus your mind exclusively on the word you're repeating. Whenever your mind wanders, bring it back gently to your chosen mantra. Continue repeating the mantra so that it drowns out all other thoughts. With practice, you'll find a vast space in your mind where you can know yourself and be at peace with yourself.

Join a class. Many centres offer basic courses that will help you to learn different techniques.

Visualise your baby

Meditation is an excellent technique for clearing away jumbled thoughts, and practising visualisation can teach you how to focus your mind – a useful technique during labour. Try the following exercise, which focuses on a candle. In subsequent sessions, choose other items that have special meaning, such as toys you have bought for your baby, things relating to your childhood or photos of important people in your life.

Settle into a comfortable chair. Place a lighted candle in front of you and let your eyes rest on the flame. Keep your gaze focused. You'll become aware of different colours and intensities of light in the flame, from the white-hot core, to the yellows and oranges that flicker along the outer edges. When your eyes start to feel heavy, let them close gently, but continue to see the candle in your mind's eye. Place your baby in the flame's image, surrounded by light, and let him stir thoughts in your mind.

Looking great

Pregnancy is a wonderful excuse to really lavish

attention on yourself – particularly as it will be hard

to find time for pampering once your baby is here.

Also, this is a time to pay special attention to your

hair, skin, teeth, breasts and feet.

Top-to-toe care

Coping with all the physical changes of pregnancy can sometimes be challenging, but focusing on the positive effects – rounded curves, shiny hair and glowing skin – can make a huge difference to the way that you feel.

Everyone talks about the bloom of pregnancy – the radiant complexion and lustrous hair – but they don't often mention the less flattering aspects – the painful breasts, swollen feet and flaky skin. While it can help to understand that such changes are just part and parcel of being pregnant, they can be demoralizing. That's why it's important to take proper care of yourself and your changing body.

Expensive products aren't essential to good skin; it's a thorough, consistent daily routine that's the basis of a healthy complexion and will keep you looking your best. Beauty products targeted specifically at pregnant women don't contain any magic ingredients, despite what they may claim, so use them only if you're really impressed with their results. Buying yourself the occasional luxury item as a treat, however, can give you a real boost.

Healthy hair

Your increased metabolism and circulation may mean that your hair grows faster, while hair loss slows down. This vigorous growth can result in hair that looks thicker and more lustrous than usual. Some pregnant women, however, are less lucky and find that their hair becomes greasy or unusually dry or lifeless. Don't worry if this happens to you: any changes that you experience will be short-lived and your hair will soon return to normal.

Hair care tips

Be gentle with your hair during pregnancy. You may find the following useful:

◆ *Use special shampoos on greasy hair* Wash hair frequently with a specially formulated shampoo and try not to brush your hair too vigorously, as this will encourage the sebaceous glands in the scalp to produce even more oil.

- *Condition hair well* If your hair becomes dry and flyaway, invest in a hot-oil treatment or deep conditioner to use once a week. Mousse can add volume, improve 'bad-hair days' and keep your style in place. Again, don't brush your hair too much as this will encourage the hair to split.
- *Invest in a good cut* As your pregnancy progresses, and certainly once your baby is born, you probably won't want to bother with a complicated hairstyle, so go for an easily managed style. This will keep your hair looking and feeling healthy throughout your pregnancy and beyond.
- *If you catch head lice,* avoid all chemical, herbal and 'natural' treatments; just remove the eggs using conditioner and a special nit comb.

Hair treatments

Although some health professionals are cautious about dyeing or highlighting hair during pregnancy, there's no evidence that these pose any risk to your baby. Today, most dyes lack potentially worrying substances, such as formaldehyde. However, if you're at all concerned avoid colouring hair during the first trimester and, after that, use only vegetable-based products. Premixed pure henna comes in many different colours. One proviso: be aware that pregnancy hormones may make your hair react differently to dyes, so you could end up with a colour you weren't expecting.

There's also no evidence to suggest that the chemicals in perms are harmful to you or your developing baby. However, your hair may react unpredictably to them and you could end up with frizzy rather than wavy hair.

Hair relaxers contain strong chemicals and although there is no evidence that they are dangerous during pregnancy, there is no proof that they are completely safe, so their use is best avoided.

A radiant complexion

The greater volume of blood circulating in your body – 50 per cent more by the time your baby is ready to be born – combined with the slight rise in your body temperature, may give your skin the characteristic pregnancy 'glow' and a soft, velvety texture as it plumps out and retains more moisture. Don't be surprised, however, if your skin becomes a bit unpredictable – it may get unusually dry or greasy, and you may even develop spots or acne.

You also may notice some other changes, such as spider angiomas (tiny broken blood vessels) on your cheeks, and chloasma – known as the mask of pregnancy – across your nose and cheeks (see page 66). Most of these marks will fade after delivery and your skin type will return to normal, but if you wish to even out your skin colour, use a good quality concealer rather than lightening fluids, which contain bleach and could damage your skin.

Sun protection

Hormones make your skin more susceptible to the effects of the sun, so that it may burn much more quickly than before. Apply a foundation or moisturizing cream containing sunscreen daily, and cover all exposed skin with sun cream with a sun protection factor (SPF) of at least 15 before you leave the house. Don't forget to take care of your lips, too. They may seem drier than usual, so use a moisturizing lip balm regularly – on its own or under lipstick – to stop them from cracking.

Your facial care

Adapt your daily skincare routine to accommodate any changes to your complexion and be prepared to keep making minor adjustments as your pregnancy progresses. In all cases, follow these guidelines for a healthy-looking complexion:

- *Cleanse your face at least once a day* Use a non-soap product suitable for your current skin type. Soap can be too harsh for your face and strip your skin of its natural oils. If you develop spots, scrupulous attention to hygiene is even more important, to keep the pores clear.

- *Use a mild astringent* This will tone greasy skin and clean out clogged pores.
- *Lavish moisturizer on dry skin* Allow it to sink in and rehydrate your complexion. If your skin becomes dry only in patches, treat it like combination skin: apply more moisturizer to the drier areas.

If you have regular facials as part of your skin-care routine there's no reason to stop while pregnant. And they are a great way to relax. Facials won't worsen any pregnancy-related skin changes, but your skin may be more sensitive than usual, so always check that any products being used are suitable.

Anti-wrinkle creams

Although anti-wrinkle creams containing vitamin A don't seem to pose a problem, it may be best to avoid using them during pregnancy, as it's possible that the nutrient can be absorbed through the skin and enter the bloodstream. There is strong evidence to suggest that vitamin supplements or medications containing vitamin A can cause birth defects (see page 106). If you're at all in doubt about what's safe to use, discuss it first with your healthcare provider.

Strong teeth and gums

It's even more important than usual to maintain good dental hygiene throughout pregnancy. The pregnancy hormones circulating in your body will probably cause your gums to swell slightly, making them more susceptible to bleeding during brushing and flossing. They also will make the gums more susceptible to plaque and bacteria.

Daily dental care

If you don't do so already, start to brush your teeth at least twice a day, and ideally after every meal. This may mean taking a toothbrush to work with you.

- *Use a soft-bristled brush* This is less likely to cause your gums to bleed. Massage your gums gently with your fingertips after brushing to encourage blood circulation.

SAFETY FIRST

SUNBEDS Although there's no conclusive evidence to show that they are dangerous in pregnancy, sunbeds can raise your body temperature dangerously high. Skin is normally extra-sensitive in pregnancy and a bed's UV radiation can worsen pre-existing chloasma and damage the skin. Some studies suggest that exposure to the UV rays used in sunbeds may cause the breakdown of folic acid in the body. It would be sensible, therefore, to avoid using them in the first 12 weeks of pregnancy, when folic acid protects the developing neural system.

Brush at least twice a day and use a soft-bristled brush, as this is less likely to damage soft gums and cause bleeding.

- *Floss daily* But floss gently, and throw out your toothbrush as soon as it shows signs of wear.
- *Chew gum* When you can't brush after eating, chew a stick of sugar-free chewing gum, as this will help to prevent plaque build-up.
- *Visit your dentist regularly* You'll need to see him or her more regularly than normal during pregnancy – once every six months is advisable. NHS dental treatment is free while you are pregnant and for a year after your baby's birth. Tell your dentist that you're pregnant, as he or she may want to avoid using X-rays at this time although limited x-rays with abdominal shielding are safe. It's probable that you may be advised that any extensive treatment should wait until after your baby is born.

Teeth whitening

Although no major studies have been done on the effects of using whitening systems – many of which use peroxide or ultraviolet light – until more is known, it's recommended that teeth whitening should be avoided during pregnancy.

Taking care of your skin

Your increased blood flow will probably make you feel warmer than usual and, as a result, you'll sweat more easily than you usually do. Make time for a daily, or even twice daily, bath or shower – use warm water rather than hot, as hot water will open your pores and make you even more likely to sweat. If your skin is feeling dry, a light aqueous cream can be used as a soap substitute or as a moisturizing skin cream, which should be applied after washing, while your skin is still wet.

You also can help to prevent sweating by choosing cotton rather than synthetic underwear, and if you wear tights, opt for types with cotton-lined gussets. Wear clothes made of natural rather than synthetic fibres to help you to stay cooler.

Keeping skin soft and supple

You probably won't need reminding to pay particular attention to your abdomen and breasts. The skin in these areas is being stretched considerably and, as a result, may feel particularly dry and itchy. Massage your tummy with a moisturizing cream or oil – a nice way to communicate with your developing baby as well as supplying a well-earned period of relaxation. If your

ways to minimise stretchmarks

1   Eat sensibly and avoid gaining too much weight. If you gain a great deal of weight in a short space of time, your skin won't have a chance to adapt and will have to stretch to accommodate your new shape.

2   Wear a well-fitting bra throughout your pregnancy. Keep your growing breasts adequately supported as they become heavier.

3   Wear a sleep bra if your breasts are large. Looking after your breasts during the day isn't enough – they need 24-hour care.

4   Keep your skin supple and itch-free. Massage cream into your breasts and tummy to elasticise the skin. Cocoa butter or almond oil extract – available from pharmacists – have proved effective for some women as have some new creams (see page 66). Try a morning and evening massage. Pure vitamin-E oil applied locally can also moisturise areas of your skin.

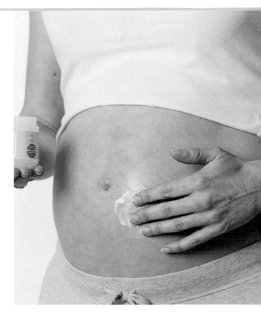

breasts are dry, apply moisturizer here, also. However, avoid over-moisturizing your nipples – if they become too soft and damp they may feel sore. If you do experience any discomfort from sore nipples, expose your breasts to the air occasionally while you're relaxing at home.

Along with your thighs, your stomach and breasts are the most likely places to develop stretch marks. There's no certain way of preventing them, nor any miracle cure for them once they have arrived, but there are some things you can do to make their appearance less likely (see page 133).

Like many women, you may enjoy massages and during pregnancy these are fine, as long as care is taken with aromatherapy oils (see page 74). Many massage therapists now offer pregnancy massages and some use special tables with a cut-out centre so you can lie face down and rest your bump.

Hair removal

Bikini, leg or facial waxes, which use a hot wax that is applied to the skin, allowed to cool, then removed from the skin along with the unwanted hair, are topical preparations that contain no substances harmful to a developing baby, so there's no reason why you can't have waxing done during pregnancy.

Although there is no known risk of depilatories or bleach harming the baby, your skin may not react well to them, and there is a possibility that their chemicals can get into the bloodstream. Electrolysis is also not recommended, even though there is no proof that it could harm the baby. Shaving and plucking unwanted hair are safer alternatives.

Tattoos and body piercing

Even if you attend a reputable parlour, tattoos and piercings should not be undertaken during pregnancy because of the high risk of infection.

Breast implants

With all the changes that are going on in your body, pregnancy is not the time to get implants for the first time. In any case, most doctors would not be prepared to perform unnecessary surgery on a pregnant woman.

If you already have silicone or saline breast implants, pregnancy will not affect their integrity but as breast tissue stretches and shrinks during pregnancy and breastfeeding, this can impair the overall effect and some future surgery may be needed. Some women have increased breast tenderness as their own breast tissue grows, and that growth combined with the increased size present from the implants stretches the overlying skin to an uncomfortable degree.

Caring for your hands and feet

You may find that your fingernails split and break more easily during pregnancy; if so, keep them short and wear rubber gloves for washing up and doing housework. You also should use gloves to protect your hands when you're working in the garden and to avoid picking up soil-borne infections (see page 257). Apply hand cream regularly, ideally the type with nail strengthener.

Pregnancy places additional strain on your feet, both through the extra weight they have to bear and through potential swelling (see page 73). You may find that it helps to soak your feet in a bowl of water in the evening and to massage with peppermint foot cream after a bath or shower.

Keep toenails short, but not so short that they may ingrow, and cut them straight across. If you can't reach your toes in the later stages of pregnancy, you may need to ask for some help or have a professional pedicure. It makes sense to go to a reputable beauty salon where the equipment is properly cleaned.

HEALTH FIRST

SEMI-SURGICAL PROCEDURES Because they use concentrated chemicals whose effects on the unborn baby are not known, chemical peels and botox and collagen injections are not recommended during pregnancy, and possibly not during breastfeeding.

Your maternity wardrobe

In recent years, glossy images of sexy, heavily pregnant celebrities have turned pregnancy into a fashion statement. This glamour and chic has filtered down to the woman on the street, so, from a fashion point of view, there has never been a better time to be pregnant.

You may feel the urge to buy a whole new wardrobe once your pregnancy is confirmed, but try to resist until your clothes become uncomfortable. Your pregnant state probably won't become obvious until about week 20 – week 14 in subsequent or multiple pregnancies. If you wait until you have to wear maternity clothes, you're less likely to be sick of them by the time your baby's born.

As your bump grows, your clothes will start to feel uncomfortable if your tummy is squeezed. Tops also may start to feel tight as your breasts grow. You can adapt many of your existing clothes for a while with a few simple adjustments. Try covering open zips on trousers with loose shirts or use suspenders to keep your trousers up. This is a good time to start 'borrowing' from your partner's wardrobe. You can replace the elastic in tracksuit bottoms with cord to give you room for expansion – sewing buttons on with elastic thread also can give valuable extra space. But if you want to wear any clothes again after your baby is born, don't wear them for so long that they're permanently stretched out of shape.

Time for a change

Inevitably, you'll need to add to your wardrobe at some stage. If you choose carefully from regular high-street shops, the clothes you buy will have a second lease of life in the first few weeks, or even months, after the birth while your figure gradually reverts to something like its pre-pregnancy state. If you plan to breastfeed, make sure that you choose tops, dresses and nightdresses that give easy and discreet access to your breasts – those with ample material or ties or buttons down the front are ideal.

5 useful pregnancy accessories

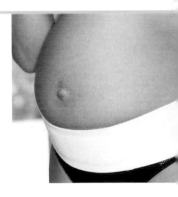

1   Bra extenders may be useful in the early stages if your chest size has increased but your cup size hasn't. The extra fastening attaches to the hooks and eyes on your existing bra to create more space.

2   Maternity tights have extra material in front to accommodate your bump and the waistband sits high enough to keep your tights up. If you have problems with aching feet or varicose veins (see page 73), maternity support tights – available in light, medium or firm – can be helpful. Slip them on in the morning, even before you get out of bed.

3   Mini maternity knickers fit snugly under your bump, while full briefs have ample material to fit over it. If you suffer from backache, maternity support knickers incorporate a semirigid back panel.

4   Support belts are special belts that fit just below your bump to provide support, relieving aching legs and a strained back. They are especially helpful if you are carrying larger or multiple babies. If you do buy such a belt, avoid wearing it all the time, as it can weaken your abdominal muscles.

5   Swimming is one of the safest and most effective forms of exercise for a pregnant woman. Maternity swimsuits grow with you and your baby.

Styles to suit you

There's no need to change your image just because you're pregnant – if you didn't like flowery prints or big bows before, why should you now? Equally, if you didn't flaunt your figure before, pregnancy may not be the best time to start.

Long, loose tops and dresses will drape your bump gracefully, while tracksuits can make comfortable everyday wear. Check that, as well as being loose around the waist, your clothes have enough material around your bottom. If not, your growing bump will pull the fabric forwards, causing it to bunch rather unattractively at the back. If you prefer more figure-hugging clothes, choose those containing plenty of stretchy fabric.

Throughout pregnancy, avoid skirts, trousers, knickers or tights that have tight elastic waistbands. Apart from being uncomfortable, the elastic may restrict your blood flow. Similarly, hold-up stockings, garters or tight knee socks may affect blood flow in your legs and could lead to varicose veins (see page 73).

Choosing maternity clothes

The main advantage of maternity clothes is that they have been designed specifically for pregnant women. Skirts and dresses are usually longer at the front than the back so that your growing bump does not cause a wavy hemline. Tucks and darts are positioned to ensure that clothes continue to hang well as your bump grows. Ribbed panels and special stretch material can accommodate your expanding bump without distorting more fitted styles. Fastenings are usually adjustable, often with several holes and buttons sewn on with elastic thread. As a result, the clothes will grow with you and continue to look good until the end of your pregnancy.

As well as specialized maternity wear shops, many department stores sell maternity clothes, and they are also available by mail order. Though your choices can seem bewildering, you needn't buy all that much – just a few carefully chosen items will keep you looking stylish during pregnancy and beyond. If you work in an environment where you need to look smart, a suit with a selection of tops may be the best

During the first months you don't need to buy special maternity clothes – purchase clothes you would normally wear in a larger size.

answer, plus some weekend wear. Simple, elegant items that can be dressed up or down, depending on the occasion, offer great flexibility. Easy-care, minimum-iron fabrics will save time if you're tired. Some mail-order companies offer 'wardrobes-in-a-box', consisting of a selection of mix-and-match items, often a dress, skirt, top and trousers, which can be combined in various ways. It's also worth looking out for shops that sell good-quality, second-hand maternity wear, as these often have tremendous bargains. However, never buy second-hand bras, as your bra needs to be well-fitting to give you support. Once your baby is born, clean and properly store any special maternity clothes for your next baby or for a good friend.

Well-supported breasts

As an expectant mother, it's vitally important to look after your breasts. Breasts themselves contain no muscles and so are supported by the muscles on the chest wall. Unsupported or badly supported breasts are more likely to develop stretchmarks or to sag, so even if you have never felt the need for a bra before, you should wear one now.

Invest in good fit

Check the fit of your existing bras or bra tops, and if they don't offer good support or if they squeeze your breasts in any way, measure yourself and invest in some new, well-fitting ones. By the end of nine months, your breasts may be up to two cup sizes larger than before, and your bra size (see below) will probably increase as your ribs expand to accommodate your growing baby. After the birth – and once you have stopped breastfeeding – your breasts will reduce in size, but probably won't be the same size and shape as they were before pregnancy. You won't need special maternity bras for most of your pregnancy, but you should buy a new bra each time your breast size increases so much that you feel uncomfortable and cramped inside your existing

one. Some women find they need new bras around week 8, others don't need to change until about week 24. Most women need a larger size again at about week 36 – these bras will also be useful for the first weeks after the birth, so you may want to buy a nursing bra, suitable for breastfeeding. Every woman develops differently, however, so be guided by the changes in your size and shape, not by the calendar. If your breasts become particularly large and heavy, you may find that a sleep bra (a lightweight maternity bra worn through the night) will help to make you feel more comfortable.

Consider the following points when buying a bra to wear during pregnancy. Choose a bra with:
- *Wide, adjustable shoulder straps* These are more comfortable than narrow straps – which can dig into your skin – because the weight is distributed more evenly.
- *A high proportion of cotton* Natural fibres allow your skin to breathe.
- *A broad band of elastic under the cups* This will support your breasts as they become heavier.

HOW TO size up for pregnancy
● ● ●

Keep your breasts comfortable by ensuring that they're properly supported at every stage of your pregnancy. You may find it easiest to

be measured professionally when you buy a new bra, but there is a good range available by mail-order, for which you'll need to know your size.

First, take a tape measure around your ribcage directly below your breasts. This is your bra size.

Next, put the tape around the fullest part of your breasts while wearing a lightweight bra. The difference between this figure and your bra size will determine your cup size. Use the box, left, to see how this difference translates to the sizes you see in shops.

FINDING YOUR CUP SIZE		
0 cm (0 in.)	=	A
3 cm (1 in.)	=	B
5 cm (2 in.)	=	C
8 cm (3 in.)	=	D
10 cm (4 in.)	=	DD
13 cm (5 in.)	=	E
15 cm (6 in.)	=	F
18 cm (7 in.)	=	G
20 cm (8 in.)	=	H

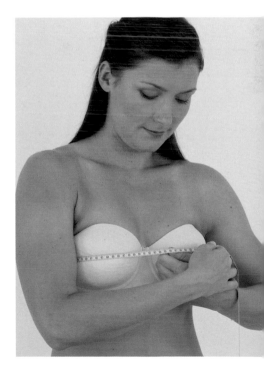

- *An adjustable back* The ideal is to have four hook-and-eye fastenings so that you can loosen your bra as your ribcage expands.
- *No underwiring* The stiff wire can pinch and damage your breast tissues, so go for a softer fit.

Choosing a nursing bra

If you're planning to breastfeed, the bras you buy around week 36 should be specially designed nursing bras. A good nursing bra has all the features listed above, and also allows you to expose one breast at a time to feed your baby.

Several types are available, including: drop-cup, where each cup unhooks from the shoulder strap; zip-cup, where the bra unzips under the breast; and front opening, where each cup is attached to the centre of the bra by a hook-and-eye fastening. If you prefer bra tops, these are also available with all the maternity features. Try on different types to discover the one you find most comfortable. Whichever you choose, make sure that you can open and close it easily with one hand – the other will be occupied holding your baby.

Breathable underwear

Itching and yeast infections are common during pregnancy so choose cotton or microfibre pants, which allow your skin to breathe. Bikini styles will sit comfortably under your bump.

Shoes and socks for comfort

It's not unusual for your feet to swell, so you may need larger sized shoes (feet can remain slightly larger after the birth). Whether or not you buy new shoes, always bear the following in mind:

- *Avoid shoes with high heels* Apart from being uncomfortable, they'll also throw your posture out, making you thrust your bump forwards and possibly leading to backache.
- *Wear comfortable, low-heeled shoes* These should be in a material that allows your skin to breathe. Avoid completely flat styles, as these don't help your balance either.
- *Avoid wearing lace-up or buckle styles* In the later stages of pregnancy you won't be able to bend easily to do them up so slip-ons and pumps are your best choice.
- *Alternate your shoes* As a rule, it's best not to wear the same pair of shoes two days in a row, but to swap between at least two pairs to allow each pair time to breathe and dry out.
- *Choose cotton socks and tights* Cotton or cotton-rich materials are preferable to synthetic, as they allow your skin to breathe. Make sure also they aren't too tight for your feet. Shorter socks, such as ankle socks, ensure that the veins in your legs aren't compressed but, ideally, you should go barefoot in the house as much as you can, to exercise the muscles in your feet and improve your circulation.

Many pregnant women find that trainers are the most comfortable form of footwear, particularly those with good foot and ankle support.

7

CHAPTER

The secret life of your unborn baby

It takes nine months for a baby to grow – and these

nine months are a period of intense activity for your

baby, as he masters all the skills he needs to survive

in the outside world.

The safety of the uterus

Protected by the amniotic sac, and supplied with oxygen and nutrients from the placenta, your baby is in the ideal environment for growth.

Advances in research have greatly increased our understanding of life in the uterus. As early as 8 weeks, when she's about the size of a grape, your baby's starting to move; from about 9 weeks she's practising how to breathe; and by 12 weeks, she's showing off her acrobatic skills with somersaults and back flips. In later pregnancy, this movement will be in response to sounds – and possibly even smells and tastes – she begins to experience via her senses.

Your baby's life-support system

From the moment your baby's conceived, your body provides her with everything she needs for complete and normal development. Initially, the uterine lining, where nutrients have been stored for nourishment, supports the developing embryo. Meanwhile, your body is hard at work preparing a more efficient life-support system: the placenta.

Chorionic villi

During the first few weeks, spongelike protrusions sprout from the wall of the fertilized egg. From these, capillary-filled tissue called chorionic villi grow. By the 8th week the chorionic villi have developed blood vessels, which carry nutrients and oxygen to the fetus. These blood vessels gradually join to form a system of blood vessels and finally the umbilical cord. At the site where the embryo implanted, the chorionic villi multiply to form the placenta, which has the job of helping your baby to survive and grow throughout pregnancy.

The placenta

Responsible for nourishing your baby, supplying her with oxygen and removing waste products, the placenta is an incredibly efficient organ. The placenta is also responsible for generating vital

THE STRUCTURE OF THE PLACENTA

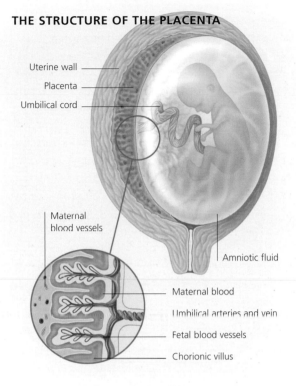

Uterine wall

Placenta

Umbilical cord

Maternal blood vessels

Amniotic fluid

Maternal blood

Umbilical arteries and vein

Fetal blood vessels

Chorionic villus

pregnancy hormones such as progesterone, so it plays a key role in stimulating your body to adapt to and maintain pregnancy (see page 60).

Attached to your uterine wall, the placenta contains blood vessels that belong to both you and your baby. In the event of identical twins, the placenta may be shared; nonidentical twins or triplets will each have their own placenta. Your baby is connected to the placenta via the umbilical cord, which is made up of a vein and two arteries. The blood vessels in the placenta intertwine but remain separate, so your blood and that of your baby never actually mixes. Everything that needs to be exchanged between the two bloodstreams is carried

out by a process of diffusion. The nutrients, antibodies and oxygen that your baby needs are passed from your bloodstream into your baby's and flow into her body along the umbilical vein. Waste products and blood that's low in oxygen are removed from her body along the umbilical arteries. These waste products pass into your bloodstream and are excreted via your kidneys.

The diffusion process means that your baby's growth and development are totally dependent on you – everything you take in, your baby takes in as well, which is why it's so important to eat a healthy, balanced diet and to avoid any substances that could harm your baby. Some research suggests that even flavours and smells from food you eat may be transferred across the placenta (see page 142).

The placenta reaches its prime at about 34 weeks, after which it begins to age. Two or three weeks later it has become less efficient in transferring nutrition to your baby. It also becomes fibrous instead of spongy, and blood clots and calcified patches appear – a sign that the blood vessels are aging. After 40 weeks, the placenta begins to deteriorate and there's a risk that it won't produce an adequate supply of nutrients and oxygen for the baby.

MORE **ABOUT**   the amniotic sac

During her time in the uterus, your baby grows inside the amniotic sac. This is filled with amniotic fluid, which cushions and protects her while also providing room for growth and movement within the uterus. The amniotic fluid is made up of fluid from the placenta, as well as fetal urine and lung fluid from your baby. At 40 weeks, your baby is surrounded by between 0.5 and 1.5 litres (1 and 3 pints) of amniotic fluid.

Your baby's senses

Far from floating dreamily in a watery world unaware of what's happening around him, your baby is hard at work developing his senses – and, surprisingly, there's plenty to stimulate them.

Your unborn baby's senses of touch, taste, smell, hearing and sight are stimulated by what is going on in your body as well as by sensations that filter through from the world outside. And learning to recognize your voice or smelling and tasting the foods that you eat may give him a sense of familiarity and security after he's born.

Touch

Your baby's sense of touch is the first to develop. About the same time he starts to move – at about 7 to 8 weeks – he becomes responsive to touch. At first, only his lips are sensitive, but soon he'll show a response in his cheeks and forehead. By about 10 to 11 weeks, the palms of your baby's hands become touch-sensitive and he'll start to feel his face, perhaps beginning to explore what he looks like. By 14 weeks, your unborn baby's whole body, with the exception of the back and top of his head, responds to touch in a similar way to newborn babies.

Plenty to explore

As your baby grows bigger, parts of his body will also touch the wall of your uterus and he'll have to curl up to fit inside you. In addition, your unborn baby is constantly brushing against his umbilical cord, and ultrasound often shows babies holding onto their cords or 'playing' with them.

DID YOU KNOW...

TWINS REACT TO EACH OTHER

As well as being in close physical proximity, twins often jostle for position. If one twin reaches out and touches the other, his brother or sister reacts to the touch and often reciprocates. This may be the beginning of the affinity that most twins have throughout life. Often one twin is more active than the other and reacts to a stimulus more readily with a faster heartbeat or harder kicking; again, this difference seems to continue in later life.

Interestingly, your baby's initial response to a touch on the cheek is to move away from the stimulus; if his hand touches his right cheek he'll turn his head to the left. This early response to touch is a result of the immaturity of his central nervous system. Later on in pregnancy, this response changes so that your baby turns his head toward the touch. This is possibly the start of the rooting reflex, which will be important in breastfeeding.

A sensitive mouth

Your baby may suck his thumb in the uterus, although he hasn't yet connected sucking with satisfying hunger. In a baby's immature body, the tongue, with its hundreds of nerve endings, is one of his most sensitive parts, and sucking is an excellent way of getting a feel for things. This can be seen in the behaviour of young children who put unfamiliar objects in their mouths to get an idea of proportions and textures, rather than feeling them in their clumsy hands. As your baby sucks his thumb in the uterus, he discovers the feel of his skin and the shape of his thumb and may receive the same sense of comfort from sucking that babies do after birth.

Taste and smell

Your baby starts to swallow amniotic fluid – the fluid surrounding him in the amniotic sac – from about 12 weeks and continues to do so throughout pregnancy. Some experts have suggested that it is through this swallowing that your baby begins to learn about taste and smell, because the amniotic fluid contains the flavour and smell of the foods you eat.

When you eat garlic, for example, your baby may taste and smell it through several routes: from your bloodstream the garlic enters your baby's, where it could stimulate the sensory receptors within your baby's nose. Second, the garlic disperses directly into the amniotic fluid and, as your baby 'breathes' and swallows, he may smell and taste the garlic. Third, as the garlic is 'expelled' from your baby's body when he urinates into the amniotic fluid, he might get a second chance to experience taste by swallowing the amniotic fluid. So while the taste of a garlic meal may be with you for a few hours, it may last some 24 hours or longer for your baby.

Developing likes and dislikes

Research has shown that unborn babies seem to be able to tell the difference between sweet and sour tastes, swallowing more when they taste a sweet substance, but less when they taste something bitter. So it may not take long before your baby starts to recognize your diet. As your breast milk is flavoured in much the same way, a radical change in diet after the birth could mean that your baby may take longer to get used to breastfeeding.

Hearing

The way that your baby responds to sounds has been extensively studied, largely because hearing is the easiest sense to stimulate in the uterus. Your baby starts reacting to sound at around 24 weeks and the louder the sound, the stronger the reaction.

Your baby's environment is full of rich and varied sounds: your heartbeat and the blood pulsing through your arteries and veins form a sound backdrop, and he also can hear intermittent gurgles from your stomach and intestines. Sounds from the world outside your body, such as voices, music and TV, also carry through your abdomen and are heard by your baby. These sounds, however, are much quieter for your baby than they are for you. This is because as a noise travels towards you, many of the

sound waves are bounced back or absorbed by your clothes and skin – only a small amount of noise penetrates through the wall of your abdomen to reach your baby's ears. Sounds with a high frequency are reflected more easily, so your baby hears mostly low-frequency sounds.

Favourite sounds

Of all the sounds your unborn baby will hear, your voice is the one that will stand out most. This is because your baby hears you in two ways: first, through the sound waves that come out of your mouth and travel through the air; and second, from the vibrations that travel through your body when you speak. This is similar to the way that you hear yourself speak, which is why your voice sounds different when you hear a recording of it – you're listening to only the airborne sounds and not the

When you're having a bath, you can try experiencing what your unborn baby hears by immersing your ears in the water. Hear how the sound changes.

internal vibrations. Your body's vibrations transmit your voice to your baby very efficiently, so whenever you speak, sing or shout, your baby hears you. It's not surprising, then, that at birth your baby will know your voice better than anyone else's. Babies don't usually recognize their father's voice at birth, although they usually can tell the difference between male and female voices.

Your voice isn't the only sound that your baby learns before he's born. Researchers have used ultrasound to observe how babies react to familiar and unfamiliar tunes played through headphones placed on their mothers' abdomens. At about 26 to 27 weeks, babies tend to increase their movements on hearing a familiar tune, almost as if they're dancing to their favourite tracks. But when they hear music that they don't recognize, they tend to stop. In some cases, familiar music may have a soothing effect on your baby after he's born, calming him down when he is crying. But use this tactic sparingly or its effects could wear off.

Sight

Your baby's sight is the least stimulated sense in his watery world and the last to develop. His eyelids remain closed until about 27 weeks, at which stage his eyes open and begin to blink, possibly practising for this reflex that he'll need after his birth.

However, inside the uterus, your baby's world is essentially a dark one. This is because the skin of your stomach and the material of your clothes prevent any light from reaching him. If you were to sunbathe on a bright sunny day wearing a bikini, he might experience a diffuse, orange glow through your skin – similar to what you see when you put your hand over a torch. Studies have shown that babies' pupils can constrict and dilate from week 33 onwards and they can perhaps even distinguish dim shapes at this stage.

ways to stimulate your unborn baby

1   Give your baby a gentle nudge and see if he gives a nudge in response. Praise him if he does – he may learn to do it again.

2   Place some headphones on your bump and play some music just for your baby. Feel him moving or 'dancing' inside you.

3   Talk and sing to your baby. He loves the sound of your voice, so read him a story or sing him a lullaby. Get your partner to join in, too – he may react differently to his voice.

4   Open up an inner dialogue with your baby. Lie down in a quiet room and visualize your baby inside you. Communicate your love for him with your thoughts.

5   Go swimming. Both you and your baby will enjoy the feeling of weightlessness that it gives you.

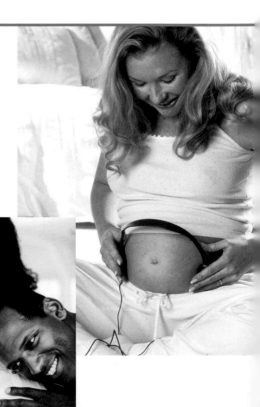

Your active baby

Your baby is like a little acrobat in the uterus and, by the time of birth, she's mastered a range of movements essential for her new life.

Your baby's movements play an important part in the normal development of her joints and muscles. The continual movement of her developing joints moulds the surfaces to each other's contours, so the bones can move together smoothly and easily. Moreover, just as you exercise to keep your body in shape, so does your baby; her movements are a kind of keep-fit programme to help her muscles to develop. She needs to be in good shape to get down the birth canal on her birth day.

First movements

Your baby first starts to move when you're about 7 to 8 weeks pregnant. At this stage, she's only about 2.5 cm (1 inch) in length, but she already has muscles along the length of her spine. As she's so small, you won't be able to feel anything yet, but these movements are just discernible on ultrasound, and researchers have described them as looking like 'twitches' or 'rippling'.

By the 12th week your baby is rolling and flipping over, even frowning, and, over the next few weeks, she'll develop an amazing range of movements. Over 20 different types have been identified in the early part of pregnancy, including sucking, yawns and hiccups. Between 13 and 17 weeks your baby is hard at work practising her full range of movements.

Patterns of activity

Your baby's movements may occur in bursts that continue for as long as 7 minutes, but more commonly, these activities last for 1 to 2 minutes, from the age of about 9 weeks. Your baby is likely to have a favourite resting place, too, where she will always return after a bout of activity. Usually this is at the lowest part of the amniotic sac.

Gaining control

Your baby's first movements are produced solely by electrical activity in her muscles: her brain is not instructing her muscles as yet. In this early part of pregnancy, her movements may be continuous and vigorous. However, as your baby's nervous system develops, her spinal cord, brain stem and then the higher centres of her brain, take over the control of her movements. The bigger movements, such as back flips and rolls, make way for finer movements, such as moving her eyes or stretching one leg. Moving her arm, for example, is a more complex action than a somersault, because each joint in the arm has muscles that allow it to extend and flex. Your baby must learn how to master both of these sets of muscles before her movements can become more graceful and controlled.

Will your baby be left-handed or right-handed?

Some of your baby's earliest movements are single, independent arm movements, which appear at about week 10. At this time, about 90 per cent of babies

DID YOU KNOW...

YOUR BABY PRACTISES BREATHING Your baby can't breathe air in her fluid-filled uterine environment – the oxygen that she needs for life is transferred from your bloodstream into hers via the placenta. However, she'll make regular and rhythmic breathing movements with her diaphragm and ribcage from about 9 weeks; by about 30 weeks, she is 'breathing' about 30 per cent of the time. These movements are essential for developing the physical structure of your baby's lungs, and they are the beginnings of the automatic reflex that will be essential for survival in an air environment.

move their right arms more, while the remaining 10 per cent prefer to move their left arms – the same proportion as for adults. This preference remains throughout pregnancy – right-handed babies at 10 weeks are still right-handed at 36 weeks – and statistics suggest that this preference lasts for life.

It used to be thought that the differences in structure between the left and right halves of the brain caused the individual to be left or right handed, but this preference in your baby's movements occurs before the two halves of her brain develop any differences. It may well be that by choosing to move her left or right arm, your baby actually causes the differences in brain structure between the two halves of the brain. In other words her physical movement could be shaping her brain.

What you feel

Feeling your baby move for the first time is one of those unforgettable pregnancy milestones. If this is your first pregnancy, you may not feel any movement until about 20 weeks, possibly as late as 24 weeks. Known as 'the quickening', these early movements will feel like flutterings or butterflies in your stomach and you might even wonder if it's wind at first. If you've been pregnant before, you may be able to identify movements slightly earlier, as you'll have learned the signs from your first pregnancy.

A lot of what you feel depends on how quickly your baby grows, and, to make you aware of her presence, she needs to be big enough to nudge and poke at your insides. When you do feel movement,

PATTERNS OF SLEEP AND DREAMING

By 36 to 38 weeks your unborn baby's activity is well coordinated, with definite periods of activity and rest, and, just like a newborn, she spends much of the time asleep.

Research has shown that during some of this sleep, unborn babies exhibit rapid eye movement (REM), which in adults is an indication of dreaming. This has led some scientists to believe that babies could be dreaming in the uterus, consolidating their experiences of

the day. Perhaps your baby might be dreaming of stretching out her limbs, listening to your voice or playing with her cord.

Research has indicated that your baby may spend much of her time in the following states:

QUIET SLEEP For about 40 per cent of the time, your baby's almost inactive, moving only occasionally, as if she's sleeping.

ACTIVE SLEEP For about 42 per cent of the time your baby seems to

be sleeping but also moving and making some random, sweeping gestures with her limbs, perhaps while she's dreaming.

ACTIVE AWAKE Your baby moves around most vigorously in this active awake state – and you'll notice it. Although it occurs only about 10 per cent of the time, it usually happens at night when you're trying to sleep.

QUIET AWAKE For about 2 to 3 per cent of the time, your unborn baby doesn't move her body much, but her eyes move constantly. This is similar to the way that newborns behave when they're quiet but appear to be paying attention to what's going on.

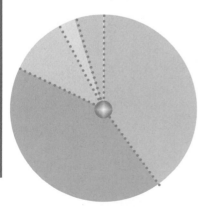

- ● QUIET SLEEP
- ● QUIET AWAKE
- ● ACTIVE SLEEP
- ● ACTIVE AWAKE
- ● CHANGING STATE

you're not actually feeling it on the lining of your uterus, as the uterus doesn't contain the necessary sensory receptors. But when your baby kicks, the uterus is knocked against muscles or organs such as the abdominal wall or bladder, and this is what provides the sensation of movement. The position of your placenta can influence this sensation. If your placenta is on the front of your uterus rather than at the back, you probably won't feel the movements of your baby as much.

Later movements

As your baby gets larger, she won't move so often, but you'll feel it more distinctly when she does. In late pregnancy, you may feel quite strong kicks to the ribs and bladder as your baby makes her presence felt. Although this reduction in activity is partly due to your baby's increasing size, it also occurs because more refined movements are required to strengthen and develop the nerve connections in your baby's neurological system.

Patterns of activity

You might notice that your baby becomes more active in response to food you've eaten – sugary food will give your baby a hit of energy resulting in a burst of movement – or to your emotions (see box, above), or simply to get comfortable when you change position. You'll probably feel her moving more at night when you're free from the distractions of the day and you're lying down, relaxed and quiet. Research has shown that unborn babies' levels of activity tend to peak around midnight, possibly foreshadowing the periods of sleep and wakefulness they will exhibit as newborns.

Learning a sense of self

Movement also teaches your baby a sense of self, an understanding of herself as a separate entity.

Through her own movements – and yours as well – plus the restrictions of her uterine environment, your baby gains a sense of what the various parts of her body are, how they're connected, and where her body starts and finishes.

We all need to know where our limbs are at any particular time. To pick up a cup, for example, we need to know the position of our arm and hand, the position of the cup and how to move our hand from its current position to the cup. For your baby, the very act of brushing a leg against the walls of the uterus, for instance, floods her system with vital information. Every movement activates sensory pathways and fuels a growing sense of self.

It's also believed that babies learn a sense of where they are in space. By about 25 weeks, most babies show a 'righting reflex', which enables them to adopt a head-down position in the uterus. Your baby will also experience gravity in her watery world. As you move around, your baby experiences this motion, so she goes through something of a roller-coaster ride as you go about your business in the world. Sitting, lying down, walking, running and bending over – everything you do will be experienced by your baby.

The birth instigator

The processes leading up to the birth are a carefully choreographed set of interactions between you and your baby. Almost like the most graceful of waltzes, your and your baby's bodies respond to each other to ensure that each step carefully follows the preceding one.

A variety of studies on animals and humans have found that it's your baby who first indicates that he's ready to be born, probably about three to four weeks before labour begins. Exactly how your baby 'knows' when it's time is a mystery, but the events that follow are better understood.

Getting ready for birth

Before he's born your baby needs to be sufficiently mature to be able to survive outside his uterine environment. In the uterus, he has relied on you to provide him with oxygen and nutrients, and to deal with waste, but as soon as he's born, his own body will have to take control of these vital functions. So, once your baby's body is mature enough, his brain sends hormone signals to the placenta to produce enzymes, which will help his vital organs to mature and then stimulate labour.

A chemical reaction

Research has shown that as the time of birth approaches, your baby's brain stimulates his pituitary gland to release the chemical adrenocorticotrophin (ACTH), which, in turn, stimulates the release of another chemical, cortisol. These chemicals are passed from your baby's body to the placenta, which reacts by converting progesterone into oestrogen. This is a significant stage, because progesterone is the hormone that keeps your powerful uterine muscles from contracting during earlier pregnancy, whereas oestrogen is responsible for triggering birth contractions. You may notice this change in hormone levels as a tightening in your uterus in the days before you go into labour.

As your baby's head presses against your cervix, a signal is sent to your brain to stimulate your pituitary gland to release the hormone oxytocin. Oxytocin stimulates the muscles of your uterus to contract, forcing your baby's head farther into your cervix and so continuing the cycle of contractions. Moreover, oxytocin stimulates the release of chemicals called prostaglandins into the bloodstream, and these intensify uterine muscle contractions. This self-perpetuating process escalates during labour, becoming more forceful and eventually resulting in the birth of your baby. It's an astounding, incredible process, with you and your baby working in perfect harmony with each other.

Preparing the birth canal

Your cervix also has to undergo changes in order to facilitate your baby's birth. Up until birth, the fibrous, tendon-like tissues of the cervix have kept your uterus tightly closed. For birth to happen according to plan, the cervix must soften and dilate, enabling the muscle contractions of the uterus to propel your baby down the birth canal.

Approximately three to four weeks before birth, as the placenta produces more oestrogen, your cervix begins to loosen and soften in preparation for birth. Finally, when labour begins, your cervix changes dramatically, becoming much thinner and shorter and dilating (opening out) to enable your baby to be born. Again, the chemical signals sent out by your baby seem to be responsible for starting this process.

These hormonal changes also stimulate your breasts to prepare for the production of milk to feed your newborn baby – a process rounded off when your baby begins to suck at your breast.

8

CHAPTER

Managing your emotions and intimacy

If you have mixed feelings about your changing

body, are worried about the impending birth, or feel

overwhelmed with the idea of becoming a parent,

then you're certainly not alone – these are natural

responses to pregnancy. Don't worry though. You'll

be able to cope.

Your response to pregnancy

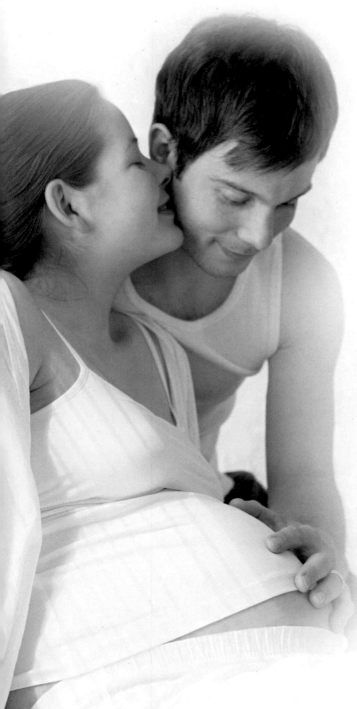

It's partly due to your hormones, partly to the huge physical and emotional adjustment you need to make, but your emotions can run riot during pregnancy, affecting every aspect of your life.

When you first discover that you're pregnant, you might feel sheer delight that you're having a longed-for baby, a sense of triumph that you're fertile or tender closeness with your partner, since it was your physical union that created this baby. Alternatively, pregnancy may loom as an enormous problem; if you don't feel ready for a baby, your natural response may be anxiety or even panic.

Early reactions

Even if you've known for a while that you wanted a baby, it's absolutely natural for some less positive feelings to creep into the picture: you may feel that it's happening too quickly; you may feel trapped; you may wonder how your body will cope with being pregnant and feel frightened about the birth; or you may be overwhelmed by the sense of lifelong responsibility for another human being.

Initially, your emotions may be working overtime to process all the changes that are taking place, but over the following weeks, some of this turbulence simmers down. Like many women, you may gain a new respect for your body, and even if early discomfort threatens to undermine this satisfaction, you'll probably be amazed by the work your body is doing to grow a new life. If this is your first pregnancy, you might be feeling grown up in a new way – you're joining the community of mothers.

Adapting to changes

The waiting period before your baby's arrival can sometimes seem like forever, but these nine months provide time for you to adjust to the huge changes that are taking place – not only will you be getting used to the effects on your body (see page 151), but also adapting to an altered lifestyle. Suddenly you might feel that it's more important to take care of your safety in order to protect the tiny human being within you. You may find that you drive more cautiously and take greater care to avoid accidents. You'll probably make changes in your eating habits, limit your alcohol or give up smoking. Even your social life might alter.

Such changes in the way you think and act can make you feel like quite a different person – a sensation that's intensified if you give up work and can no longer define yourself by your career but don't yet consider yourself to be a mother. You may find it easier to take on this new aspect of your identity if you spend time daydreaming and visualizing yourself with your new baby. Also, consider keeping a diary to help you to work out your changing moods.

Respect your body

Pregnancy is a time of continuous physical change. Some of these changes are expected and visible to the outside world, such as the enlargement of your breasts and the filling out of your belly, while others are less visible and may be unexpected, such as your hair becoming a little greasy or your feet swelling.

Emotional reactions to pregnancy are highly individual and unpredictable, but it's almost impossible not to have a strong reaction to your changing appearance – you may love your new look or hate feeling bulky.

Some women who are conscious of their figures feel disturbed by their increasing size during pregnancy. If you begin to feel like this, try not to feel embarrassed about your bump: you aren't

getting fat, you're growing a baby – a physical task that draws continuously on your energy and on every system of your body.

Accept your new image

As the months go by, you'll come to terms with your changing shape. At first, you may feel frustrated that there's nothing to see. In the second or third month, as your clothes begin to feel tight, you may experience impatience, because you're no longer the

MORE**ABOUT**   the effect of hormones

The hormones oestrogen and progesterone play a vital role in orchestrating all the physical changes needed to initiate and maintain a pregnancy (see page 60), but they also have a profound effect on your emotions. Hormones can cause some women to experience a newfound serenity, their focus turning inwards to form a protective cocoon around their babies. Other women experience a roller coaster of emotions: sadness turning into floods of tears; a new sensitivity to the sufferings of others; and joy so intense that it, too, spills over into tears. It can be difficult to judge whether these ups and downs are due to your hormones or simply an emotional response to your new lifestyle. But whatever happens, accept that for the next nine months, you may be less in control of your emotions than usual. It's as if your hormones are opening up the emotional part of your psyche and preparing you to be receptive to your newborn baby.

shape you were, but neither are you recognizably pregnant. Around the fourth month, you'll probably be relieved that your protruding tummy is clearly visible. With your pregnancy public knowledge, you may find that people openly scrutinize your shape or even want to touch your bump. Some women resent the invasion of their personal space; others enjoy people's involvement. In the later months, you may hardly believe that your body can go on growing and that your bump is so firm. You may feel unwieldy and be inwardly shocked by the struggle of getting out of an armchair. This is the time to take it easy and to look forward to meeting your new baby.

Acknowledge your worries

It's difficult to be completely relaxed all the time about the well-being of your baby, even if you have no rational reason for concern. You may worry about miscarriage during the early months (see page 278), particularly if you have miscarried before. In these instances, it's perfectly natural to feel anxious until you're safely past the date at which your other baby was lost. Hard though it might be, try to stay relaxed and trust your body.

It can be tremendously exciting to see your tiny but complete baby moving around or sucking his thumb during an ultrasound scan, but antenatal testing (see page 236) is a common source of worry for expectant parents. Even though it's designed to provide reassuring information, testing can prompt new anxieties. Bear in mind that testing is designed

to detect problems early so that your baby has the best chance of being born healthy. But if you feel pressured about taking a particular test, make sure you discuss your need for it with your doctor.

If any problems are picked up during testing, try to stay positive. If you are told, for example, that your baby has a one-in-ten chance of developing Down's syndrome (see page 249), turn the statistic around – your baby has a nine-in-ten chance of not being born with Down's syndrome.

You may have concerns, too, about the impact of your lifestyle on your unborn baby. The damaging effects of smoking, alcohol and exposure to other hazards (see page 75) are widely publicized. The best way to limit your anxiety is to adjust your lifestyle so that it provides a healthier environment for your growing baby. If you think that you've taken any risks – for example, if, like many women, you believe you were drinking too much before you discovered that you were pregnant, tell your healthcare provider; he or she will probably be able to discuss any possible risks and provide reassurance.

5 ways to quell anxiety

1   Talk to other expectant parents. Most are keen to share their feelings and experiences with others, and many join antenatal classes primarily for this reason (see page 172).

2   Try to find an antenatal teacher who puts a high priority on discussion. You shouldn't feel that you have to know everything, nor should you be afraid to ask questions – that's what your teacher is there for.

3   Read up as much as you can about pregnancy. The more informed you are, the more in control you'll feel and, consequently, less worried.

4   Visit your healthcare provider. If you have any symptoms that worry you, don't put off going for fear that something is really wrong. It will probably be nothing, but it's best to put your mind at rest.

5   Remember, while awareness of potential problems is greater than ever, there's never been a safer time to have a baby. Medicine and society haven't eliminated all problems, but for healthy women who receive good antenatal care the outlook for their babies is excellent.

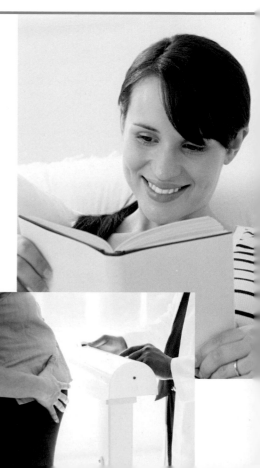

Get close to your family. Expectant mothers can also feel the need to be looked after, and your parents' commitment to you and your baby can be very comforting.

Thinking about parenting

You may anticipate parenthood with confidence, or you may feel distinctly nervous about this untried role. If marriage or moving in with your partner seemed a huge step, the addition of a baby is an even more momentous change.

It takes time for an individual to grow into a parent. Being a good mother or father certainly doesn't happen as soon as your baby is born. Pregnancy, besides being a period of waiting, is a time of preparation for parenthood. Talk to other parents, and use every opportunity to get close to newborns. The best way to learn is by hands-on experience, so ask to baby-sit for a friend with a baby. Practise holding, changing and playing with him or her. Your friend may be kind enough to return the favour after your baby is born and you need a break.

Look to your relatives and friends

Pregnancy often brings women closer to their parents, in-laws and siblings. You may feel a need to ask your mother how you were born or to look through baby photos of your partner for clues as to how your baby will look. Families often give much needed support during pregnancy, particularly if you don't have a partner around to help (see page 154).

However, if you're going through pregnancy without the support of your own mother, you may find yourself feeling a particular kind of loneliness. If this leaves a gap in your life, an aunt or a friend who is a mother will probably be happy to be there for you. In addition, you may be able to find a self-help organization in your area or on the Internet.

At this time, you also might find yourself thinking back to your upbringing: which aspects of your childhood do you want to replicate for your child and which would you rather not repeat? Experts believe that open discussion with your partner about how you were each brought up helps to replace negative patterns with positive ones. Consider how the expectations you and your partner bring from your family backgrounds can be meshed into a cohesive philosophy of parenting. But, bear in mind that it's impossible to work out a complete strategy before your baby puts in his appearance – part of the fulfilment of parenthood is learning from new situations and from your child himself.

Expecting a second baby

If this is your second pregnancy you will have learned a lot. However, there are extra considerations when having a second child. Most mothers find that they're a lot more tired during the second pregnancy, as they have a child to look after at the same time. There are also the practicalities of caring for two children – two require extra work and extra expense.

Some parents expecting their second child worry about whether they'll love their new baby as much as their first. It can seem almost like a betrayal to bring another baby onto the scene. However, once the baby is born, parents are surprised to discover in themselves a new fount of love for the youngest member of the family.

Your older child may feel insecure when she realizes that there's another child on the way, so make time to prepare her for the new arrival. She might, for example, be secretly afraid that you'll have less time for her, that you might not love her as much or even that the baby might have to sleep in her bed. These fears are very real in the mind of a child, so talk to her as soon as your pregnancy is noticeable. Calmly explain that she'll soon have a new baby brother or sister who will love her very much. Give her lots of cuddles and smiles so that she adopts a positive attitude, too.

Include your older child in your pregnancy. Let her feel and talk to the baby or read him a story (see page 352) – it will help her to accept him more when he's born.

HOW TO face pregnancy alone

Whether or not your pregnancy was planned, facing pregnancy on your own can be very hard – and the prospect of having sole responsibility for a baby overwhelming. The absence of a partner to share in the care and decision-making can leave you feeling isolated and lonely. This is why it's vital to enlist as much support as you can. Many single mothers find that their families prove to be enormously supportive. Indeed, a baby can positively benefit from growing up in the protective, loving environment of an extended family.

If you don't have a family to fall back on, local or Internet-based self-help organizations can put you in touch with other single parents and provide emotional and practical support. You'll probably need to draw on other people not only for friendship, but also to be with you throughout labour and, later on, to provide you with adult company and occasional time off from caring for your baby.

You and your partner

Pregnancy should be seen as a great opportunity to strengthen the bond between you and your partner. Adjusting to the changes that pregnancy makes to your life together will prepare you for the challenges of parenthood.

The arrival of a first child is a major milestone in the life of any couple. Until this time, your partner has probably been the person you put first in your life, and you no doubt spend a lot of time solely in each other's company. At the moment, you may lead roughly parallel existences – both going out to work, contributing to the income, sharing the tasks and decorating your home together. Evenings are times for unwinding, talking over your day and enjoying the support you get from each other. It's easy to go out for a meal on the spur of the moment or to meet up with friends in a bar.

Nearly every aspect of this lifestyle is likely to be affected by the arrival of your baby, and some of the changes begin during pregnancy. You may already have noticed that your roles are diverging – perhaps, to your surprise, developing into male and female stereotypes. As pregnancy advances, a woman is less able to do heavy physical work, so it falls to her partner. She stops work, becomes more home-based and may take over more of the cooking or household chores. You may both enjoy this change, but equally, you might find it difficult to adjust to some aspects of this development.

Other changes are on the horizon or nudging their way into view. Does your baby make you and your partner feel closer together than ever, or does she seem an intruder on your intimacy as a couple? Is becoming a parent going to involve some losses as well as gains? It's easy to share happy thoughts about pregnancy, but are you also making time to explore your negative feelings? By discussing these things, you'll enhance your mutual understanding and develop the trust and openness that will help you to cope with being parents together.

Changes to your sex life

Pregnancy almost inevitably affects the sex life of a couple – changes that can be both negative and positive. There are physical and psychological factors at play, and a woman's responses can be very different to those of her partner.

Is it safe?

A lot of couples worry that making love during pregnancy will harm the baby. Some parents fear that sex might cause an infection in the uterus or their baby, but unless one partner has a sexually transmitted disease, there is no possibility of this happening – the baby is protected by the mucous plug sealing the cervix as well as by the amniotic sac. Moreover, a man's penis cannot penetrate beyond the vagina. In most cases, there is no risk to the unborn baby when her parents make love. The few exceptions are listed in the box, below.

You can, however, make sex more comfortable and manageable with a few precautions. After the fourth month of pregnancy it's not a good idea to

---

SAFETY FIRST

MISCARRIAGE AND PRETERM DELIVERY

Although there is no evidence that sexual activity is a cause of miscarriage, if you have a history of miscarriages, you may be advised to avoid penetrative sex until you are beyond the danger period (see page 278). Likewise, if you've previously had a premature delivery, or are experiencing signs of early labour, it may be suggested that you avoid sex in the last trimester, as it could trigger the onset of labour (see page 208). You should also avoid sex in late pregnancy if your membranes have broken or if you have any bleeding (see page 275).

spend too much time lying on your back and you may well find this position uncomfortable when making love. But this shouldn't be a problem, as the process of finding alternatives can be fun (see box, below). You may want also to make love gently so consider using a lubricant to avoid the possibility of abrasions and soreness in your extra-sensitive vagina.

Late in pregnancy, an orgasm – or just having sex – can set off Braxton Hicks contractions (see page 211). This is perfectly normal but, if it feels uncomfortable, either lie quietly or try a relaxation technique until the contractions pass.

Sex can be better

In the early weeks of pregnancy, nausea and extreme tiredness can mean that sex is the last thing on your mind. Bed is for one thing only: sleep. As this stage wears off, however, you may enjoy a new liberation in your lovemaking, as there's no longer pressure to become pregnant or any need for birth control.

What's more, the emotional closeness that you feel can lead to particularly tender, loving sex.

The physical changes associated with pregnancy also can intensify the sensations of sex: your breasts and nipples may become more sensitive; the extra blood and fluids circulating in your body suffuse the vaginal tissues, making them more sensitive; and the pregnancy hormones promote extra lubrication to the vagina. These changes in your body also can enhance your partner's enjoyment of sex; for example, the engorged tissues of your vagina will grip his penis more tightly.

Some pregnant women describe being in an almost constant state of arousal, particularly in the middle three months, and many women experience more intense orgasms than before they became pregnant, with the vaginal tissues remaining swollen long after orgasm. This may mean, however, that you can feel somewhat unsatisfied after sex – a sensation that can be eased with masturbation.

COMFORTABLE LOVEMAKING

Your ever-growing bump may mean that some positions for sexual intercourse become uncomfortable. Any position in which your partner lies on top, is especially unsuitable once your tummy starts to protrude, unless your partner lifts his weight off your body. There are many other positions to try, however; experimentation can, in itself, make lovemaking more satisfying.

WOMAN ON TOP This involves you positioning yourself astride your partner either on your knees or squatting. Take your weight on your arms rather than your stomach. As your bump grows, you might find squatting rather than lying on your partner more comfortable.

SITTING DOWN Your partner sits on a sturdy chair or on the side of the bed and you sit astride him, either facing him or facing the other way. In this position, you can control the depth of penetration, while his arms are free to caress your body.

It's possible that your unborn baby benefits from your lovemaking, although this theory is difficult to prove. What is more certain is that such activity is likely to make you feel happy, loved and relaxed – feelings that are passed onto your baby. You may notice that she seems to respond to your lovemaking, either by becoming more lively or by calming down. But your baby's reactions are nothing to do with your lovemaking, they are responses solely to hormonal and uterine activity.

Sex can be worse

Pregnancy doesn't always mean satisfying and carefree sex, however.

You might feel uncomfortable, tired or so dislike your new shape, that you don't feel at all sexy. If your breasts are tender, particularly in early and late pregnancy, you might prefer that your partner doesn't touch them. Be prepared also that, late in pregnancy, your breasts may leak colostrum (see page 298) if they are stimulated, which you or your partner might find off-putting.

In turn, your partner may feel daunted by your changing shape or anxious about hurting you or your baby. He also might start to see you more as a mother figure than a lover, and this could disturb his usual response. Some men are put off sex by the very proximity of their babies, who seem to be 'witnessing' the whole performance. Be assured, however, that your baby will have no memory of you making love while she's in the uterus.

It's all too possible in pregnancy for one partner to feel rejected by the other – not because there's less love between you, but because the usual patterns of expressing it are disturbed. If you feel turned off sex for any reason, it's important to talk about it, to be specific about what has changed for you, but also to express all the positive feelings that are unchanged. It may be that what you both need is simply reassurance of each other's love and commitment.

ALL FOURS You kneel on all fours, supporting your weight on your arms, while your partner kneels behind you. You can lean on your forearms if you find it more comfortable. This position allows your partner to vary the depth of penetration and gives him great freedom of movement.

SPOONS Easy and comfortable, this is ideal when your bump becomes really large. In this intimate position, you simply nestle together like a pair of spoons, either lying on your back with your legs curled over his, or both lying on your sides with your legs bent. Your partner enters your vagina from behind.

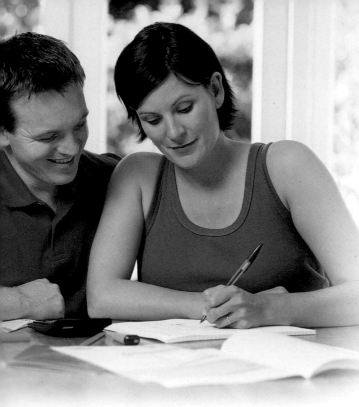

Sit down with your partner and work out your budget. If you haven't done so already, start cutting down on luxuries and putting away the money you save.

Other ways of showing affection

Sex doesn't have to mean full intercourse. If you prefer to avoid penetrative sex, then you could try extended foreplay. If your partner is masturbating you, he should use a lubricant – saliva, if nothing else – to avoid causing abrasion. Your partner should be aware, too, that your vaginal secretions may taste stronger during oral sex. He should also take care not to blow into your vagina, as there is a small risk that this can lead to an embolism (a small air bubble in a blood vessel).

Pregnancy is a great opportunity to explore other ways of enjoying intimacy; you can express your feelings with simple kisses, cuddles and stroking, or you might decide to share a bath together. Massage is a welcome luxury when you're pregnant, especially if you're feeling uncomfortable and finding it difficult to relax (see page 126).

Changes to finances

Apart from sex, another area of potential change can be in your family income. The impending arrival of a new baby might mean a reduction in money coming in – you or your partner may have to give up work, and it will inevitably entail some new expenses. It's worth thinking ahead about the impact of these financial changes before they hit home.

Consider your income

One of the important things to think about is how early or late you plan to leave work, but bear in mind this might be affected by health circumstances beyond your control. Also, you might want to weigh up a loss of income during your maternity leave against any benefits you might receive.

Although it's a long way off, there's no harm in researching your options for returning to work – when the time comes, you'll be able to make an informed decision. You could compare the costs of childcare to the money you'll get from working or think about possible alternatives to full-time work (see page 193).

Be creative with your savings

You don't need to spend a fortune on your new baby. Decorating her room may be a labour of love, but you don't have to break your back or your bank account to do it. Your baby's needs in this respect are modest. While she does need love, attention and stimulation, she's not too bothered about a super-smart nursery. If you have the time and can resist the temptations of catalogues and shops, consider the second-hand market in baby clothes and equipment (see page 196). Most items are outgrown rather than worn out, so it's quite possible to set up your baby's nursery and wardrobe with almost-new items. Contact local parenting organizations to find out if they run any sales in your area. However, certain items, such as car seats and cot mattresses, you should always buy new (see page 196).

Minimising labour worries

At some stage in your pregnancy, the inevitability of giving birth will suddenly strike you, and you may well have qualms about how you will cope with the challenge.

Excitement, fear, anticipation, bewilderment and uncertainty about recognizing the start of labour – all these emotions and more will probably fill your mind in your last trimester, as your due date looms. Childbirth is always a journey into the unknown and this is particularly true of first births. But, however many babies you have, there is always an element of unpredictability about how this particular delivery will go.

All women experience a mixture of feelings when approaching labour and delivery, but some women can draw on a lot more confidence in the face of this challenge than others. Your confidence will be influenced by a number of factors:

- Your past experience of coping with particularly stressful events.
- Your trust in your own body and the process of childbirth itself.
- The extent of your knowledge about what childbirth involves.
- The love and support of those close to you.
- The respect and encouragement of all your healthcare providers.

DREAMING YOUR FEARS

Many women experience unusually vivid dreams during pregnancy and it's possible that these are caused by hormone changes. Dreams often feature the forthcoming labour or the baby himself, and can be so vivid that they disturb your sleep and are difficult to forget about.

The following common dreams bring certain fears to light. You may dream that:

- The pregnancy isn't real and that you will give birth to nothing, or simply deflate.
- You give birth to a baby animal, or even some mundane household object.
- Your baby is damaged or deformed in some way.

Such nightmare-like dreams can be disconcerting, if not plain upsetting. They do, however, allow you to express anxieties that are normally suppressed during waking hours. Such fears may stem from the fact that, despite antenatal scans and examinations, the human being growing inside you is a shadowy figure, not fully seen or known.

If you're prone to disturbing dreams, try to spend some time daydreaming about your baby in a positive way, imagining yourself holding him, thinking about names or picturing him in his cot. Experts agree that this is an excellent way to 'practise' relating to your baby. Compare your dreams with those of other pregnant women – discussing what they may mean might help to relieve your anxieties.

THE KEY TO DREAMS
Some common themes and what they might refer to:

- Sex in a positive or negative light: normal sexual confusion during pregnancy.
- Loss and forgetfulness: fear of the responsibility of motherhood.
- Pain and hurt: a sense of vulnerability.
- Being trapped: concerns about loss of freedom.
- Losing your partner: worry about your body image.
- Dramatic changes in weight: concerns about your diet.

Will you manage the pain?

A good antenatal teacher won't have concealed the fact that labour is a physically intense experience, and that it can range from discomfort to excruciating pain. Strong messages about labour come from other sources, too, and these can influence your expectations, for example, listening to the birth experiences within your circle of family and friends. However, your antenatal teacher will have provided you also with skills to ease the pain – such as relaxation, breathing, massage and mobility (see page 218) – and should have helped to reinforce your confidence in your ability to give birth.

If you're worried about the pain, or you are concerned about your ability to cope when the time comes, think now about the pain-relief options that you have (see page 178). The way that you envisage labour will affect your response to it, so you might find it comforting to practise visualization techniques. When you think about contractions, imagine the muscles of your uterus opening up your cervix. See in your mind's eye your baby moving down the birth canal and remind yourself that each contraction will take you a step closer to his birth. Remember, too, that it's easier to cope with pain when you think that it's a sign that the body is working naturally and efficiently.

Will you lose all control?

Many people feel inhibited about showing strong emotions in public, or even in private, so don't be surprised if you find yourself feeling uneasy about crying, shouting or simply being helpless in the presence of others. Being in hospital, away from your home environment may add to your anxiety, particularly if this is your first baby, as you may have little real experience of the extent of your strength and inner resources.

It helps if you can accept the probability of some loss of emotional control. Many women find that making a noise during labour – groaning or grunting – helps release tension. You'll work more efficiently through childbirth if you can let yourself go, be in tune with your body and almost forget about the people around you.

A messy business

Some women say that dignity goes out of the window during birth, and first-time mothers particularly worry about losing physical control. You'll certainly have no control over loss of amniotic fluid. At the height of contractions you may have less control over your bowels and may even vomit. Your genital area is exposed and indeed is the focus of attention. However, bear in mind that all these aspects of birth have been experienced by women throughout the centuries. Your healthcare providers will not only have seen it all before, but they will be too focused on your well-being and that of your baby to think about anything else. Moreover, you'll probably find that any personal embarrassment disappears as you concentrate on the intense physicality of your task, and you'll be filled with wonder at the miracle of bringing your baby into the world. If you're particularly worried about the physical exposure of labour, however, talk to your healthcare provider, who will guide you through the process gently and sensitively.

Will you 'make the grade'?

There's a tendency among women in their first pregnancies to perceive labour as a test in which some women do well and others don't – for instance, if a woman had planned a drug-free delivery, but later decided that she needed an epidural, she may feel that she was weak in some way. But there's nothing standard about childbirth – a woman can't know what cards nature will deal her, nor what the experience is really like for other women. The important thing when you go into labour is that you feel supported by those around you and that you're able to interact positively with every challenge with which you're presented. Aim to allow all the emotions of the birth to sink in, so that you can look back and feel that you made the most of this incredible experience.

Pregnancy for dads

Pregnancy is a partnership between two parents

working together for a baby. For a dad, this is the

time to support your partner, emotionally,

financially and physically, and to develop a

relationship with the new life you've

helped to create.

New to fatherhood

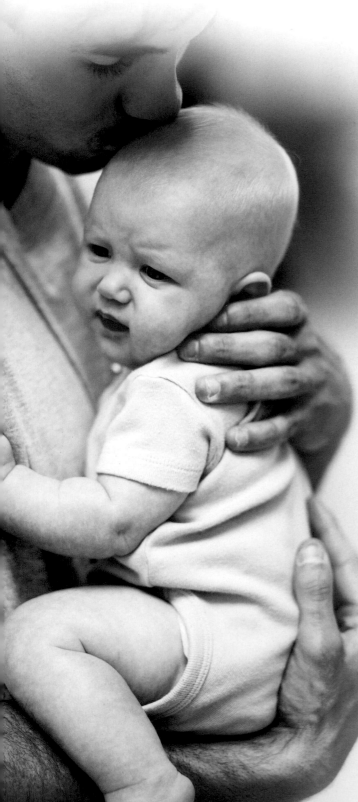

Finding out you're going to become a father can evoke a mixture of emotions. You'll probably feel delight, pride and a sense of fulfilment, but it is also quite natural for your happiness to be tinged with some uncertainty as you confront the reality that a tiny person, who is part of you, is on her way into the world.

Your feelings about becoming a father may well be influenced by past and present circumstances. If you are in a warm and loving relationship with your partner; if you've had previous good experience with babies; if the pregnancy was planned or desired; if you had a happy childhood yourself; and if your lifestyle and financial status can accommodate a child, you are likely to have a positive outlook on pregnancy and fatherhood. If some of these factors are missing, it is quite natural for you to feel some trepidation about the future. However, you should bear in mind that becoming a father is one of the most momentous events in your life. Whatever your situation, your life will never be the same again, so don't be too surprised if you find yourself feeling ambivalent about fatherhood some of the time and elated at others.

Tackling your worries

It's always best to acknowledge any concerns you have rather than bottle them up and if this is your first baby, you're likely to have a few anxieties. As pregnancy advances, your emotions may alter, just as your partner's will and you'll have to come to terms with changing feelings about your partner and your new baby. If you're finding it difficult to cope with the way you are feeling, discuss your anxiety openly with your partner.

Dealing with unexpected news

If this pregnancy wasn't planned, you might still be reeling from the shock. Contraception, whatever method you use, isn't infallible and accidents do happen. If you've been taken by surprise, you may feel frustrated or even angry about the situation in which you suddenly find yourself, particularly if you're not in a serious relationship with your baby's mother. But take time to let the news sink in and believe that you can still have a deep, lifelong relationship with your child, even without a similar commitment to her mother – and the best time for that relationship to begin is during pregnancy.

Feeling left out

Most fathers feel excluded at one time or another during pregnancy, so you're not alone if you find yourself becoming a little jealous of your unborn baby. From early on, you could feel that you're taking second place to an extremely demanding newcomer. You also might feel that your partner's family, friends and even her doctors are taking over your usual protective role and that there's no space for you. But don't feel pushed out and withdraw into the background. Try explaining what you're going through to your partner. Be careful not to demand too much of her, though – she's already receiving an emotional crash course in dependency from the baby growing inside her.

If you find it difficult to overcome your sense of alienation, consider discussing your feelings with a close friend, your family doctor, or a professional counsellor. Also, attending parenting classes will give you the chance to talk to other men in the same position as you – your doctor's surgery or local library should be able to provide you with details or you could try searching on the Internet.

Often, the best way to tackle worries about feeling left out is to throw yourself into the idea of becoming a parent. Fathers today have plenty of opportunities to be directly involved in their partner's pregnancy and there are many things you can do to join in (see box, below). Immerse yourself in this exciting time with your partner – after all, you're both expecting this baby.

5 ways to share your partner's pregnancy

1   Attend antenatal checks. You'll learn more about what's happening to your partner and to your baby.

2   See your baby. Ultrasound scans will offer you exhilarating glimpses of your baby. Ask for pictures.

3   Listen to your baby. From about week 30, you can press your ear to your partner's tummy and hear your baby's tiny heart beating.

4   Feel your baby moving. From five months into the pregnancy, you'll be able to feel your baby shifting position – you may even be able to identify tiny hands and feet.

5   Talk, read, and sing to your baby. She can hear your voice from within the uterus, so bond with her and entertain your partner in the process.

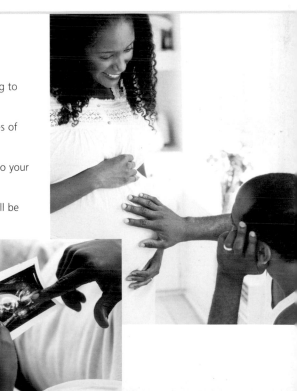

Redefining your relationship

Gaining an understanding of your partner's changing body will help you to appreciate how she is feeling. Remind yourself that while she's carrying your child, you have a key role to play too, part of which is adapting to her needs.

A sense of security will be vital to your partner at this time and this will be influenced by the way you communicate. If you avoid intimacy and don't discuss your emotions, she may feel that she's on her own. But if you share your feelings, she is more likely to want to confide in you. Try to be sensitive and encourage her to discuss her hopes and fears.

Expect changes to your sex life

It's not uncommon for a man to be turned off by his partner's pregnant body. Often this is not so much due to physical changes, but anxieties the man has about the growing baby inside. If you find yourself losing interest in sex, it can help to find out more about what's happening to your partner physically, so that you become more at ease with the changes. Don't lose sight of the fact that after the birth, her body will begin to return to normal.

It's more likely, however, that you'll be turned on by your partner's softer curves and find the voluptuousness of pregnancy extremely sexy. This

EVERYDAY HELP

Your relationship with your partner will be affected profoundly by how you handle these crucial nine months. It certainly will be a challenging experience, but if all goes well, you'll be closer than ever.

There is also ample evidence to suggest that if your partner is happy, relaxed and relatively stress-free during pregnancy, your baby will experience long-term emotional and even physical benefits. What's more, a supportive relationship between parents may make delivery less stressful, postnatal depression less likely (see page 328) and breastfeeding easier—and it should enable you both to bond with your baby more readily.

Aside from attending scans and medical check-ups, there is a wide range of everyday 'services' you can provide to make your partner's life more comfortable.

EXERCISE TOGETHER Join your partner in the pool or go for a brisk walk – getting into shape is a good way to spend time together and to tone up both of your bodies.

MASSAGE HER As your baby grows, your partner may experience discomfort in her back, feet and legs. A gentle massage can ease the

---

POSITIVE REINFORCEMENT

Just as you can help your partner by doing a few thoughtful things, you also can do a lot of good by avoiding some things:

- Cut down on smoking or smoke away from your partner. If she's a smoker, it helps her to quit (see page 75) and it avoids the possibility of cigarette fumes 'passively' filtering through to your baby.
- Reduce your alcohol intake. It will show your support at a time when your partner shouldn't drink excessively (see page 111).
- Avoid junk food and eat healthily together. Choose from a selection of mouthwatering ideas on page 104.
- Resist pressure to go away on business or with friends during the last month of the pregnancy – some babies decide to arrive early.

may increase your desire for intercourse at a time when your partner's sexual drive is erratic. In this case, you will need to adapt to her needs and desires, which could mean finding new ways to express your feelings, such as through cuddling, kissing, massage and non-penetrative sex (see page 157).

Encourage family support

During the pregnancy, you'll probably see more of your partner's mother than ever before. This is a time when the bond between mother and daughter is stronger than ever. Try to encourage this closeness, as your partner will need that special support. When your baby is born, your in-laws, as well as your own parents, will be anxious, no doubt, to get involved with the new family member. Don't see their enthusiasm as interference – it's important that your child gets to know all his grandparents. By including them in your family life, you'll be doing far more than acquiring willing baby-sitters: you'll be offering your child the experience of another generation and encouraging him to develop a sense of respect for older people.

tension and it's a great way of showing you care. See page 126 for ideas on how to give her a relaxing massage.

DO THE SHOPPING Your partner should avoid lugging around heavy shopping bags, particularly in late pregnancy. She also may find walking supermarket aisles tiring, so, if you're not already doing the shopping, now's the time to start. Of course, if you do the cooking some of the time, that's something else she'll appreciate.

GET YOUR BABY'S ROOM READY Your partner shouldn't be climbing ladders, so decorating your baby's room could be your job. Discuss colour schemes together and then start painting. You also could help to shop for baby clothes and equipment (see page 195) so that the room is 100 per cent ready for its new occupant.

LET YOUR PARTNER SLEEP LATE She needs more rest than before, so encourage her to get a few extra hours in the mornings. You could also serve her breakfast in bed – a thoughtful gesture that can help morning sickness (see page 67).

ATTEND ANTENATAL CLASSES You'll not only be supporting your partner, but you will also learn a good deal yourself, particularly about the physical side of labour. Both you and your partner will gain a lot of confidence through meeting other parents-to-be.

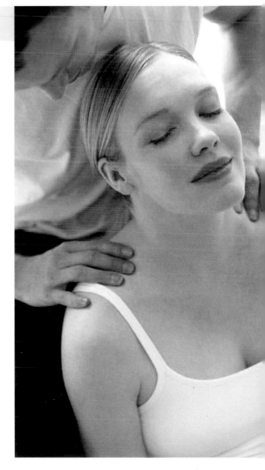

Your role at the birth

It's likely that you'll play the role of primary birth partner, which means that you'll need to be ready, alert and most important, available when her waters break or contractions begin.

Until the 1970s, fathers were routinely banned from most delivery rooms, so they didn't have the opportunity to see their children's arrival into the world unless it was a home birth. Today, about 90 per cent of fathers in the Western world are present at the births of their children.

Prepare yourself

If you and your partner decide that you'll be present at your baby's birth, you should have a clear idea of what to expect – although there are bound to be a few surprises. During the course of the pregnancy, you may have attended antenatal classes, had a tour of the hospital and read a book or two on the subject, but when it comes down to the birth you may still find yourself shocked by the blood, mucus, excreta, moaning and screaming involved. While most labours aren't particularly complicated, things

often don't go precisely as expected: the onset of labour seldom happens on the due date; there may be false alarms; it may be over within an hour, or last through the day, the night and beyond. Events may not proceed in the order you anticipated, but keep a cool head, try to remain sensitive to your partner's needs and, if possible, retain your sense of humour – you're not her instructor but you're there to help her and to share an unforgettable experience. There are few events in life that approach the joy of seeing your own child being born. Don't be surprised if you burst into tears when your baby finally arrives – and make sure that you hold her as soon as possible.

Help to create the birth plan

Fear, pain and anxiety don't create the ideal environment for rational decisions, so it's a good idea to get to know your partner's birth plan (see page 185) well before the due date. You may eventually discard it, but the sense that things have been worked out beforehand will reassure you both as you prepare for labour. The birth plan should include details of how your partner hopes to handle her labour through to delivery. It will answer questions such as: is she happy with a 'normal' hospital birth or does she want to try for a water birth or another form of 'natural' birth (see page 174); what is her preferred birth posture – perhaps on her back, squatting, or kneeling? It will also include details of what sort of pain relief she wants, if any. It should stress whether you both have objections to any procedures during delivery, such as episiotomy. You'll need to be fully versed in the details of the plan and make sure the birth

---

MORE **ABOUT**　　　sympathetic pregnancies

Some men become so emotionally involved in their partner's pregnancies and labours that they share certain physical symptoms. This is known as couvade – from the French word couver, *meaning 'to hatch' – and is usually a sympathetic response that emerges from a man's extremely close identification with his partner. Men who experience couvade may gain weight, become constipated and suffer from morning sickness. Occasionally a difficulty arises during labour when the father finds himself becoming more than usually distressed at the pain of childbirth and even experiencing labour-type pains himself. If you find yourself suffering from such symptoms, you should seek professional advice.*

attendants are familiar with it. You may have to adapt the plan and make some on-the-spot decisions if anything unusual occurs during labour or delivery.

Your role in labour

There's plenty you can do to assist your partner during labour: holding and supporting her; massaging her lower back, neck, inner thighs and feet; and reminding her of relaxation and breathing techniques. See page 182 for specific advice on how to help. Antenatal classes will provide further ideas.

Be prepared, however, that when the moment comes you may find that your partner wants something quite different. For instance, you may have been practising breathing techniques together, only to find that all she really wants is for you to hold her hand or wipe her forehead with a cool cloth. Or, after the first contraction, you may find that she no longer wants a natural birth and asks for an epidural injection instead. Don't discourage her if

she does ask for pain relief – she's the one going through the pain and it's better for her and the baby if she's not distressed.

Be prepared, too, for the unexpected in your partner's emotional response. During the transition phase, for example, (see page 216) it's not uncommon for the surge of adrenaline and pain to prompt her into outbursts of the 'get out – I never want to see you again' variety. In most cases, the best option is to ride it out without leaving her side. As the moment of the birth draws closer, you may find her suddenly expressing terror and she will need you there for comfort and to reassure her about the options available. Try to be clear-headed, flexible and sensitive to your partner's needs.

Will I be able to cope?

It's not at all unusual for men to worry that they'll feel faint or sick in the delivery room. Be reassured, however, that it's highly unlikely that either of these

---

7 things to remember

1 Alert your employer to the impending birth and negotiate your leave (see page 170). Remember that flexible arrangements are best, as only 1 in 20 babies arrive on their due dates.

2 List your contacts. Compile a list of emergency telephone numbers, including your partner's caregivers and the hospital. Don't forget to list family and friends you'll want to call with the good news.

3 Within the final month, get to know the community midwife or visit the hospital so that you understand the techniques and machines used in labour and delivery rooms.

4 Keep talking. In the final three weeks before the birth, keep in regular contact with your partner when you're at work – it will reassure you both.

5 Arrange transport. If you're using your own car, make sure that you keep the petrol tank full and work out the most reliable route to the hospital. If you're using a taxi, contact a reliable company and make sure that it is expecting your call.

6 Check, check and recheck. Before leaving for the hospital, make sure that you have: your partner's bags (see page 206), snacks, the birth plan, your list of phone numbers and change for the phone – mobiles can be used only outside the hospital.

7 Take charge. When you reach the hospital hand the birth plan to the midwives and explain it to them if they don't know it already.

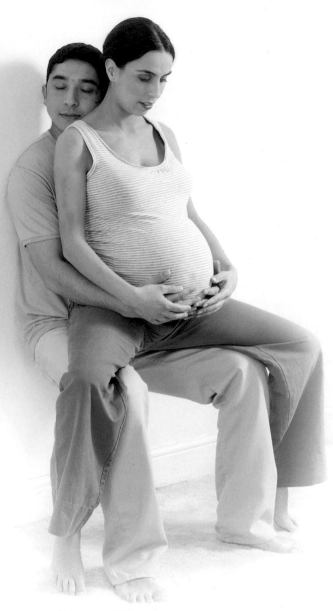

Practise birth positions together. If your partner wants to squat, for example, you will need to support her weight. Remember to try several alternatives (see page 220).

fathers. Remember, if there's anything you're unsure of during the birth, you can talk to the doctor or midwife. The more you understand, the better you'll be able to play your vital supporting role. However, if you're still concerned about how you'll cope, talk to your partner about the possibility of having a doula at the birth (see page 184). The doula will be able to support your partner, explain procedures to you both and take some of the pressure off you.

If you're not planning to be at the birth

You may prefer not to be present at the birth: you may simply have no desire to be involved in the process, or there may be cultural reasons – men in some societies, for example, are traditionally excluded from the delivery room. Some men worry that witnessing a bloody vaginal delivery will make it difficult for them to see their partners in a sexual light afterwards; others fear that the pain and mess will make them fall apart. If you don't want to be there when your baby physically arrives, you may consider being present to support your partner during labour, but withdrawing from the process during the birth. Not being at the birth shouldn't make any difference to the bond you have with your baby – you'll still experience the feeling of delight and fulfilment when you first set eyes on her.

On the other hand, some women prefer that their partners don't attend the birth, perhaps because they think they will feel inhibited by them. If your partner feels like this talk to her about her feelings and respect her wishes – it's not a reflection on you.

will happen. When the moment comes, not only is it unlikely you'll feel squeamish, but you'll probably be fascinated by the miracle of your baby's birth.

If you do feel you have to look away at any stage, focus on your partner's face and help her with her breathing – you'll probably find, however, that you can't resist watching. And don't worry if you need to go outside to get some air. Sit with your head between your knees until you're ready to return.

The best way to combat your fears is to find out as much as you can before the birth. Read all the books, visit the hospital labour and delivery rooms, attend antenatal classes together and talk to other

HOW TO DEAL WITH AN EMERGENCY BIRTH

It's extremely unlikely that your partner would have to give birth outside of the hospital. Even if she does go into labour quickly, there's usually time to get help. However, for your peace of mind, here's how you can help your partner should medical help be unavailable:

DON'T PANIC Call an ambulance, making sure that you tell the operator the expected due date, the name of the hospital and any special medical needs.

HELP GET HER COMFORTABLE Reassure your partner and help her to lie down on a bed or the floor, with her knees bent and apart.

SCRUB UP Wash your hands with soap and water – don't use disinfectant. Cover the area where she's going to have your baby with clean sheets or towels.

TELL HER WHEN TO PUSH Don't let your partner bear down until you can see your baby's head. Get her to pant or blow if she wants to push too soon. Only when your baby's head 'crowns' (when it can be seen at the entrance of the vagina) should you tell your partner to push during each contraction for a count of ten.

SUPPORT YOUR BABY'S HEAD Rest your hand very gently on your baby's head so that it doesn't come out too quickly. Don't pull on her head; it will come out naturally.

HELP YOUR BABY TO BREATHE As the head is delivered, hold it with your hands. Once it's free, ask your partner to stop pushing. If the umbilical cord is around your baby's neck, check that it's loose and gently hook it over her head. Clear any mucus from your baby's nose and mouth with the corner of a clean towel.

DELIVER YOUR BABY'S BODY Put your hands either side of your baby's head and very gently direct it down towards the ground. Ask your partner to push at the same time, until the top shoulder comes out. Now direct your baby upward and support her head and shoulder as the rest of her body emerges, which should happen quite quickly. If your baby's shoulders **are** stuck at any stage, ask your partner to push hard – don't pull.

DRAIN ANY FLUIDS Immediately after the birth, lay your baby across her mother's stomach, with her feet higher than her head, to drain any fluids from her mouth and nose.

WRAP UP YOUR BABY Use clean towels or blankets to wrap her and lay her back on her mother's stomach. Don't wash her at all and don't cut or pull the umbilical cord.

DELIVER THE PLACENTA If an ambulance still hasn't arrived, your partner may have to push out the placenta. Once it's out, put it in a plastic bag. Gently massage your partner's stomach, just below the navel, to encourage the uterus to contract and stem the bleeding from the site of the placenta.

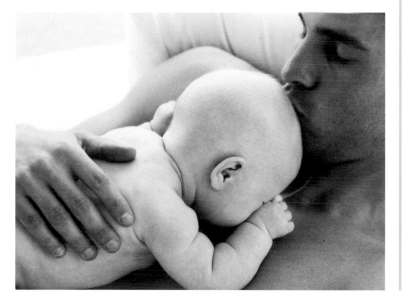

Thinking about the future

Your baby will change you in ways that you could never anticipate. Not only will he depend on you for love, companionship, learning, discipline, life skills and financial support, but for the rest of your life, you'll never stop caring about his well-being and trying to do your best for him. So it's worth thinking now about the kind of relationship you would like to have with your child.

Consider parental leave

A lot of fathers today take time off to develop a loving relationship with their child from the start. Many fathers are now legally entitled to one or two weeks paid paternity leave on the birth of a child – some companies offer their employees a longer period of paid leave. However, employees need to meet certain requirements to be eligible. For more information about your rights contact your local Department for Work and Pensions. Your local Inland Revenue Office will be able to give you details of Statutory Paternity Pay. If you have the option of paid leave, take it; not only will it help you to form a lasting relationship with your child, it will be a very good way of offering support to your partner in the crucial first weeks.

DID YOU KNOW...

FATHER-BABY BONDS ARE STRONG The Aka pygmy men, from the northern Congo in Central Africa, remain within arm's reach of their infants about 47 per cent of the day, hold their babies close to their bodies for up to two hours a day and sometimes provide their own nipples as pacifiers. And like most fathers, the more time they spend with their babies, the stronger the bond between them becomes.

Changing notions of fatherhood

Nurturing was once considered the terrain of mothers, but today there is far more flexibility in the way men relate to their children and the kind of families into which children are born. For example, over a third of children in the United Kingdom are born to unmarried parents and the proportion of single parents is growing – single fathers now represent 10 per cent of UK single parents. Mothers are earning increasing proportions of the family income, while fathers are increasing the amount of time they spend with their children. If it's financially viable and you and your partner agree, then why not consider becoming a stay-at-home dad?

Making the most of your time

If you're planning to continue working full time there are still plenty of things you can do to make the most of your time with your baby. Help with evening and night-time feeds, give him a bath, or sing him a lullaby at bedtime – you can enjoy time with your baby and give your partner a break. If you usually work long hours, you may want to consider cutting down when the baby's born. The more time you spend caring for your baby, the better you will get to know each other.

Remember, however, that you're not just a parent but part of a couple. It's important for you and your partner to set aside time to be alone together, perhaps in the evenings, when your baby is asleep – your mutual support will be invaluable.

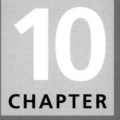

10

CHAPTER

Choices in childbirth

What sort of childbirth class should you attend?
Where's the best place to have your baby? How do
you make a birth plan and what, if any, pain relief is
best for you? These are all important considerations
that will help to give you and your baby the best
possible birth outcome.

Childbirth classes

Birth is such a natural part of life that it may seem unusual that you need to prepare for it, but childbirth classes have an important role to play in helping you to understand and make informed decisions about the type of birth you want.

The growing use of complex medical equipment and the variety of pain relief available are both good reasons to know the benefits and risks of all the available procedures. You may find yourself having to make a quick decision during labour, and you'll want to be able to make an informed choice.

What a class can do for you

First and foremost, a childbirth class gives a great opportunity for you to discover more about your pregnancy. Visits to your healthcare providers rarely include leisurely chats – they're over before you know it – and questions you meant to ask can remain unanswered. Childbirth classes provide an environment in which you can ask almost anything,

and if you forget to ask, the woman next to you will remember. The central goal of childbirth education is to prepare you for the experience of birth. Your instructor will outline what happens physically and emotionally, and there will be demonstrations and practice sessions for specific coping mechanisms.

Meeting in a group can be very supportive. The other women in the class are in the same situation, so they fully appreciate everything that's going on in your life. An antenatal class is also a great place to make new friends who share a common interest in babies and children. Many 'graduates' go on to form new-parent support groups or playgroups.

An antenatal class will be good for partners, too. It will help your partner to understand his or her role in the birth and become involved in the pregnancy and childbirth preparations. Becoming a new parent is a period of intense emotional growth, for you, your partner and your relationship – a good class instructor will recognize this and suggest ways to help you to make the most of these changes.

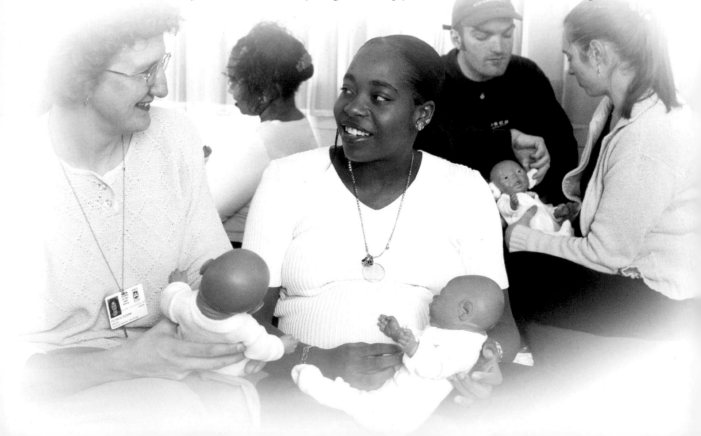

What you'll learn

Childbirth classes usually begin at around 28 to 32 weeks. Depending on what you feel you need, you can attend classes spanning a number of weeks, or brush up your knowledge at a one-off refresher session. Classes are often held in the evenings and at weekends and are usually conducted by a midwife. Although the emphasis can vary, all classes cover the basics: what happens during labour and birth; when to call your healthcare provider; relaxation and breathing techniques; medical pain relief; Caesareans; and care of your newborn.

Choosing a class

Ask doctors, midwives, friends or family for recommendations, and find out what classes are available in your area. Health service classes are usually offered by hospitals, healthcare centres and doctors' surgeries. They are run by midwives or health visitors, sometimes with input from a doctor if there is something medical on the agenda. They are free, but are often conducted in large groups, possibly making it harder to make friends with other prospective parents.

Private childbirth classes are usually held in someone's home, or a community setting of some sort, and are run by a teacher trained by the organization offering the classes, who may or may not be a health professional. Some will allow you to sit in on a session so that you can decide if it's right for you. An ideal class size is around five to seven couples – large enough to provide good discussion but small enough for everyone to get individual attention during sessions.

Finding the right teacher

Many private childbirth teachers approach the subject from a specific angle or philosophy, so it's important to find a teacher who shares your views on childbirth. At the same time, approaching different classes with an open mind will help you to

learn about different approaches to labour and birth so that you can make informed choices, which really suit you.

- *National Childbirth Trust (NCT)* The classes are taught by NCT-trained antenatal teachers and take place in the last three months of pregnancy. The classes are for small groups of couples and offer practical information and a chance to talk through your feelings .
- *Active Birth* Specializing in yoga and relaxation for pregnancy and water births, these classes focus on preparing you for birth in a modern birthing environment.
- *Lamaze International Inc* Childbirth teachers with Lamaze certification encourage active birth and specific breathing patterns to distract from the pain of labour.
- *Bradley Certification* These classes focus on husband-coached, 'natural' childbirth with emphasis on diet, antenatal exercise, and inner focus to cope with the pain of labour.

Most private classes are run over six to eight sessions, in the last few weeks of pregnancy. In some areas you may find 'labour and birth' weekends or days, where you attend for one or two long sessions.

Deciding where to give birth

You may want to have your baby in hospital to take full advantage of medical technology. Or you may want to give birth in a more relaxed setting, such as a midwife-led unit or your own home. But it's important to know all the options so you can make the decision that's right for you.

Research has shown that women achieve the greatest satisfaction in childbirth by having a good relationship with their healthcare providers and by being involved in decisions. Start these early on and you're laying the foundations for a positive birth.

Hospital care

In the United Kingdom 97 per cent of babies are born in hospital. A hospital birth means you have instant access to potentially life-saving technology, which can be very reassuring, particularly if you are a first-time mother. Specialists are available to address any complications; you can have partial or total pain relief; and a Caesarean can be performed, if necessary. If you want all the benefits of a hospital birth, yet prefer as little medical intervention as possible, opt for midwife-led care in a hospital unit.

Choosing a hospital

Most pregnant women in the United Kingdom who have uncomplicated pregnancies will receive the majority of their antenatal care from their community midwife and GP. You will only be referred to a local hospital for any scans, one or two antenatal checks and for the birth. You are free to choose which hospital you attend, so visit the local maternity units and ask advice from your GP,

ALTERNATIVE WAYS TO GIVE BIRTH

Recent years have seen a move away from hospital births with pain relief, and women now have greater choice about the circumstances in which they give birth.

NATURAL BIRTH

Those who favour giving birth without drugs believe that birth is a natural, healthy process, which women's bodies are equipped to deal with on their own. Natural childbirth gives a woman a great deal of control over her labour and delivery. You can choose: how mobile to be; which birthing positions to try; and which labour aids, such as meditation or a warm shower, you want to use.

You can have a natural birth in hospital or at home, but, while it's perfectly possible to have a natural birth in a hospital, it's important to find out your midwife's views on this. Some are happy to let women dictate certain practices, such as leaving membranes un-ruptured or not inducing labour, while others feel that while it's important to consider a woman's feelings, medically they must do what they think is right.

HOME BIRTH

Until the 20th century, most babies were born at home. But then a change in medical philosophy meant that birth moved to hospital and changed from being considered a natural experience to a medically managed condition. Today, approximately 2 per cent of UK babies are born at home.

Mothers who choose a home birth tend to do so because they want: continuity of care; a familiar environment; and the ability to make their own decisions and avoid medical intervention. In contrast, women who choose a hospital birth may place a higher value on access to pain relief and not needing to be transported if a problem arises.

Opinion is divided over the safety of home births. Some healthcare providers are reluctant to support home births, believing that it is safer midwife and friends who have recently had babies, before you decide. Bear in mind the distance of the hospital from your home or work, not just for the delivery but for antenatal visits. If you already have a relationship with an obstetrician or midwife, so you'll be more inclined to have your baby in the hospital or unit to which he or she is affiliated.

Many hospital births occur in special birthing rooms in obstetric units. These are rooms where you go through labour, give birth and recover all in one room. In some hospitals you may even be able to stay in the same room until you check out.

Questions to ask at the hospital

It's important to find out as much as you can about the hospital where you'll give birth. You should ask about Caesarean rates and attitudes at the hospital towards induction. You'll need information about parking facilities, maps to the hospital and important phone numbers. It's also worth taking a tour of the hospital's maternity units. Questions you could ask include:

- ◆ Can I move around during labour, or do I have to stay in bed?
- ◆ Do you tend to use fetal monitoring intermittently or continuously?
- ◆ Will you manually break my waters at a certain stage of labour?
- ◆ Can I eat and drink during labour?
- ◆ How many people can I have in the birthing room to support me?
- ◆ Can I choose the position I give birth in?
- ◆ Is a TENS machine available or does one have to be hired?

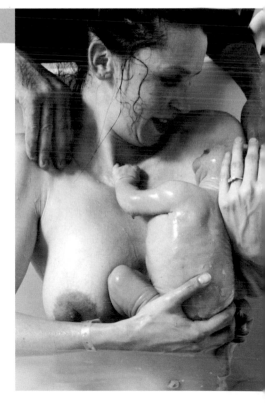

and easier for mothers to give birth in hospitals. On the other hand, studies in the United Kingdom have shown that home births are as safe or even safer than hospital births for healthy women who have normal, low-risk pregnancies, where there is adequate support. It was also found that babies born at home had significantly better APGAR scores.

Home births are usually overseen by midwives who have GPs or hospital obstetricians to consult with, or to refer patients to, if complications arise. Throughout your pregnancy, your midwife will keep a close eye on you and your baby, to keep the birth as risk-free as possible. If complications do arise

during labour, your midwife would call an ambulance to take you to the nearest hospital delivery unit.

WATER BIRTH

You can spend part of your labour, and sometimes give birth, in water. Warm water helps your muscles to relax, which often speeds up labour, and being in a pool can help you more easily assume a comfortable upright position. However, being in water isn't suitable if there are any complications or you want an epidural (unless you come out). Most water births are carried out by midwives in midwife units or in the home, but some hospitals provide birth pools.

Establishing a good relationship with your healthcare provider during pregnancy can lead to a better-than-expected experience of birth.

- Have you got a birthing pool and midwives experienced in water births?
- Do you have a 24-hour epidural service?
- Will medical students/student midwives be involved with the birth?
- What are your induction/Caesarean rates? How do these compare with other local hospitals?
- How long will I stay in hospital, and what are the visiting hours? Can my partner visit me outside these hours?
- Is there help available for breastfeeding?
- What facilities are there for sick babies?
- What security measures are in place? Systems vary, but many hospitals have electronic systems with security tags on the newborns' wrists or ankles that set off an alarm if someone takes the baby out of the building.
- How are newborns identified so that they don't get mixed up? Most hospitals put identification bands on the mother and baby, and often on a third person, too, such as the baby's father. Hospital staff have to check these ID bands every

time the baby leaves or enters the mother's room or the nursery.

Birth centres

Many low-risk midwife-led deliveries now take place in special birth centres, located in hospital obstetric units. The philosophy of these units is to provide care as much like home as possible, focusing on natural birth. Relaxed decor with subdued lighting, and easy access to birthing pools are all provided. These are 'low-tech' options for women who don't want to give birth in a hospital environment, but don't like the idea of a home birth.

Home birth

You may prefer the idea of giving birth in familiar surroundings, with your partner and maybe other family members present. Some women choose home births because they want as little medical intervention during the birth as possible.

Although you are legally entitled to have a home birth, a shortage of midwives in some areas can make this difficult to achieve. If you are considering a home birth you will need to talk to your GP as he or she is the person responsible for organizing your maternity care. Some GPs are against home births because they feel both mother and baby are safer in hospital, but a number of studies have concluded that home births are safe for women who have normal, low-risk pregnancies, where there is adequate infrastructure and support.

If your GP isn't supportive of home births – and your pregnancy is normal – contact one of the supervisors of midwives at your local hospital, or the community midwife manager, who may be able to arrange a home birth for you. In most areas, midwives are supportive of a woman's choice to have her baby at home and will do their best to provide a home birth service. The National Childbirth Trust also run home birth support groups and can supply you with information.

Birthing pools can be rented for home confinements.

Support measures for labour

Although it's impossible to predict the type of labour and birth you'll experience, there's plenty you can do to turn the experience into a positive one – it's just a question of doing your homework.

You need to decide who want to deliver your baby, what sort of pain relief you might like, and who's the best person to be with you and support you through the birth.

Your birth attendant

Who will attend the birth and deliver your baby will depend largely on where you choose to give birth, whether you have had any complications during pregnancy, and how straightforward your labour and delivery turns out to be.

Obstetrician

An obstetrician is a specialist in the field and heads a hospital-based team of midwives, nurses and other doctors who will provide your antenatal care and deliver your baby. One will usually only attend difficult or high-risk births, for example, if you require a Caesarean or develop pre-eclampsia. You may be referred to an expert in high-risk pregnancies – also known as a maternal-fetal medical specialist.

General practitioner/family doctor

Your general practitioner (GP) may be qualified to attend you during the birth of your baby, either at home or in a local hospital unit. However, many GPs have stopped being involved in births. They feel that community midwives are better experienced than them, as well as having more time to devote to an individual woman's labour and delivery.

Midwife

The belief that women's bodies were designed for birth is at the core of midwifery, which tends towards the natural rather than the interventionist approach to labour and birth. UK studies have shown that healthy women with straightforward pregnancies who chose midwifery care had very good outcomes with fewer interventions and lower Caesarean rates.

Private care

Maternity care is also available privately at your own cost, usually in private maternity units in general hospitals, or in private maternity hospitals.

Pain relief in labour

All women use one or more pain-relieving strategies during labour. What is important about the one(s) you choose, is that you remain positive and are able to communicate with your caregivers to ensure that you feel in control and confident. It is important to remain flexible about what you want.

If you haven't prepared for childbirth, fear of the unknown can be a major problem; this is because fear leads to the stress response, which can lead to pain. Finding out what to expect in labour and birth can be very helpful to reduce this fear. The more you and your partner know about what happens in labour – asking questions of your caregiver to allay your anxieties – the more likely you are to find it manageable. If the fear is deep-seated, or, if you have seen or heard frightening experiences of childbirth, you may find it useful to discuss your concerns with your healthcare provider.

Analgesics

These drugs are injected into a muscle or given intravenously to relieve pain. They can make you sleepy if narcotic based. Pethidine is the most common analgesic used in labour. It is given either by injection in the buttocks or intravenously when labour is established, and takes about 20 minutes to kick in. It can be particularly helpful when early labour is prolonged and uncomfortable, helping you to rest and taking the edge off strong sensations. It can make you feel sick, so it is often given with an anti-sickness drug, and can make you feel drowsy, which may help you to cope with the passage of time in labour.

On the negative side, analgesics can hinder your ability to get up and walk about during labour, because they can make you unsteady on your feet. Also, you may dislike feeling drowsy and out of control. If given close to delivery, pethidine can make your baby drowsy and slow to feed and interact. It also may impair his breathing and he may need extra oxygen. The effects on your baby can last a day or two, as his immature system is less capable of clearing the medication from his body, and can cause difficulties with early feeding, Medication can be given to the baby after birth to reverse these effects.

Anaesthetics

These medications produce a loss of sensation and are excellent at taking away pain. Many hospitals run obstetric anaesthetic clinics where you can meet an anaesthetist to discuss what type of anaesthetics are available. This is useful if you have any medical issues that may affect the type of pain relief you can have in labour. For example, very overweight women need to be aware that it may be difficult for them to have an epidural or spinal anaesthetic.

Local anaesthetics are commonly used for epidural insertion and pudendal blocks, and can be given at the time of birth and for episiotomies. Regional anaesthetics such as epidurals blocks pain in a wider area.

- *A pudendal block* This method is given at the time of delivery, by a needle inserted through the vagina. As these anaesthetics numb only this perineal area, you'll feel less pain, but you'll still feel contractions. It's usually given with forceps or vacuum extraction and its effect can last through an episiotomy and subsequent stitching.
- *Epidural* The most popular choice for pain relief during labour, an epidural blocks most pain sensations in the abdomen, although you can still feel pressure. Only an anaesthetist, a specialist in anaesthesia, can administer an epidural. This is

vital questions about pain relief

1   Does your hospital have a 24-hour anaesthesia service? With certain types of pain relief, such as an epidural, an anaesthetist (a doctor with specialised training in anaesthetics), must be present to administer anaesthetic medications and perform the necessary procedures. You may wish to ask for an interview with the anaesthetist before your labour. It's important to know the department's availability and philosophy of pain relief in childbirth.

2   Will you be given clear and concise written and spoken information regarding the risks versus benefits of pain relief measures?

3   What are the side effects, short- and long-term, for both the mother and the baby, of the different pain-relief measures on offer?

4   Does your healthcare provider's philosophy of care agree with yours? If you prefer a more natural approach to pain relief, does he or she know and support your wishes?

5   Does your healthcare provider have experience in different types of pain-relief techniques such as imaging, massage, or specific childbirth preparation techniques, for example Lamaze?

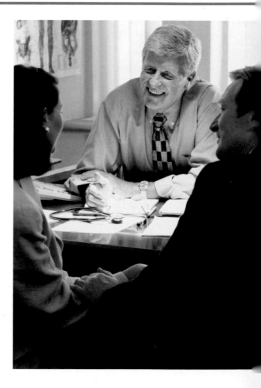

done by placing a small needle into the epidural space, in the lower part of your back. The needle passes between the bones of the lower vertebrae, below the location of the spinal cord. A very tiny, sterile tube is threaded through the needle. The needle is then removed, leaving the tiny tube in place. Medications are injected or pumped through the tube, and these include: narcotics, such as morphine and fentanyl, which take away pain; and, sometimes, local anaesthetic drugs, such as lidocaine, that block pain but cause numbness. Once the medication reaches the tube, you may feel relief from any pain in ten minutes. Whereas injections tend to wear off after some time, a pump is designed to provide a continuous low dose of the drug.

♦ *Walking epidural* Narcotics given with low doses of local anaesthetics may reduce pain without the loss of sensation. If lower doses of drugs are used, you are able to be up and about, and can choose the position you want in which to deliver your baby. If you are not numb, you are more likely to be able to push effectively, as well.

♦ *Spinal* This is similar to an epidural, but instead of being put into the epidural space, the needle and tube are inserted directly into the spinal fluid, also below the spinal cord. Medication injected into this area results in profound pain relief and numbness. This is desirable if immediate anaesthesia is needed, such as for an emergency Caesarean. Because it penetrates the dura (the membrane around the spinal fluid) it is possible to get a spinal headache, which can be treated with a blood patch (see below).

♦ *Combined spinal-epidural* This combines the two procedures of a spinal anaesthetic with an epidural to accomplish very rapid pain relief. It is particularly useful when pain is most intense – usually towards the end of labour or if a medical intervention is needed.

When epidurals include a local anaesthetic drug, which causes numbness, you may experience little or no feeling, which means that it can be difficult to urinate. A small catheter or tube will be inserted through the urethra into the bladder so that the

An epidural is a regional anaesthetic injected into the space at the lower end of the spine to provide pain relief in the abdominal area.

Spinal cord

Epidural space

Vertebra

bladder can be emptied automatically. An epidural may also make it difficult to push at the end of labour. Sitting in a relatively upright position for delivery – at a 45- to 90-degree angle – and concentrating on pushing can help.

Epidurals also can lower your blood pressure. Since it is essential to keep your circulation going so that your baby gets enough oxygen, your blood pressure will be monitored frequently before and after an epidural is inserted. In addition, you'll be given fluids via an IV to keep your circulating blood volume stable. Your baby will be monitored by an electronic fetal monitor.

It used to be thought than an epidural increased the risk of having forceps, but if the second stage is managed by delayed pushing, this is not so. However, labour is generally longer if one is given.

While some women complain of backache after birth, it is more likely that this comes from the inability to move around a lot in labour and the passage of the baby through the pelvis. Research has found no link between epidurals and long-term lower back pain. Some women, however, experience headaches after an epidural. This happens if there is a leak of spinal fluid after the epidural is inserted. If the headache persists, it can be treated with a 'blood patch', which involves a small amount of blood being taken from a vein on the woman's arm, and injecting it into the epidural space, sealing the leak.

There has been very little research into the effect epidurals have on babies. A recent study linked their use to the reluctance of newborn babies to breast-feed. In this study, women given epidurals were

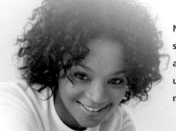

Natural forms of pain relief, such as using a birthing ball and other postures are often used in conjunction with medications.

twice as likely as those giving birth naturally to give up breastfeeding.

Tranquillisers

These are muscle relaxants, which can relieve tension. They are usually given with a narcotic to maximize the effect of a small dose of narcotic.

General anaesthesia

This is anaesthetic gas mixed with oxygen and is only given if medically necessary, in particular during an emergency Caesarean. When you awake, you may feel drowsy. It may have the same sedative effect on your baby.

Gas and air

Entonox (50 percent nitrous oxide and 50 percent oxygen) is a rapid acting pain reliever, which you inhale via a mask from a cylinder on a mobile support. It will take the edge off pain, and can be used as and when needed. It does not cross the placenta so cannot harm the baby. It can, however, cause nausea and lightheadedness.

TENS

Transcutaneous Electrical Nerve Stimulation is the application of low-voltage electrical pulses to areas of pain. A hand-held unit delivers tingling levels of electrical stimulation to various points on your body via wires attached to pads and taped to your skin. It's thought that it works by blocking the transmission of pain signals to your brain. It also may stimulate the production of endorphins, your body's natural analgesic.

The success of the method depends on the positioning of the pads; it works best if the pads are attached to acupuncture points on the back. Although it can only be used in first stage labour, many women find it helpful, and this may demonstrate that the experience of pain in labour has a psychological component as well as a physical one. It perhaps shows that mums-to-be, whilst in labour, need distraction and to feel in control.

Natural pain relief

Many women, as soon as labour starts, begin to feel anxious because they anticipate it to be painful. As a reaction to this stress, adrenalin is pumped round the body causing blood to be diverted from the uterus to the legs, and breathing to become rapid and shallow. Such anaerobic breathing produces lactic acid, which attaches itself to pain receptors and sends pain messages to the brain, resulting in yet more stress and the cycle repeats.

Relaxation techniques (see page 219) can reduce anxiety levels and thus block this stress/pain cycle.

Pain also can be reduced by changing your position – walk, kneel, or use a birthing ball – whatever makes you feel most comfortable. An added benefit of a change in position is that it can help to encourage a baby who is facing the 'wrong way' – towards your back (occipital posterior) – to assume a better position for birth. In the occipital posterior position, your baby's head fits less well in your pelvis and stronger than normal contractions are necessary to move him down (see also page 204).

You might also like to consider visualisation (see page 128) and breathing techniques (see page 218).

Support that your partner can give during labour, such as massage and warm or cold compresses (see page 182) can help the body to relax and distract you from pain. Massage, particularly in the first stage of labour, has been shown to help women experiencing backache, which can occur if baby isn't positioned properly or is lying with his or her back against the mother's back.

Alternative therapies such as hypnosis or reflexology (applying pressure to a specific part of the foot has been shown to dull pain experienced in another part of the body) are also becoming increasingly popular during labour. Some birth centres have trained personnel available.

Acupuncture, the insertion of ultra-fine needles into the skin at various points can be used during labour to increase or decrease the strength of contractions, for pain control, and to assist the baby's journey along the birth canal.

However, with all such therapies, you should check their use with your healthcare provider first. Always make sure that you find a qualified practitioner and visit him or her well in advance of your due date to discuss and practise techniques. You should also make sure that your hospital or birth centre will allow him or her to be with you.

MORE **ABOUT**   water for pain relief

A surprisingly effective form of pain relief, immersing yourself in water during labour or just taking a shower, can relax you, making contractions easier to bear and enabling labour to progress more smoothly. It also supports you, so you can move around freely. The use of water in the first stage of labour reduces the use of epidual/spinal anaesthesia, and reduces pain.

Water therapy seems to work best when labour is fairly advanced. Women have reported that just waiting for the pool to fill up relaxes them, as they anticipate sinking into the warm, supportive water (the temperature should not exceed 37.5° C).

Choosing your birth partner

Who you want to be present at the birth is a highly personal decision – some people are happy with a large audience and others prefer to keep it private. Bear in mind that you may need more privacy than you expect. Choose carefully; once an invitation is extended, it's hard to take it back. Make sure that your invitees are calm and supportive. Children and young people will need to be prepared for this powerful event to avoid misinterpretation, and they will need to be accompanied by an adult. Check with your hospital about visiting policies, some have limits on the number or age of participants. At the same time, find out if there might be students or ancillary personnel present; if you're not comfortable

Labouring women have five basic needs: physical care and comfort; pain relief; the constant presence of a supportive person; unconditional acceptance and reassurance; and knowledge of what is happening. A supportive birth partner can help to: shorten labour; decrease the need for medication and intervention; decrease the risk of a Caesarean and improve the outcome for his newborn. The needs of women in labour do differ, however, so try to tune into what your partner wants.

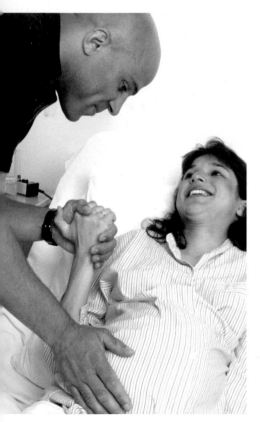

STAY CLOSE BY Some women like to be touched during labour but others don't. Touch can help to communicate caring and concern and will also stop your partner feeling isolated.

CONSIDER HER POSITION Urge her to change position frequently, as this can help to ease backache. Use pillows, rolled blankets or towels to provide comfort. If she's able to walk, encourage and assist her. Some mothers bounce on large, air-filled 'birthing balls' to relieve the pain of a contraction.

KEEP HER CLEAN AND DRY Labour may cause a woman to move her bowels or urinate, and at some point her waters will break. Help to clean her quickly.

ENCOURAGE HER TO EAT AND DRINK It's best if a woman eats, lightly and frequently during labour, although there are some situations where this is not advisable; your midwife will let you know. High-energy food that's easy to digest, such as toast with jam, bananas and soup are best. She also should keep hydrated. Isotonic drinks are more beneficial than water. Drinking may lead to some vomiting but this is not harmful to the baby.

RELIEVE HER DRY MOUTH Use of breathing techniques can dry out her mouth, so help her to drink liquids or to suck on ice chips. Use lip balm to moisten her lips. Also, help her to brush her teeth.

KEEP HER COOl Apply a cool cloth to her face, throat or other body parts. Spray her face gently with water. Alternatively, try fanning her.

APPLY A COMPRESS Contractions may cause back pain or cramp. Help her out by applying a warm or cold face flannel to her back.

MASSAGE HER LOWER BACK Ask her to lie on her side so you can give her a back-rub using lotion. This may be helpful if she's having back labour (when the pain of contractions is felt mainly in the back). However, be aware that she might prefer you to stop the massage during a contraction.

ENCOURAGE HER TO PASS URINE A full bladder may slow down labour, so remind her to go to the toilet frequently – she should try at least every couple of hours.

USE RELAXATION TECHNIQUES Ideally, practise these before labour begins. One easy technique involves asking her to tighten then relax each muscle in turn, starting with her upper body and progressing slowly down to her toes.

HELP WITH BREATHING TECHNIQUES Learn whatever breathing exercise she wishes to use in advance, and help her to focus

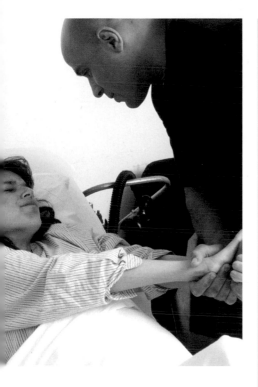

on it during contractions. It may help if you ask her to take a deep breath and sigh after each contraction to help to 'exhale tension'.

PROMOTE REST Keep her surroundings as peaceful as possible, and encourage her to rest to prevent exhaustion.

ASSURE HER PRIVACY Respect her need – or lack of need – for clothing and covers during labour.

OFFER EMOTIONAL SUPPORT Whisper words of encouragement. Praise her for her tremendous effort. Tell her 'You're doing brilliantly!'

HOW TO STAY FOCUSED ON HER NEEDS

Each woman is unique, responds individually, and has different needs in labour, so it's important to ask her if a particular technique is helpful or desirable. Be prepared to change tactics or give her a bit of space, if that's what she wants. Bear in mind these key points:

CONSIDER YOUR PURPOSE What are you trying to do with your support and comfort measures? Make sure that you focus on what your partner wants.

BE INVOLVED Your constant presence and attention to how she is feeling and the procedures that are being carried out are necessary to provide meaningful support.

BE PREPARED Pack necessary items several weeks before the due date, and plan your route to the hospital in advance.

KEEP UP YOUR ENERGY LEVELS To provide effective support you need to stay energised yourself. Be sure to get something to eat and drink during the labour. It's best to take food and drinks with you. Also, take a break, if possible. Relax in a chair in the labour room or take a short walk on the ward. But don't leave the ward – you could miss the birth.

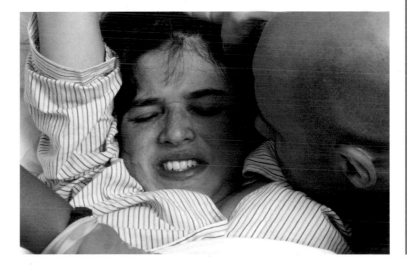

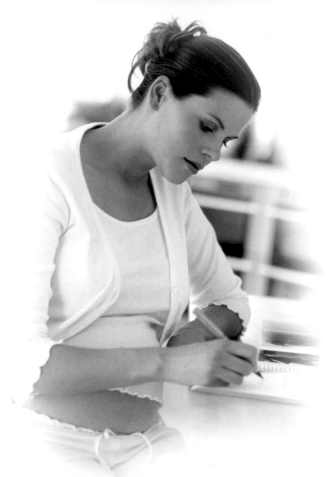

Writing a birth plan can help you to understand your options, and undergoing childbirth with an educated but open mind can help your labour.

advance of your due date. Some caregivers encourage women to make formal birthing plans, listing their preferences and even supply blank forms. A sample plan is on page 185, but bear in mind that it isn't exhaustive – you can include anything you like. You'll need to bring the plan with you for the birth.

However, it's important to be flexible. Birth isn't a predictable event: like babies and people, each birth has its own 'personality'. Even if you have had other children, this birth will be different and special, and you may have to adapt your birth plan accordingly.

All sorts of factors influence your decisions about childbirth, including how you feel at the time. For example, if you plan to take very little or no pain relief, you may find that you change your mind during the actual labour. Many women feel that they've somehow failed if things don't go according to their birth plan – maybe an emergency Caesarean was necessary because the baby was in distress – but it's no failure to accept the most appropriate medical treatment for the safe delivery of your baby.

with this, you still have time to find a solution. Warn your guests that they may be asked to leave at any point during the birth, according to your needs or at the discretion of your healthcare provider.

Professional labour support

Hiring a trained or experienced birth helper is another option that can be a great support in some circumstances. If your partner travels away from home on business a lot, you're having a vaginal birth after Caesarean (VBAC), or you want to limit medical intervention, it's well worth thinking about hiring either a doula (Greek for 'in service to woman') or a monitrice (from the French, 'to watch over'). Their services usually include visits before and after delivery, as well as at-home support during early labour. Ask your healthcare provider for more information and recommendations.

Your birth plan

After you consider your options, it's important to discuss them with your healthcare provider far in

DID YOU KNOW...

SUPPORT CAN SHORTEN LABOUR Studies show that when a doula or other birth partner is present, women have less painful labours, fewer medical interventions, fewer Caesareans and healthier babies. Recent evidence suggests that when a doula provides support, women are more satisfied with their experiences, and the mother-infant interaction is enhanced for as long as two months after the birth. Doula support has been found to have a positive effect on a couple's relationship as well.

Tick all that apply in each section

BIRTH PARTNERS

I would like the following people to be at the birth

- ☐ Partner
- ☐ Friend
- ☐ Relative
- ☐ Doula
- ☐ Other children

INDUCTION

- ☐ I would prefer not to be induced.
- ☐ I would consider induction for medical reasons only.
- ☐ I would prefer to be induced to control the time/date of my delivery.

LABOUR

- ☐ I want to be able to walk around and be out of bed if possible.
- ☐ I would like to drink fluids and/or eat lightly throughout the first stage.
- ☐ I would like to keep the number of vaginal examinations to a minimum.
- ☐ I would like to view the birth using a mirror.

MONITORING

- ☐ I do not wish to have continuous fetal monitoring unless my baby is distressed.

PHOTOGRAPHY

- ☐ I wish to have my birth photographed/videoed.

PAIN MANAGEMENT

- ☐ I wish to have a natural birth and do not want pain medication offered to me during labour.
- ☐ I would like an epidural as early as possible.
- ☐ I would like an epidural later in labour.
- ☐ I wish to have pain medication available but only given to me if I request it.

EPISIOTOMY

- ☐ I would prefer not to have an episiotomy unless it is required for my baby's safety.
- ☐ I would prefer to have an episiotomy rather than risk tearing.

CAESAREAN

- ☐ If I need to have an emergency Caesarean I would like my partner present at all times during the operation.
- ☐ I wish to have an epidural or spinal for anaesthesia.
- ☐ If I have to have a full anaesthetic, I wish my baby to be handed to (name of person) after the birth

POST-BIRTH

- ☐ I would like to hold my baby immediately after the birth.
- ☐ I want to wait until the umbilical cord stops pulsing before it is cut.
- ☐ I would like my partner to cut the cord.
- ☐ I would prefer not to have routine syntocinon after the birth.
- ☐ I plan to breastfeed my baby.
- ☐ I wish to put my baby to the breast as soon after the birth as possible.

Interventions and procedures

When considering the type of delivery you want, there may be certain procedures that you want to avoid, if possible. Your healthcare provider should respect your wishes as long as you and your baby are not at risk.

However, it can help to find out as much as possible about what the procedures involve and to be prepared, when the time comes, to allow your midwife to judge if intervention is needed.

Induction

When a woman goes into labour naturally, a series of hormonal changes and the pressure of the full-term baby on the uterine muscles help to initiate the process of labour. But labour also can be induced (started artificially) by hormones, medications, catheters or membrane sweeping (manual stimulation of the cervix). Induction is only used when vaginal delivery is the most likely outcome.

Left to nature, most women will go into labour and deliver their babies within two weeks either side of their due date. Labour is induced when it's better for the baby to be born than remain inside the uterus or when the health of mother or baby is deemed at risk should the pregnancy continue. If a baby isn't growing sufficiently towards the end of a pregnancy or if he is large or has a serious medical condition or is in breech position, or if it's a twin pregnancy, ending a pregnancy by inducing labour may be the best option. Mothers who have high-risk conditions, such as diabetes or pregnancy-induced hypertension, or who have a history of very fast labour may be candidates for induction. Other reasons include the pre-labour rupture of membranes, as induction may lower the risk of infection, and if the pregnancy is prolonged. Where resources allow, your healthcare provider should consider a request for induction if you have compelling psychological or social reasons. He or she will want to be certain that your baby is

sufficiently mature and the cervix is favourable before agreeing to your request.

No matter the reason for induction, your healthcare provider should discuss the procedure with you thoroughly beforehand. You should be told the reasons, method, and potential risks and consequences for accepting or refusing the offer. This is known as 'informed consent'.

Syntocinon

Even if your labour is not induced, your healthcare provider may help the progress of labour by using syntocinon (a synthetic form of oxytocin) to make your contractions stronger and more effective.

Syntocinon should be given in such a way as to simulate normal contractions. However, artificially induced contractions are often stronger and more frequent than natural contractions. This, in turn, can lead to abnormal fetal heart readings, so women who are receiving syntocinon are almost always on a fetal monitor to see how the baby is tolerating the contractions. If the frequency of contractions is too high, the dose may be adjusted downwards.

Fetal monitors

These devices are used to check the baby's heart beat during labour. One of the most common types is the external fetal monitor, consisting of electrodes placed on your abdomen. These are hooked up to a machine that displays or prints out readings of your baby's heartbeat and your contractions.

Some hospitals monitor all women with these monitors continuously in labour. But some studies have shown that it can lead to an increase in unnecessary Caesareans, because the readings were misinterpreted and the monitors indicated that there was a problem where there wasn't. For this reason, if you have a low-risk pregnancy and birth, you may be checked with a fetal monitor intermittently, or the baby's heart beat may be measured with a Doppler (a hand-held ultrasound device).

If your healthcare provider needs a more detailed picture of your baby's condition, he or she may want to monitor your baby internally by passing an electrode through your vagina and attaching it to your baby's scalp to measure the heartbeat. Internal monitoring is more accurate than external monitoring, but it does have some drawbacks: the use of the monitor restricts your mobility, which may slow down the progress of your labour. Because of these factors, internal monitoring is normally only carried out when there are proven benefits.

Episiotomy

This is a small cut made in the perineum (the skin between the vagina and anus) in order to enlarge the vaginal opening when the baby's head is about to be born. Episiotomies used to be performed routinely but over the last two decades, there has been a significant reduction in the percentage of deliveries involving them — from 64 per cent in 1980 down to 33 per cent in 2000. Current thinking is that there's no absolute benefit in routine episiotomies. Frequently, the skill and patience of an experienced caregiver will stretch the area and allow the baby to be born with minimal or no tears and no need for an episiotomy. A small tear is easily repaired and causes less pain than a large and invasive episiotomy.

Episiotomy is still considered valuable to shorten the pushing stage of birth because of fetal distress or if the mother has a medical problem such as a heart condition and cannot cope with a long labour, or if forceps or a ventouse will be used. An episiotomy

may be recommended to protect the delicate skull of a premature infant or to provide more space for the delivery of breech or very large babies.

Forceps and vacuum extraction

In certain cases, medical instruments are used to ease the baby out of the birth canal thus shortening the second stage of labour to reduce the risk to the mother or baby. Studies show that certain medications and labour positions may increase the likelihood that instruments will be needed. It's wise to talk to your healthcare provider about the use of forceps and vacuum extractors long before you go into labour.

Although they are traditionally associated with an increased risk of vaginal or perineal laceration, recent studies show that a forceps delivery is no better or worse than other deliveries and can reduce the chances of trauma to a baby and may prevent the need for a Caesarean birth. Forceps (metal instruments resembling salad tongs) may be used if the mother can't push effectively or if the baby has to be born quickly. They also can be used to turn a baby into a different position.

Opponents of forceps maintain that they can be used out of convenience when labour is slow and the medical team want the baby to be delivered as quickly as possible.

A vacuum extractor (ventouse) works in a similar way to forceps, but here a soft cup is placed on the baby's head and suction helps to pull the baby out as the mother pushes. Vacuum extractors can be used higher up the birth canal than forceps and cause less damage to the perineum.

Caesarean sections

Only an obstetrician or a surgeon can perform a Caesarean, as it involves making an incision in the lower part of the mother's abdomen to deliver the baby. Most Caesareans are performed for medical reasons (see box, below).

Choosing an elective Caesarean

Whether it's your first pregnancy and you are scared about the pain involved in a vaginal birth, or you had a difficult birth first time round and are having flashbacks about the experience, you may want to request a Caesarean. Since 2011, under guidelines proposed by the National Institute for Health and Clinical Excellence (NICE), if a woman requests a Caesarean section because she is anxious about childbirth, she should be referred to a healthcare professional with expertise in providing mental health support. She should be offered a planned Caesarean if, after discussion and support, she still feels that a vaginal birth is not an acceptable option.

Like any operation, Caesarean section carries risks such an increased likelihood of infection and excessive bleeding. It may limit the number of children you can have as repeated Caesareans are not necessarily advisable. Recovery after birth is longer than for a straightforward vaginal birth.

Babies born by Caesarean are more likely to have short-term breathing problems compared to vaginally delivered ones and, very rarely, can suffer a nick or cut from the operating knife. Some healthcare workers believe that Caesarean sections should only be done for medical reasons.

Talk through your concerns about vaginal delivery with your healthcare provider. A supportive midwife, reassurance that you will get good pain-relief in labour and a detailed birth plan may make all the difference in you feeling confident enough to try for a vaginal delivery. Second labours are usually quicker and more straightforward than first births so you should not let a previous experience put you off.

Vaginal births after a Caesarean (VBAC)

It's no longer true that 'Once a Caesarean, always a Caesarean.' Most Caesareans now are accomplished using the low transverse or 'bikini' uterine incision (see page 232), which is less likely to rupture in subsequent labours (there is a 0.5 per cent risk). Because each repeat Caesarean is more difficult due to scar tissue from prior surgery, VBAC after a lower segment Caesarean section (LSCS) is considered safer for mother and baby. In addition, 70 per cent of mother who attempt labour after a Caesarean will successfully accomplish VBAC.

However, opponents of VBAC maintain that even with a 'bikini cut' there are risks, including a greater risk of uterine rupture than with a repeat Caesarean. Women who have a VBAC induced with medication are at the highest risk for uterine rupture so most obstetricians prefer you to go into labour without medical intervention if you are aiming for VBAC.

7 medical reasons for a Caesarean

1   Sometimes a baby is in a difficult position for delivery – in a breech position (feet or buttocks first) or transverse (lying sideways). Many breech babies and all transverse babies must be born by Caesarean.

2   If a pregnant woman has a high-risk condition, such as bleeding, genital herpes, diabetes and pregnancy-induced hypertension or eclampsia (see page 254).

3   If there's more than one baby, it's more likely that they will be born by Caesarean, although some twins are successfully delivered vaginally if they're in favourable positions.

4   Poor growth of the baby or a high-risk condition of the mother or baby can make it safer for the pregnancy to end with a planned Caesarean.

5   The baby is very large. Some babies are just too big to be born from a mother's birth canal.

6   Fetal distress as a result of the stresses and strains of labour. This can be detected by fetal monitoring and special tests.

7   Two or more previous Caesarean sections. After an initial Caesarean a VBAC (see opposite) may be recommended.

Getting ready for the birth of your baby

As the last trimester of your pregnancy draws to an end you'll be feeling excited about the imminent arrival of your baby and you will want to make final preparations for labour. Now is a good time to plan and organise the things you need to do.

Decisions about your baby

It's well worth spending time before your baby is born thinking about some of the choices you will need to make once she arrives. Even if you change your mind later, by considering the options now you will be able to make more informed decisions.

Some things to consider before your baby arrives include: how you want to feed her; whether to save her cord blood; what will be her name(s); whether to return to work and/or require childcare.

Breast or bottle?

Deciding how you will feed your baby is a very personal matter and you should spend some time understanding the benefits and drawbacks of breastfeeding and bottlefeeding so that you can make an informed decision. There's no question that breast milk is more natural and nutritious and is easier to provide especially in the initial weeks after birth. However, there may be a reason why bottlefeeding is the better option. Ultimately, it's important to make sure that both you and your baby are comfortable, healthy and happy. See Chapter 14 for more on feeding your baby.

Breastfeeding

Women and babies were designed to breastfeed, regardless of the size or shape of the woman's breasts though if nipples are flat or inverted, a little help may be needed in learning to position your baby. Most women manage it very successfully within a few weeks of the birth, though some with the help of their healthcare provider. Natural hormonal changes within the body ensure that breastfeeding becomes emotionally satisfying. If you're unsure about it, you should aim at least to try breastfeeding; many women who don't do so wish they had at a later date. It's harder to take up breastfeeding after a baby has started on a bottle, so you may not have another chance if you don't try it from the beginning.

Even if you're returning to work soon after giving birth, it's definitely worthwhile starting breastfeeding; breast milk benefits your baby most during the early weeks by building up her immunity. You also can consider combined feeding: breastfeeding when you're at home and relying on expressed or formula milk when you are at work.

Bottlefeeding

If you have problems with or an antipathy to breastfeeding, you may decide to bottlefeed. There also are some medications and conditions, such as HIV, which aren't compatible with breastfeeding because of the risks to the baby, in which case bottlefeeding is essential. Your caregiver will advise in such cases.

Storing cord blood

Blood from your baby's umbilical cord can be obtained at the time of delivery and stored frozen in a cord blood bank. Umbilical cord blood contains stem cells, which have the potential to become many different types of cells or organ tissues. In the unlikely event your baby should need a bone marrow or organ transplant, her umbilical cord blood cells would be a perfect match and she would not experience any rejection. UK-based blood banks are for public use, however. You would need to contact a US-based cord bank who would also provide you with information about and equipment for harvesting the cells.

Choosing a name

Naming your baby can be a fun and exciting project. Discuss ideas with your partner, then make a list of your favourites and attach it to the fridge or a notice board so that you look at the names frequently and get a good feeling for each one. Some parents prefer not to divulge the name until after the birth – a beautiful new baby can help to appease a

benefits of breastfeeding

1   Breast milk is naturally designed to provide all the nutrients your baby needs in the right amounts.

2   Breast milk contains antibodies and other protective factors that help to fight infection. Breastfed infants are known to have decreased risks of respiratory and ear infections, gastroenteritis, diabetes, Crohn's disease, autoimmune diseases, SIDS and obesity, among many other problems.

3   Breast milk is easily digested and is less likely to cause stomach upsets, diarrhoea or constipation.

4   Breast milk is cheap, readily available, the right temperature and fresh.

5   Breastfeeding speeds the process of your uterus returning to its normal size and can help you to lose the weight you gained during pregnancy.

6   Breastfeeding can reduce a woman's risk of developing breast cancer

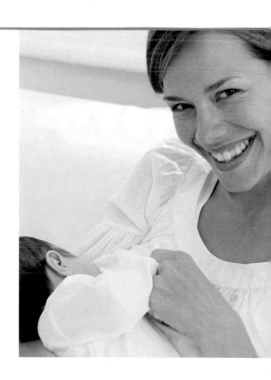

At some stage before your due date you'll need to decide whether you're going to have your baby boy circumcised and, if so, arrange for the procedure to be carried out soon after the birth. Although it's a controversial procedure, it has been shown to be protective against male urinary tract infections (especially in the first year of life), prostate cancer and the heterosexual acquisition of HIV and other sexually transmitted diseases. However, many parents decide on the procedure for religious or other reasons. The procedure is painful but relatively quick, and warrants some form of anaesthesia; there are small risks of infection, excess bleeding or scarring (although much less than in adult males undergoing the procedure). Talk this decision over with your partner and doctor.

bearing in mind you can always edit the shots later. Make sure you have extra batteries and invest in a disposable camera just in case. Check beforehand that you're allowed to film or take photographs, as some doctors and hospitals don't permit them.

Don't watch the video or pore over the photographs too soon after the event. Giving birth is very emotional and your body copes naturally with this by creating a neurochemical amnesia that softens your birth memories over the following weeks.

grandparent who thinks that the chosen name is inappropriate. Bear in mind that when your baby arrives, you may change your mind about the name you have chosen and decide on a different one that suits her better. Here are some tips:

◆ *Find out the derivation and meaning* Buy a names book or look on the Internet.
◆ *Try to think of possible nicknames* Charles could become Charlie, Alyssa may become shortened to Aly, Samantha to Sam.
◆ *Avoid 'difficult' names* Avoid names that others will find hard to spell or pronounce.
◆ *Consider fads and fashions* Will you and your child be happy to be named Star, Suri, Brooklyn, Paris, Pixie and so on?
◆ *Keep it in the family* Is there an important namesake you wish to honour – or avoid?
◆ *Pay attention to how the name sounds* And with a middle name? If you give your baby a middle name, consider what the initials spell.

Photographing the birth

This might seem a trivial thing to think about, but planning how you want to record your baby's birth can save a lot of tension on the day.

Decide whether you want the birth photographed or videoed. Arrange for someone, preferably other than your partner, to be in charge of the camera. Consider carefully what you want to be filmed,

Finding a child-friendly practice

Registering your baby with a GP who has a special interest in paediatrics can take some keen detective work. Ask your health visitor, midwife, friends and relatives for their recommendations and then conduct a telephone interview with the practice manager. The following questions will be helpful:

◆ What is the type of practice? Is it solo or group? (It may be better to choose a group practice where there'll always be someone on call.)
◆ Are there dedicated baby clinics?
◆ What are the surgery hours, typical waiting times, and on-call group policy?
◆ How are after-hours calls handled?
◆ What happens in emergencies?

If you're still interested, make an appointment to meet the GP. At this visit, try to obtain the following information:

◆ What's the doctor's philosophy on issues such as breastfeeding, supplementation, newborn jaundice, circumcision, antibiotic use, immunisation and so on?
◆ Is the waiting area welcoming and clean, and are there plenty of toys and books to keep young children entertained?
◆ Are the reception staff welcoming and friendly and how do they interact with children?

Going back to work

Another decision that you'll probably need to make before giving birth is when you plan to return to work and how you want your baby to be looked after when this happens. Bear in mind that most daycare facilities have long waiting lists and should be contacted well before the birth to get your baby's name on the list.

You may want to leave it as long as you can before going back to work – most mothers find it harder to leave their babies than they expected. And if the thought of going back to work full-time fills you with dread, consider a more flexible work pattern, such as working part-time – between 20 and 32 hours per week – or working flexibly, where you fit your job into fewer days with longer hours or more days with shorter hours.

Negotiating different hours

New guidelines have been bought in which are designed to help parents with children under the age of six years to work flexibly. To be eligible you have to meet certain criteria, so talk to your human resources department, trade union or ask your local Department for Work and Pensions for more detailed information before you make any decisions. Here are some tips that may help you when you put your case to your employer:

- *Test the reaction* Warn your employer that you're thinking about working part time and arrange a meeting to discuss the matter. Ask if he or she would like a written outline of how you think this would work.
- *Prepare your case* Describe exactly how the job would get done if you change your hours. It will help if you can satisfy your boss that you can work just as efficiently as before.
- *Explain it to your co-workers* Tell them what you're doing and try and work through any difficulties that may arise.

Organising childcare

However, whether you plan to go back to work full time or part time, you'll still need to arrange some form of childcare, and it'll be a lot easier returning to a working life if you feel happy and confident about this. Ask your health visitor, family and friends for recommendations, and get a list of

Any childcare facility should welcome you to spend time there, getting to know the staff and observing the quality of care provided.

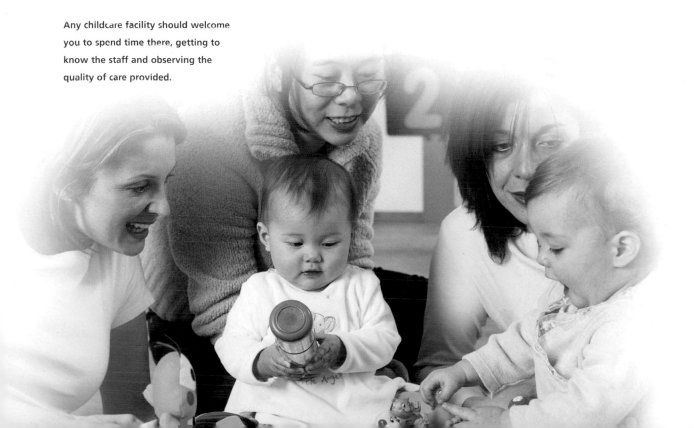

DAYCARE CAN BENEFIT CHILDREN
Studies in the United Kingdom, Europe and the United States show that quality childcare has important and lasting beneficial effects on the education, health and welfare of children, especially those from low-income families, or with development problems.

---

registered childminders from your local authority. Remember that the most important factor is to ensure the safety and well-being of your baby. Licensing, training certificates, references and any facility that you are considering should always be double-checked.

Your options

Take time to research your options. Your baby needs to be with someone that you and your partner both like and trust, otherwise the arrangement will fall apart. Your basic choices are:

- *Parent at home* Obviously this is the ideal option. One of you stays at home to look after the baby, or you both work different hours so that the care can be shared.
- *Family* Having your mother or another relative looking after your baby can be an excellent childcare solution, providing your baby with continuity of care.
- *Nanny* In-home care can be expensive, but if you have more than one child it becomes more economical. There's no doubt that one-on-one care during the first year of life is very beneficial, but that depends on having a reliable, experienced nanny who's in tune with a child's physical and emotional needs.
- *Childminder* This is offered by people who are licensed to offer childcare in their homes, possibly in combination with looking after their own children. This arrangement will provide playmates and a family environment for your child, and has the advantage of her having the same caregiver and being in a small group.
- *Nurseries* These work well for children of any age, as long as they're of a high standard. However, not all nurseries take babies under the age of 12 months.

Help once you're home

Planning ahead for your return home with your baby is important since you want to be able to get to know her and to adjust to your new role in a relaxed atmosphere. If you've had a difficult or lengthy birth, you also may be tired and in need of plenty of rest. Getting help at home for the first few weeks after the birth can be make a huge difference, but you need to make sure that you choose the right sort of help – and the right sort of person.

Be clear what you want

Helpers range from full-time professional maternity nurses, who can train you in childcare and provide breastfeeding support, to experienced mothers who are paid to come in for a few hours to help with the housework and listen to any concerns you may have. You need to be clear what you want your helper to do and how long you'll need her. Ask about fees, training and experience, check references and make sure that you're going to get on well.

Some women depend on relatives to help out, which is ideal, provided that you're on good terms with your family and are confident in their knowledge and experience of childcare.

Shopping for your baby

Nothing quite beats the thrill of buying your very first items for your baby. However, resist the temptation to buy up the whole shop. It's best to purchase the basics now, and then shop for other items when you require them.

It's easy to be seduced into getting things that look attractive but that you don't actually need. Bear in mind, too, that you will probably receive lots of presents once your baby is born.

Furnishing the nursery

It is recommended that your baby share your bedroom for at least the first few months but you may want to prepare the nursery for his daytime naps. Until he's much older, your baby won't notice his surroundings – all that will matter to him is that he's warm, well-fed and comfortable. Yet for most parents, preparing the nursery is one of the most enjoyable parts of pregnancy and provides an excellent way for them to feel that they are welcoming their new baby into their home.

Bear in mind that your baby will probably use the same room throughout his childhood and that the decorations should grow with him. Plain background colours and fashionable finishing touches, such as borders, friezes and stencils, can be quickly updated as he grows up.

Walls should be washable or at least spongeable. Paint is more practical than wallpaper. Choose a natural, water-based paint rather than solvent-based one; these don't give off chemical fumes while the room is being painted.

Your newborn won't need a lot of furniture at first, but make sure that you have enough storage

Shopping for your baby is fun, and you'll have more time now than after the birth. Try to enlist some help to carry some of the load.

SAFETY FIRST

DECORATING There are several things you should watch out for when decorating your baby's room during pregnancy:

- Avoid breathing in paint fumes – get someone else to do the painting.
- If you suspect that old paint may be lead-based, get someone else to sand and paint over it. Lead-based paint can be toxic.
- Remember that your balance has altered, so be extra careful on stepladders and never attempt to reach too far, even when you are standing on the floor.
- Stop before you become exhausted – you are more likely than usual to have accidents.

space, especially around the changing area. Unless you plan to replace the furniture as soon as he's crawling and trying to stand up on his own, furniture should be solid and have smooth, rounded edges. You also might like to include a comfortable chair for your own use at feeding times.

A night light or dimmer switch fitted to the main light can help you find your way in the dark (darkness won't worry your baby) and a baby monitor will allow you to hear him when he starts to cry. Thick curtains or blinds will help to prevent him being woken by light outside. The room's temperature needs to be kept at 18°C (65°F), which is sufficiently warm but can't cause overheating.

A place to sleep

As your newborn should sleep in your bedroom, you may prefer to put him in a smaller first bed such as a Moses basket, crib, carrycot or hammock before progressing to a cot when he's about 4 months old, or you could use a cot right away. Smaller first beds create a soft, comforting environment for a tiny baby; however, they are an extra expense, need their own bedding and are soon outgrown. Cots are more practical, as your baby can sleep in a cot up until the age of 3 years, but a cot may not be suitable at first if there's insufficient space in your bedroom.

Choosing a first bed

Moses baskets are light, small and portable; some can be purchased with a stand. A carrycot is similar to although plainer than a Moses basket; it often comes as part of a pram. Cribs can accommodate a slightly older baby and some have rocker feet or can be suspended from a frame. Hammocks either fasten to conventional stands or may be suspended.

Make sure any first bed you buy is robust enough to withstand the weight of a healthy, fast-growing infant and bear in mind that you'll need to move your baby to a cot once he reaches the upper weight limit given by the manufacturer, or if he seems squashed or restless. Consider also the following:

- *Locks on legs/wheels* Make sure that any first bed with folding legs and/or wheels have locking mechanisms to keep them stable.
- *Hoods that fold back* If hoods won't fold back it can make it tricky to pick up your baby.
- *Rounded edges and corners* Make sure that any woven or wicker baskets don't have any sharp edges that could hurt your baby.
- *Avoid quilts, cords and ribbons* If the bed comes with a quilt, discard it; soft bedding has been linked to SIDS (see page 309). Remove cords and ribbons as these could strangle your baby.
- *A firm mattress that fits snugly* If you can fit two fingers between the mattress and the side of the bed, the mattress is too small.
- *A good base* Cribs, carrycots and Moses baskets should have strong, wide bases.

Choosing a cot

Whether you intend to put your baby in a cot from birth or later, it's worth shopping around for one now, as you may have to order it in advance. There's

5 tips on shopping for baby

1 Consider the practicality of major items before you buy. For example, when choosing a pushchair, make sure it is suitable for getting on and off public transport, or that it will fit into the boot of your car.

2 Think about buying or borrowing some second-hand items or clothes; baby slings, for example, can be in good condition because newborns outgrow them so quickly. However, car seats and mattresses, must always be bought new.

3 Only purchase a few outfits in newborn size; not only will your baby outgrow them very quickly but you'll probably be given a lot of first-sized clothes once he's born.

4 If you don't know the sex of your baby, choose neutral colours – yellows, greens, greys – and plain patterns, which can work for both.

5 Many mail order and Internet companies specialise in baby clothes and equipment, and their prices can be very competitive.

a few options to consider. In addition to a standard cot, a bedside cot, can enable you to share your bed safely with your infant and make breastfeeding easier. It has one side that drops down and a base that adjusts level with your mattress. A cot-bed, which is larger than a standard cot, transforms into a junior bed. Bear in mind, however, that you will need a single bed eventually and the cot may be needed if you're planning to have another baby.

The more expensive brands of cot tend to offer more features, such as adjustable mattress heights. Some have drop sides, which can be operable with one hand, and a quiet mechanism. Lockable casters make moving and cleaning under the cot easier.

When buying a cot, it's very important that it conforms to safety standard BS-EN 76-1, carries a Kitemark tag and has the following safety features:

- *Narrow enough gaps in the side rails* The gap between the side rail slats should be no greater than 45–65 mm, to prevent your baby getting stuck between them.
- *Dual releases on the side rails* There should be a catch on each end to prevent your child lowering the rail. When lowered, the rails should also be at least 23 cm above the mattress support to prevent your child falling out. When raised, the top of the side rails should be at least 66 cm above the mattress at its lowest position. Before buying a cot, raise and lower the sides of each model to see which one is easiest to operate.
- *Well-assembled joints and mechanisms* Check that all the parts of the assembled cot are securely fastened and the cot is sturdy. The moving parts should work smoothly so that fingers or clothing do not become trapped.
- *A snug-fitting mattress* There should be no chance that your baby can become stuck between the mattress and the cot. The mattress itself should always be new and needs to be firm, plastic covered and with reinforced corners and sides.
- *Plain, practical designs* Avoid cut-out designs in the end pieces, as your baby could trap his arm or head in them.
- *A clean safety record* Never buy a used or old cot, as you won't know its history.

Choosing a mattress

Whether or not your cot is new, you will need to purchase a new mattress. The mattress must be firm, fit the bed snugly and have a waterproof covering – look for a 'breathable' one. Foam mattresses are relatively cheap, lightweight and non-allergenic but they are not as comfortable for older babies and must be kept covered with a waterproof layer. Sprung mattresses, made with foam, coir and sometimes lambswool, are more comfortable and supportive for older children but also more expensive and heavier. Coir (natural coconut fibre) mattresses usually need separate waterproof mattress protectors but are a popular 'green' choice.

Getting about

Your baby will need to be comfortable and safe when you take him out. If you are walking you will need a pram, pushchair or a carrier; if you are driving, an infant car seat is essential.

Prams and pushchairs

One item you will not want to be without is a pram or pushchair. There's a huge range to choose from – traditional prams with a spring-suspension chassis, two- and three-in one combinations (chassis with a carrycot and a single- or double-facing pushchair seat), all-terrain pushchairs, standard-size pushchairs, travel systems (pushchair with infant car seat), umbrella and telescopic folding buggies, and double pushchairs. To help you to decide on the right model, think about your lifestyle. If you're going to use it every day around town, a traditional pram offers a comfortable ride and will be long lasting; if you're active and keen to maintain fitness, an all-terrain pushchair, which you can jog with might be the answer (but only when your baby is older). Check the recommended age range for the pram or pushchair before you buy, to make sure it is suitable for use from birth. Newborns should lie flat.

Slings and carriers

Both slings and carriers (the former having a simpler structure, less fastenings and are without a seat), enable you to 'wear' your baby, usually close to your chest. Both can be used indoors as well as out. When transporting a young baby, cotton, padded and machine-washable versions are best. Some styles leave the legs and arms free; others cover the whole baby. Before you buy, make sure that the item offers good head and back support, has wide shoulder straps, so that it is comfortable for you, and you can put it on easily without help.

You will carry your young baby on your front facing inwards until he can support his head by himself, when he can be carried facing outward.

Before you buy a carrier, make sure that stitching is free of any faults. Triple stitching gives the most strength and durability. All buckles, zips and fasteners should work smoothly and the shoulder straps should sit comfortably and be well-padded. Check that the fabric is washable and shrink-proof and that it carries a safety standards logo.

Infant car seat

This is an essential buy before the birth, as you'll need a car seat when you take your baby home from hospital. Only use a second-hand car seat if it is relatively new, has its manual and you know for certain it has not been in an accident.

A first-stage car seat (depending on whether its group 0 or 0+) can be used from birth until your baby weighs 10–13 kg (22–29 lbs), or around nine months of age. The most convenient have a three-point, one-pull harness, a one-pull handle, a head-hugger to keep a very young baby's head steady, and deep, padded sides. Ones with an Isofix base (which fixes to the car's chassis) can attach to this base, ones with a non-Isofix base must be secured by the car's seat belt. An infant car seat should be rear facing and positioned in the middle rear seat. It's vital that the seat you buy fits your car and is properly installed. Infant car seats can be used as comfortable baby seats outside the car – but not for more than two hours a day as this can cause an infant problems with breathing and spinal development.

Feeding

The sort of equipment that you'll need will depend on whether you're planning to breast- or bottlefeed.

Even if you want to breastfeed your baby exclusively, you'll still need some equipment for expressing milk and bottles for feeding.

Bottles and teats

Bottles can be standard or wide-necked, have a graspable shape, and a straight or angled top (to prevent baby swallowing too much air, which can lead to wind. Bottles can be glass or plastic (today's bottles are BPA [bisphenol A]-free). There are also bottles with disposable liners on the market; these are expensive but handy for travelling.

For a new baby, the 115 g (4 oz) size is large enough, but it's more practical to buy larger bottles that will be suitable for when he's older. Most sterilisers take standard and wide-necked shapes, but some travel bags take only standard bottles.

There are a variety of shaped teats available, made from clear silicone or yellowy latex; silicone teats can last up to a year, latex teats begin to deteriorate after about a month but are softer and more 'skin like'. Natural or orthodontic-shaped teats mimic sucking at the breast and may be the best choice if you're planning to mix breast- and bottlefeeding. Anti-colic teats allow air into the bottle as the baby empties it, which minimises the amount of air he will swallow while feeding. Choose either the smallest hole or variable flow types at first.

Breast pumps

Whether you're a working mum or are keen for your partner to be able to feed your baby as well, a breast pump can help you to extract milk to be stored for future use. You can choose between electric and manual models depending on your needs.

Changing and bathing

Although not essential, a purpose-made changing table can help to prevent back strain; choose one that will hold nappies and cleaning materials. However, you can just use a changing mat on a waist-high surface. Changing mats should be wipe-clean and slightly padded to keep your baby comfortable. When you're out with your baby, a smaller travel changing mat will be invaluable;

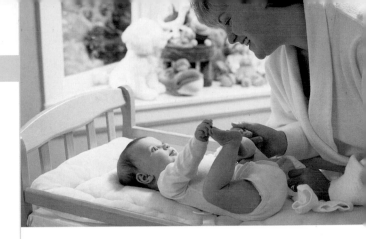

YOUR BABY'S STARTER KIT

FEEDING

Breastfeeding

- 2 bottles and teats
- Breast pads – non-plastic backed
- Pump for expressing milk (optional)
- Breast milk storage containers/bags (optional)
- 2 or 3 breastfeeding bras

Bottlefeeding

- 6 bottles and teats
- Formula
- Formula dispenser

Both methods

- Steriliser
- Bottle brush
- 6 burp cloths
- 2 or 3 dummies

CHANGING

- Changing mat
- 6 towelling squares (to line changing mat)
- Cottonwool pads or baby wipes
- Nappy cream
- 70 first-size disposable nappies or 20 cloth nappies (4 wraps if using two-piece system)
- Lidded nappy bin or nappy disposal unit (for disposables)
- 2 laundry nets (for cloth nappies)
- Nappy sacks (for disposables)

CLOTHES

- 6 all-in-ones (in newborn or 0–3 months size)
- 2 or 3 sleepgowns
- 6–8 short-sleeved bodysuits (in newborn or 0–3 months size) or vests
- 2 cardigans (lightweight in summer; medium-weight for winter)
- 2 or 3 bibs
- 4 pairs socks
- 2 hats – type depending on season
- 2 pairs scratch mitts
- 2 pairs mittens (winter baby only)

BEDTIME

- 3 fitted bottom sheets
- 3 top sheets or 2-3 newborn swaddles or sleeping bags
- 2 or 3 lightweight blankets
- 2 mattress protectors

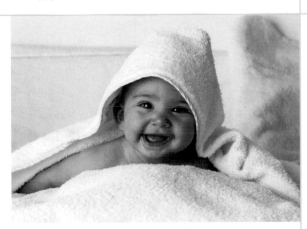

BATHING

- Newborn bath support or baby bath
- Baby toiletries
- 2 large soft towels
- Flannel or sponge
- Baby hairbrush
- Baby nail clippers or scissors

disposable or fold-up mats are inexpensive and fit easily into a baby's travel bag.

A special baby bath isn't essential but it can make bathing baby easier. But whether you use a sink or full-size or baby bath, a bath support should be used to hold your baby in a lying position with his head above water, leaving both your hands free to wash him. These come in various shapes and materials including moulded plastic, foam and fabric.

Nappies

The type of nappies you choose will depend on what you prefer and what suits your lifestyle. Keep in mind that you don't have to stick with one type, but you can mix and match to suit your needs.

Disposables are popular with many parents, because they're more convenient, labour-saving and easy to use. You don't have to wash and dry them or worry about buying separate wraps, liners or clips. They are particularly useful if you're out for the day or travelling. Advances in design have meant that disposables are also very good at drawing moisture away from your baby's skin, helping to prevent skin irritations and nappy rash.

However, disposables can end up being very costly if you rely on them all the time. They're also thought to be harmful for the environment, because they're usually made from wood pulp treated with chemicals and most end up in landfill sites, where they take hundreds of years to decompose. If you do choose disposables, non-chlorine bleached nappies are more environmentally friendly. Disposables come in a range of sizes and styles, so you may need to try a few brands to find nappies that fit your baby well.

Cloth nappies may eventually be cheaper than disposables, as they are a once-only purchase. They can even be used for another child. Many are now shaped so that they're easy to change, have Velcro® fastenings and incorporate a waterproof layer, which helps with both nappy-changing and cleaning. If the ones that you buy don't have this layer, you'll need to buy some waterproof wraps. Consider getting nappy liners, too. These can draw moisture away from your baby's skin and prevent staining of the nappies.

Clothes

Baby clothes are generally sold according to age or in centimetre sizes starting at 50 cm. A big baby may not get any wear out of newborn size clothes, so if your baby's weight is projected to be 4.5 kg or more, you may want to start with a 3-month size. There are special ranges for premature babies.

Your baby will probably dislike being dressed and undressed, so choose clothes that are easy to put on and take off. Avoid buying clothes that you need to hand-wash, iron or dry clean. Choose natural fibres; these minimise sweating and irritation. Always check that there are no raised seams or scratchy labels.

All-in-ones and nightwear

The most practical all-in-ones have poppers up the front and around the crotch to give easy access for nappy changing. Your baby's bones are very soft and it's essential that all-in-one suits have plenty of room in the legs and feet for proper growth.

Most baby sleepgowns have drawstring bottoms but if not, your baby's feet may become cold so you will need socks. You may prefer to put your baby in an all-in-one or appropriately sized sleeping bag, or if it is warm, put him to bed in a vest and nappy.

Vests

These should have wide or envelope necks so that they can be slipped easily over the head. Many brands of vest fasten under the crotch with poppers (also called body suits), providing extra warmth and keeping the nappy securely in place.

Outdoor clothes

Your baby loses a lot of heat from his head, so a hat is essential in winter and may be advisable in spring and autumn. A sun hat is needed in summer if you plan to spend a lot of time in outdoors.

If it's very cold and your pushchair doesn't provide much protection from the elements, you will need a sheepskin or footmuff. Shawls, cardigans and mittens are all useful when cold and should be close-knitted to prevent tiny fingers getting trapped.

If it gets very hot, invest in a few lightweight romper suits.

Preparing for labour

As your due date approaches you'll want to prepare yourself for the birth – both physically and emotionally. Now is the time to look at things you can do that will help you to be comfortable, and to address concerns you may have about giving birth.

Although you may be feeling excited about having a new baby in your life, you may not feel quite so enthusiastic about the birth itself. This is very natural, since the act of giving birth involves a highly sensitive and private part of your body, which carries with it a wealth of emotional feelings. Be prepared to react emotionally to the process of giving birth as well as physically, and try to work through any fears beforehand so that the birth can be a positive, unproblematic experience.

Emotional fears can affect the birth in a very direct physical way. A woman who isn't prepared for the pain of normal contractions may believe that something is wrong and become frightened. This can disrupt her breathing, increase the tension – and therefore pain – in her muscles, and may even decrease the flow of oxytocin, the hormone that causes the uterus to contract. Learning about labour and good birth support can help a woman to work with contractions rather than resist them.

The best way to avoid this is to try to find and resolve any emotional problems that you might have buried deep in your subconscious mind. It's no coincidence that your fantasies and fears rise to the surface in late pregnancy to help you to face problems before the birth and you can use this opportunity to chase these out of your life for good. If you have had especially difficult and traumatic experiences, such as a history of sexual abuse or a previous negative birth experience – or if you have strong control issues – it may be beneficial to seek out some professional counselling.

tips to help you through late pregnancy

1   Wear light, loose clothing. You'll be feeling hotter than normal, mostly because of increased fat deposits and an increased metabolism.

2   Try to get as much sleep as possible. Supplement your nightly sleep with naps, especially if you're being woken by trips to the toilet.

3   Keep your body hydrated. Drink plenty of fluids so that you cope better with your faster metabolism and to relieve swelling feet and legs.

4   Take a break whenever you can. If you have swelling in your feet and legs, sit down and put your feet up on a stool for 10 to 15 minutes, three times a day.

5   Increase your intake of protein. Plenty of milk, eggs, meat and fish can alleviate some of the problems with late pregnancy.

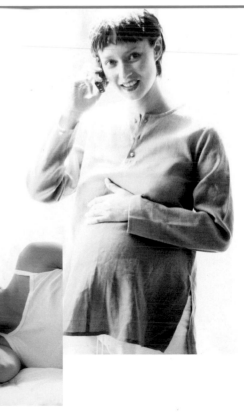

From about 28 weeks you can add some exercises that can help with labour to your daily exercise (see page 117).

TAILOR SITTING This position helps to improve pelvic flexibility in preparation for the birth. Place pillows under your thighs to support them and sit with your back straight and the soles of your feet together **1**. Draw your heels towards your perineum, using your arms to push down on your thighs. Relax your shoulders and the back of your neck and breathe deeply. Hold the stretch for a count of 12 and repeat daily.

As you get more flexible, you can remove the pillows from under your thighs **2**, and push your knees closer to the floor.

PELVIC FLOOR

At around 28 weeks start building up the intensity of your pelvic-floor exercises (see page 122). Start to hold each squeeze for a count of 10, and repeat four to six times, at least three times a day.

Vary your technique. Try changing the speed you do the pull ups in order to acquire greater flexibility and control. Count quickly to 10 or 20, alternately contracting and relaxing your pelvic floor each time you say a number. Or, do it slowly, contracting for a slow count of 4, waiting for a count of 10 and then slowly releasing the muscles for a count of 4.

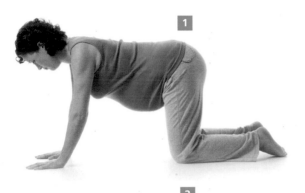

MODIFIED SQUATS Deep squats should be avoided at this stage, but modified squats strengthen your thigh muscles and can encourage the baby to descend properly into the pelvis. Stand with your feet hip-distance apart about 60 cm (2 ft) from a wall. Place your hands on the wall. Keeping your back flat against the wall, slowly lower yourself until your thighs are almost parallel to the floor. Make sure that your knees don't go beyond your toes. Hold briefly, then slowly stand. Repeat 12 times, twice a day.

PELVIC ROCKS This exercise can ease backache during late pregnancy and labour. Get down on your hands and knees, with your knees about hip-width apart. Begin with your neck in line with your spine and your back flat – don't let it sag **1**. Slowly round your shoulders and back and let your head drop down **2**, tightening your abdomen and buttocks as you do so. Hold briefly, then gradually return to the start position. Repeat 10 times, twice a day or whenever you feel tension.

PERINEAL MASSAGE

You can use this technique daily, from around 34 weeks, to stretch the tissue around your vagina and perineum in preparation for the birth.

Always wash your hands before and after this exercise. Use a hand-held mirror to locate your vaginal opening, perineum and urethra.

Sit or lean back comfortably, with a towel under your hips. Using a non-petroleum lubricant, such as K-Y jelly, coat your thumbs and perineal area. Place your thumbs 3 to 4 cm (1 to 1½ inches) inside your vagina. Press gently down and to the sides. Stretch until you feel a slight tingling sensation. Hold this pressure for about 2 minutes.

Maintaining the pressure, gently massage back and forth over the lower half of your vagina for 3 to 4 minutes. Take care to avoid your urethra during the massage because of the risk of urinary tract infection.

Many women find taking a tour of the delivery suite beforehand very helpful. By doing this, you may be more able to picture yourself giving birth, and can emotionally prepare for the actual event.

Your body in late pregnancy

During the last weeks of pregnancy, you'll probably find it increasingly hard to get comfortable, as your baby takes up more and more space, and you're likely to experience a number of minor problems. For more information, see Chapter 2.

Indigestion is one of the most common discomforts of late pregnancy. While hormones relax the sphincter between your stomach and oesophagus, your growing baby puts pressure on your abdomen, causing a reflux of wind and gastric juices into your oesophagus. You can help to ease this by avoiding large meals, not eating close to bedtime, and sleeping with extra pillows to prevent acid from rising up. Antacids containing calcium carbonate aren't generally effective as they cause an increase in stomach acidity.

Abdominal stretching can cause an uncomfortable burning sensation over your taut tummy. Sometimes called hot spots, these are quite common and are superficial pains – if the pains are deeper within your abdomen you must inform your healthcare provider. Hot spots can be irritated by tight or heavy clothing, so avoid tights and stick to loose clothing, and apply an ice pack to relieve the

WHAT POSITION IS YOUR BABY IN?

HEAD DOWN

This is the best position for birth, and more than 95 per cent of babies naturally adopt it before labour. If your baby's back is facing your abdomen, this is called occiput anterior; if her back is turned towards your spine, this is called occiput posterior. This position can cause severe backache during labour.

BREECH PRESENTATION

As many as 4 per cent of babies settle bottom or feet first. This is known as a breech presentation. There are small, but significant, risks to the vaginal birth of a breech baby, especially for first babies, and some doctors will only deliver breech babies by Caesarean. However, you can carry out exercises to move the baby into a head-down position (see opposite).

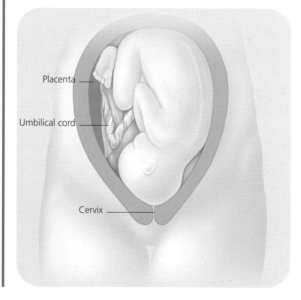

Placenta

Umbilical cord

Cervix

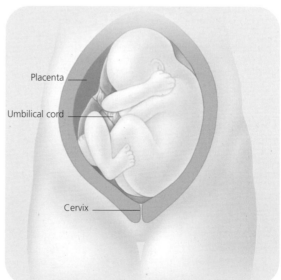

Placenta

Umbilical cord

Cervix

burning. Worn occasionally, an abdominal support designed for pregnancy is helpful for backache, especially for women whose abdominal muscles have been stretched by frequent or closely spaced pregnancies. For an exercise to strengthen abdominal muscles, see page 123.

Helping a breech baby to turn

When the baby is still relatively small, before about 32 weeks, she has room to change positions frequently. After this most babies settle into their preferred position (see below), and it's important to know what this is, since this can profoundly affect the birth. Your healthcare provider can tell the position of your baby by palpating (gently pressing)

TRANSVERSE LIE

Less than 1 per cent of babies are positioned across the uterus. This is known as a transverse or oblique lie, and it makes a normal vaginal birth impossible. It is sometimes possible to change these positions using the breech tilt after 32 weeks and external version after 37 weeks.

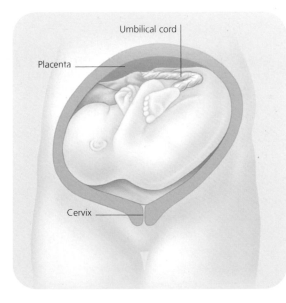

Umbilical cord

Placenta

Cervix

your abdomen. If your baby is in a breech position or a transverse lie, it may be possible to help her to assume the head-down position with the following.

Breech tilt

Lie on your back with your knees flexed and place four plump pillows or cushions under your buttocks so that your pelvis is higher than your stomach. Alternatively, kneel down on the floor with your buttocks raised as high as possible while your head rests on your folded arms. Remain in this position for a minimum of 10 minutes twice a day. Because your pelvis is higher than your stomach it will allow your baby's head to float, which will encourage her to turn so that her head moves up into the pelvis.

Visualisation

On an empty stomach, concentrate on relaxing your abdomen while visualising your baby turning. Repeat for 10 minutes twice a day. This technique was developed by Dr. Juliet DeSa Souza, who found it to be successful in turning 89 per cent of breech presentations, usually within two to three weeks.

External version

If a breech baby fails to turn before you are 37 weeks into your pregnancy, some obstetricians will perform an external version – manipulating the mother's abdomen so that the baby slowly turns. This procedure is not without risks, which your obstetrician should discuss with you. An external version is carried out ideally at 37 to 38 weeks, when there's enough amniotic fluid to allow for a small amount of movement. Success rates vary from 50 to 70 per cent.

Position of the the baby's head

Another aspect of positioning that affects the birth involves how your baby's head rotates as it descends through your pelvis. Since the top opening of a woman's pelvis is oval, with the long axis from side to side, babies enter the pelvis facing sideways. But the lower opening of the pelvis is oval with its long axis from front to back, with the largest part at the front. This means that the head must turn during its

BAG FOR LABOUR

- About 3 changes of loose and comfortable clothes.
- Change for telephone calls, parking and snacks.
- Mobile phone.
- Phone numbers for when labour begins: birth partner, doula, doctor/midwife, relatives.
- Phone numbers for after the birth: friends, relatives, maternity nurse, nappy service.
- Camera or video equipment.
- Magazines, books, MP3 player and other distractions.
- Snacks for you and your birth partner.
- Watch with a second hand for timing contractions.
- Lotion for massage.
- Cold and warm packs for back relief.
- Slippers and heavy socks for cold feet.
- Toothbrush, toothpaste and mouthwash.
- Hairbrush, clips and bands.
- Pillow.
- Dressing gown.

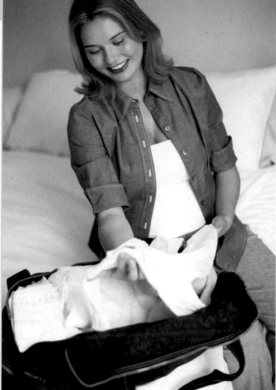

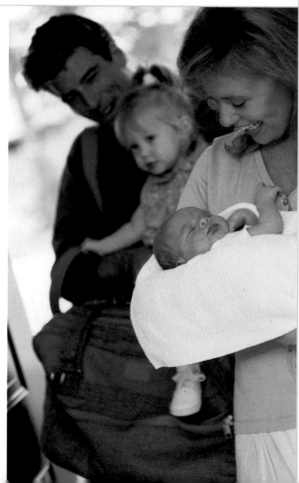

BAG FOR AFTER THE BIRTH

- Dressing gown, 2 nightgowns (front opening, if breastfeeding) and underwear (at least 2 bras (maternity or breastfeeding) and 6 pairs knickers).
- Maternity sanitary pads (about 24).
- Breastfeeding pads and purified lanolin for nipples.
- Changing bag and nappies for your baby.
- Baby clothes.
- Toiletries.
- Birth announcement cards, address list and a pen.
- Baby book for footprints and signatures.
- Extra camera batteries and memory card.

BAG FOR GOING HOME

- Loose outfit, including comfortable shoes.
- Bag for carrying home gifts and hospital supplies.
- Infant car seat.
- Going home outfit for your baby: vest, nightgown, and socks or all-in-one suit; shawl and hat (warmer hat and shawl if cold).
- Nappies and baby wipes.

descent so that the baby faces the mother's tailbone, known as the occiput anterior (OA) position. Unfortunately, 20 per cent of babies rotate into an occiput posterior (OP) position, facing forwards. This may lead to prolonged labour (see page 250).

Monitoring your baby's well-being

Once you can feel your baby's movements – from around 20 to 22 weeks – it's good to pay attention to her levels of activity. Your baby is capable of making many different movements including jumping, kicking and hiccoughing, which will lessen over time as space in the uterus becomes more constricted. While there isn't a set number of kicks you should feel, you should try and become familiar with your baby's pattern of movements during waking hours. Every baby has a different pattern of waking and sleeping, but you'll come to know what is normal for your baby. As your pregnancy progresses, it becomes easier to learn this rhythm.

You probably won't be advised to keep a written record or chart of your baby's movements, as used to happen, as today, practitioners don't believe such charts are helpful for telling whether or not a baby has a problem. It's easy to forget to fill them in and if they are inaccurate, you can become unnecessarily concerned.

What is important, however, is if you notice a change in your baby's pattern, to always tell your midwife or doctor straight away. You should always report a significant decrease in your baby's movement immediately, whether you are keeping a kick chart or not. After 30 weeks of pregnancy, if you think your baby's movements are lessening, lie on your left side and focus on the movements for two hours. If you don't feel 10 or more movements, contact your doctor or maternity unit immediately.

A decrease in your baby's movements could be a sign that he's not getting enough nutrients or oxygen through the placenta. If this is suspected, you're likely to be referred to a maternal or fetal assessment unit in hospital. If tests show that your baby is not growing well in the uterus, your healthcare provider may recommend early delivery by induction of labour or caesarean section.

Getting ready to go

As the excitement builds up towards the delivery date, you need to make sure that everything is at hand when you need it. At least four weeks ahead of time, you need to pack your bags, leaving room for last-minute items, and make final preparations for your trip to the hospital. If you're having a home birth, special preparations must also be made, so check with your healthcare provider.

Travel plans

Decide how you want to get to the hospital; are you confident about your transport arrangements? It's a good idea to have a backup plan. If you ask a friend or neighbour to take you, make sure to keep the number of a reliable cab service handy in case he or she is suddenly unavailable. Or, your maternity unit may be able to arrange an ambulance to pick you up if you call them.

Map out the easiest route and try it out; you may find that you need a different one during rush hours. It may also be necessary to find a cheap car park. Find out which entrance of the hospital you need and where to go when you get there.

If you already have children, you'll need to book a babysitter to stay at your home or collect your children straight away. Once again make sure that you have a couple of backups available.

> **HEALTH FIRST**
> *CHANGE IN BABY'S MOVEMENTS* If your baby doesn't start to move in response to noise or some other stimulus (a cold drink) or there's a big decrease in your baby's movements, or a gradual one over several days, contact your midwife or doctor right away.

Going overdue

A pregnancy that extends over the due date is considered 'post term'. However, this may enable crucial extra resting time before the birth. Only 5 per cent of women deliver on their due date, with the majority giving birth a little late.

The main reason for due dates rarely being accurate is because the due date is an estimated time around 40 weeks from the start of your last period. Your baby is expected to be born within two weeks either side of the due date, so a pregnancy is only considered officially overdue after 42 weeks.

It's also common for a baby to be overdue if it's a mother's first pregnancy, which is prolonged, on average, eight days past the due date. The average second baby is born three days late. Poor positioning of the baby's head can also delay the baby's descent.

Many women prefer to avoid the concern of friends and family by giving a general time span for when the baby is to be born, such as the middle of June. It also helps you to prepare for continuing beyond your due date. If your pregnancy approaches 41 weeks, your healthcare provider will discuss a membrane sweep and at 12–14 days post term, will arrange induction to start labour (see page 186).

Monitoring your overdue baby

A small number of pregnancies outlive the placenta's ability to nourish the baby. Since this can cause problems for the baby, your midwife may suggest special precautions after 40 weeks to ensure that your baby is doing well:

- *Kick-count sheets* You may be asked to keep track of baby's movements and to call your midwife or go to the hospital if your baby seems less active than normal.
- *Fetal heart rate monitoring* This is usually carried out by your midwife at the clinic or in the hospital delivery suite.
- *A biophysical profile* This is an ultrasound that measures your baby's heart rate and breathing movements, and the amount of amniotic fluid.

6 natural ways to encourage labour

1 Exercises for positioning of the baby (see page 205) can help to avoid a prolonged pregnancy.

2 Sexual intercourse can help to prepare your cervix for labour. Semen is rich in prostaglandins, hormones that are known to soften the cervix. Orgasm also stimulates uterine contractions.

3 Nipple stimulation causes secretion of the hormone oxytocin, which stimulates your uterus to contract. Occasionally, nipple stimulation can cause strong, lengthy contractions and may result in decreased blood flow to the baby. This technique should be used under the supervision of a trained professional.

4 Emotional readiness is a component of labour that is rarely discussed. Women who are emotionally unprepared may subconsciously forestall birth. If you have any concerns about the effect your new baby will have on your life, discuss them with your partner or healthcare provider.

5 Certain herbs and homeopathic remedies may stimulate uterine activity. There haven't been any scientific studies to determine how safe or effective these herbs are, so don't take anything without professional advice.

6 Sweeping the membranes involves introducing a gloved finger into the cervix and teasing the membranes away from the edge of the cervix. In some, but not all, studies this procedure has been shown to reduce late births. This should only be done by your healthcare provider.

Your labour and birth experience

Very soon now, you will go through the process of labour, culminating in the birth of your baby. It's an awesome prospect, but finding out as much as you can about what happens during labour and birth is invaluable. It will make you feel more in control, a lot more confident, and more able to enjoy this special event.

Recognising labour

Before real labour can begin, your body has to undergo certain changes. For most women, these pre-labour preparations take place some time during the three weeks before or two weeks after their 'due dates' – only 5 per cent of women actually deliver on their due dates.

Your emotions can veer wildly before labour. You may feel thrilled by the anticipation of your baby's arrival one minute, and totally unprepared for labour, birth and motherhood the next. All these feelings are entirely natural. It's common also to feel a little down during these last weeks of pregnancy – your baby may seem to have taken over your life and your body completely. If you feel like this, try to keep your emotions positive by treating yourself to a baby-shopping spree or lunch with a friend.

Signs that labour is approaching
In the days or weeks before your baby's birth you may have a number of symptoms of your body's preparation for labour. If you are a first-time mum,

these physical changes can begin weeks before true labour. With subsequent babies, these changes are more likely to happen closer to the birth.

Engagement
As the lower part of your uterus softens and expands, your baby's head descends lower into your pelvis. This is known as engagement or 'dropping', and when it happens you'll find that you have more space to breathe. Any heartburn symptoms you've had may be eased, and you won't feel uncomfortably full after a meal. Engagement usually occurs between two and four weeks before labour starts if it's your first baby; with subsequent pregnancies it often occurs as labour is about to begin.

Pelvic pressure
Once your baby's head is settled in your pelvis, you may experience some minor discomforts. You'll probably need to pass water and have bowel movements more frequently because of the pressure that your baby is placing on your bladder and

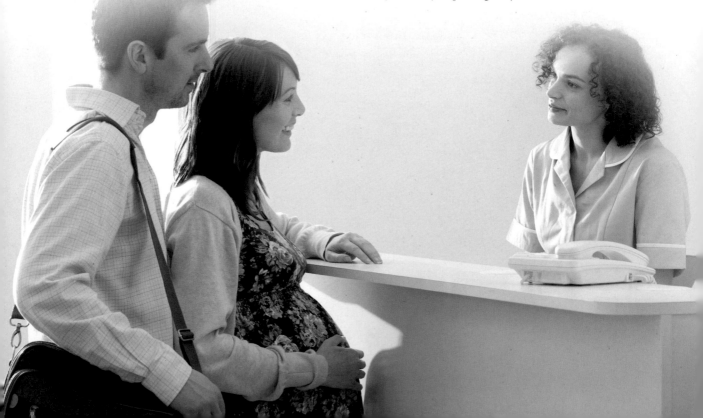

HOW THE HEAD ENGAGES

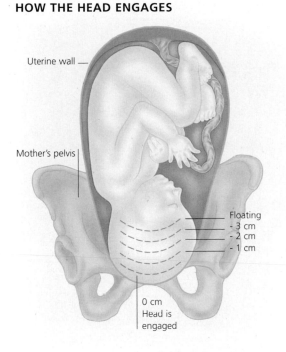

Uterine wall

Mother's pelvis

Floating
- 3 cm
- 2 cm
- 1 cm

0 cm
Head is
engaged

bowels. The relaxation of your joints and ligaments may make your pubic bones and back ache, and you may experience sharp twinges as your baby presses down on your pelvic floor. Compression of pelvic blood vessels can cause your legs and feet to swell. Pelvic rocks (see page 203) and lying on your left side can help to relieve some of this pelvic pressure.

Vaginal discharge
Many women experience increased vaginal secretions as the cervix softens. This discharge is usually like egg white, but it can be tinged pink. A yellow or frothy discharge may signal an infection, so you should report it to your healthcare provider.

Nesting instinct
If in the last month you find yourself seized with a sudden desire to empty drawers, clear out closets, and scrub the house from top to bottom, you're simply experiencing what's known as the 'nesting instinct', an inbuilt maternal urge to prepare the home for the imminent arrival of the baby. While you may want to make the most of this burst of energy, take care not to overdo it. You need to conserve your strength for labour.

Braxton Hicks contractions
Named after the doctor who first identified them, Braxton Hicks aren't true contractions, but 'practice' ones, designed to stretch the lower part of your uterus – enabling your baby's head to settle into your pelvis – and to soften and thin the cervix. In the run-up to labour, these practice contractions can intensify, giving you a tightening or 'balling up' sensation in your abdomen. Lying down usually helps to ease any discomfort.

Shivering or trembling
You may find yourself shivering or trembling for no apparent reason when labour or pre-labour symptoms arrive – often without any sensation of cold or weakness. This can be a result of stress hormones or an alteration in progesterone levels.

Diarrhoea
Prostaglandins, which are the body chemicals released in the process of early labour, may trigger episodes of loose bowel movements.

Signs that labour is imminent
The exact cause of the onset of labour remains unknown. The most widely held theory is that your baby will produce substances that result in a change in pregnancy hormones. Alternatively, you may develop an increasing sensitivity towards the end of pregnancy to substances in the body that produce uterine contractions. So how do you know you're in labour if there's no clearly defined start to it? This is the question that every pregnant woman worries about, but you can rest assured that when the time comes, you will know.

Although the only true sign that labour has started is the onset of regular contractions, which cause your cervix to dilate, there are other signs that labour is imminent.

Mucus plug and bloodstained show

As the cervix softens, shortens and begins to dilate, the mucus plug that has sealed the cervix for most of your pregnancy is dislodged. This is called a bloodstained show – or sometimes just a 'show' – and usually appears as a small amount of bright red or brownish mucus. A show may also appear as a heavier discharge or it may simply be unnoticeable. Though a show can be a sign that labour's imminent, it can occur as much as six weeks before the birth. However, if you have a show, you should contact your healthcare provider for advice.

Rupture of membranes

The amniotic sac containing the fluid around your baby usually ruptures – known as the 'waters breaking' – at some point during labour. Occasionally, however, it may rupture before contractions begin in earnest. Most women go into labour within 24 hours of their waters breaking, as the rupture causes the release of prostaglandins, contraction-stimulating substances. Sometimes a woman may have been having contractions before her waters break but has not been aware of them. Once the waters break, contractions can intensify, as the baby's presenting part (the part that will be born first) now presses directly onto the dilating cervix.

If your waters break at home, make a note of the time it broke and its consistency, and notify your healthcare provider. Amniotic fluid is usually clear and odourless, and once the bag of water has ruptured at term, it will go on leaking until delivery.

TRUE OR FALSE LABOUR?
Contractions are the one sure way to tell if you're in labour or not.
Use this chart to find out if your contractions are the real thing.

TRUE LABOUR	FALSE LABOUR
Contractions have a regular pattern – coming every 5 minutes.	Contractions are irregular – coming every 3 minutes, and then every 5 to 10 minutes.
Contractions become progressively stronger.	Contractions don't intensify with time.
Contractions don't abate when walking or resting.	Contractions may recede with changes in activity or position.
Contractions may be accompanied by a show.	Contractions usually not accompanied by increased mucus or bloodstained show.
Progressive cervical dilatation.	No significant cervical change is detectable.

If you're preterm, or if your baby was felt to be un-engaged or high in the pelvis at your last examination, your healthcare provider may recommend that you go into the hospital to be assessed before contractions start.

Once your waters break it's important not to put anything into your vagina as there is a possible risk of infection. Showers are preferable to baths until active labour has begun and your baby has been assessed by your healthcare provider.

If you're aware of something pulsing in the vagina after your waters break, this may be a prolapsed cord, so call your healthcare provider immediately and go to the hospital right away.

Regular contractions

Identifiers of true labour are that the cervix steadily dilates (opens out) and there are regular contractions. Early contractions are sometimes called 'false' labour, because they occur only intermittently as they prepare the uterus for true, progressive labour. These early contractions stretch the lower uterus to accommodate the baby as she moves down into it. They also soften the cervix, but do not result in cervical change as regular contractions do. Labour aids or narcotic analgesia may help your body to relax and allow the uterus to work more efficiently.

At some point, any brief, irregular contractions are replaced by ones that have a rhythmic pattern and longer length. These contractions are likely to be progressively contracting the upper uterus while stretching the lower part and opening the cervix. By this mechanism, the powerful upper uterus muscles push the baby through the stretchable lower uterus.

Sometimes back labour occurs (see page 251). If you experience back pain every 5 minutes, call your healthcare provider and go to the hospital.

When to go to the hospital

The early part of labour can take hours. If you're not in any real discomfort, it's best to stay at home in familiar surroundings where there's plenty to do to distract yourself. If you're in a lot of discomfort, however, you may want to go to the hospital sooner. As a rough guide, aim to go to hospital when

Time your contractions at home. If they've been occurring regularly, 5 minutes apart, for over an hour, it's time to go to hospital.

contractions are so intense that you're unable to hold a conversation during one and if you've been having regular contractions for over an hour – 5 minutes apart, each lasting 45 to 60 seconds. Intense contractions that are less than 3 minutes apart are often a signal that birth is very near. If you've given birth before, bear in mind, that, on average, second babies arrive in half the time that first babies take.

If your waters break in the midst of regular contractions, this may be a signal to go to hospital. If your waters break before regular 5-minute contractions occur, call your healthcare provider for advice. If you aren't sure whether it's false or real labour, don't feel embarrassed about going to the hospital to be assessed or asking your midwife to check you. It can be easy to misinterpret the signs of labour, especially with a first pregnancy, and it's better to err on the side of caution.

What happens when you arrive at the hospital

While admissions procedures for hospitals vary greatly, the same things still have to happen once you're admitted. Generally, most women are asked to go to the maternity ward or delivery suite at once, although at a few hospitals you may be asked to go to the casualty department so you can be taken to your room in a wheelchair. Remember to take your pregnancy records with you. You may then be taken to a labour and delivery suite, or the room where you will give birth, where a midwife will assess your progress by carrying out the following procedures:

- *Vital signs* Your pulse, blood pressure, breathing and temperature will be checked repeatedly throughout labour. You'll also be asked about your contractions, whether your waters have broken, and whether you've recently eaten.
- *Monitoring* Your contractions and your baby's heart rate will be monitored in some way.
- *Internal examination* You'll have an internal examination to see whether your cervix is dilated. If you're in early labour and everything's fine, you may be sent home until you go into active labour.
- *Brief history* You'll be asked what sort of pregnancy you've had and what sort of pain relief you want to have if you make that decision.

You'll probably be given a hospital gown to change into, although some hospitals will allow you to wear your own clothes if you want to.

- *An intravenous line* You may have an intravenous line (IV) inserted if you have had a previous Caesarean or could be at risk of bleeding after the birth. An IV is also needed if you have an epidural later. You may have a blood sample taken for your blood group and an anaemia test.

When you're admitted to the hospital, the midwife may ask if you have a birth plan. You may talk it through when you hand it over.

The stages of labour

Childbirth is divided into three stages. During the first stage or labour, uterine contractions work to fully dilate the cervix. The second stage is the passage of the baby out of the uterus, down the birth canal and delivery into the outside world. The third stage is the delivery of the placenta.

While every woman's experience of childbirth is unique, all women giving birth will go through these three stages. The whole process takes, on average, up to 18 hours for a first baby and up to 12 hours for later babies. Some labours, however, progress more slowly during the first stage and then speed up at the beginning of the second stage. There are a variety of reasons why labour may slow down:

◆ *The baby is in the wrong position* Most babies fit best down the birth canal with their heads flexed and downwards, facing the mother's side when passing through the pelvis, and facing her back when emerging from the pelvis. If your baby isn't in this position already, it can take a while for him to get into it. By changing position yourself and staying upright as much as possible you can help your baby to adopt the best position for birth.

◆ *More moulding and stretching is needed* Your baby's head needs to mould and your pelvic tissues need to stretch as he moves through the birth canal. This moulding and stretching can take time.

◆ *Your contractions are weak* Contractions can be inefficient especially if it is your first baby. Your healthcare provider may help to strengthen your contractions with syntocinon (synthetic oxytocin) injected through an IV line.

The first stage

Labour is often divided into three phases: early or latent labour, active or established labour and transition or hard labour. For many women, these stages are distinct and noticeable. Other women may not notice such clear-cut differences.

Early or latent labour

While usually the longest part of labour, this is generally the easiest. During this time, the cervix continues to efface (thin out) and progressively dilate to 3 or 4 cm. At this stage, you may be aware of contractions, but they're usually manageable, and you may be able to sleep through them.

Contractions are usually short, lasting from 20 to 60 seconds. Initially they may be as far apart as 20 minutes, becoming increasingly stronger and closer over a six- to eight- hour period. This may be the point at which the mucus plug is dislodged or membranes rupture. Unless there's a medical reason for you to go early to the hospital, you'll be much more comfortable staying at home in early labour.

If you first notice the contractions at night, continue resting as much as possible. If you can't

---

MORE **ABOUT**   active management of labour

Many hospitals follow a policy of active management of labour (AMOL) for first-time labours. This means that your labour is expected to proceed within a certain time-frame and your healthcare provider helps it along if it seems to be taking longer. Once labour is diagnosed – with regular painful contractions, dilation (opening up) of the cervix and, sometimes, ruptured membranes – women are expected to deliver within about 12 hours. Frequent vaginal examinations are used to check that your cervix is dilating at a rate of 0.5 to 1 cm per hour. If your labour appears to be slowing down, the membranes will be ruptured artificially (see page 228) and a dose of syntocinon is given. In hospitals that practise AMOL, it has helped to shorten the length of first labours and reduce the Caesarean rate.

---

rest, find a distracting, but not taxing, activity. Don't forget to eat light snacks during this early stage. Women used to be advised not to eat at all in labour in case they needed a general anaesthetic, in which case it was thought that they might breathe in food. But studies have shown that this risk is very small, while eating light solids in labour can actually improve labour outcome – labour is hard work and your body needs energy in order to cope.

Your symptoms in early labour may be similar to those of pre-labour – cramps, backache, increased urination and bowel movements, increased vaginal discharge, pelvic pressure, and leg and hip cramps. Many women also experience a burst of energy, but try to conserve this energy for later on.

Active labour

This stage is reached when the cervix begins to dilate rapidly. For first-time mothers in this stage, the cervix usually dilates at a minimum of 1 cm an hour. Contractions become noticeably more intense, and if a cervical check is performed, you'll probably be 4–6 cm dilated. Contractions now last 45 to 60 seconds, getting progressively stronger and closer together, from occurring about every five to seven minutes to every two to three minutes.

As contractions become stronger and longer, you may need to work harder to relax through and between them. Try moving around and changing your position to relieve muscle tension. The sheer physical effort of labour can lead to increased breathing, heart rate, perspiration and even nausea. It's important to drink plenty of isotonic drinks to guard against dehydration.

As contractions strengthen, you may experience increased aches and tiredness. Your membranes may rupture if they haven't already. You'll probably feel a lot less sociable now as you focus in on yourself.

MORE **ABOUT**	latent labour

If this is your first baby you may get backache and bouts of painful contractions that last for several hours, or even days, before proper labour begins. You may be convinced that your baby is on her way only to find that it all wears off again, or your midwife says your cervix is still closed despite what seems like many hours of painful contractions. This is more common if your baby is lying with her back towards your back, or in the occipito-posterior position. If you can, stay at home during this phase as you will feel more comfortable there. Keep active to take your mind off the discomfort. A warm bath or back massage from your partner may help. Practise any breathing or relaxation techniques you have learnt in your ante-natal classes. Make you sure you keep energy levels up by regular light snacks. Do not get too disheartened; your cervix is softening and your uterus limbering up in preparation for the great event of labour.

Women in this stage sometimes feel that labour is never going to end. Try to remember that this phase is usually rapid and the cervix will be dilated soon, and that every contraction is one nearer your baby. You also may worry about how well things are progressing, so ask your midwife about anything that's bothering you. If you find this difficult for any reason, you may prefer your birth partner to ask on your behalf.

Transitional labour

Lasting between around one and two hours, transition is labour's most difficult and demanding period, during which the cervix fully dilates from 8 to 10 cm. Contractions now become very strong, lasting from 60 to 90 seconds and coming every 2 to 3 minutes. Where you might have made rapid progress though the active phase, everything can seem to slow down during transitional labour. Be assured, however, that the end is in sight.

Because of the intensity of this phase, dramatic physical and emotional changes can accompany it. As your baby is pushed into your pelvis, you'll experience strong pressure in your lower back and/or perineum. You may have the urge to push or move your bowels and your legs may become shaky and weak. Significant stress reactions aren't uncommon, with perspiration, hyperventilation, shivering, nausea, vomiting and exhaustion all possible. Without meaning to, women can reject the help of their birth partners and find every touch or labour aid unacceptable during this phase.

Many women lose all inhibitions, and may verbalize their distress uncharacteristically by shouting and swearing. Keep the goal in sight. The pushing stage will come soon and your discomfort will be much more controllable. Bear in mind that stronger contractions bring the phase to an end faster. Don't be afraid to express yourself – make it clear what helps and what doesn't. Try also to relax; it's the key to conserving strength and the best way to help contractions to accomplish their goal.

Dealing with pain during labour

Labour is just what its name suggests – hard work. It's work that's performed by a very powerful muscular organ. Because the uterine muscle is a smooth muscle like the heart, most of your sensation of its activity comes from the muscles and nerves surrounding the uterus. The neighbouring muscles in the abdomen and pelvis need to relax so that the uterus can accomplish its work efficiently, pushing your baby past these muscles and out of your body. The accompanying sensation can be felt as anything from serious discomfort to extreme pain.

Why pain occurs

Hard work requires adequate oxygen and nutrition to keep the muscles being used pain-free. Muscles forced to work without oxygen or food, or that become tense will produce pain. The experience of pain in the first stage of labour (see page 215) may indicate that your body needs extra oxygen or nourishment or to be relaxed. Just as you would change an activity if you suddenly developed pain

MONITORING YOUR BABY

Being squeezed through the birth canal is a stressful, although natural, experience for your baby, so your healthcare provider may want to monitor his well-being. The least invasive way of doing this is to check his heartbeat with a Doppler, a hand-held ultrasound device. Tests should be carried out at regular intervals of 15 to 30 minutes during labour and then every 5 minutes during delivery.

Alternatively, you may be fitted with an external fetal monitor that has two devices – one detects your baby's heartbeat, the other measures your contractions – used intermittently, so that you can move around during labour.

If your baby appears to be in distress, his progress may need to be monitored internally. After the membranes have ruptured, a small electrode is passed through your vagina and attached to your baby's head to monitor his fetal heart rate.

If your healthcare providers feel that they need more information, they may carry out a fetal blood sample. A small tube inserted through your vagina collects a few drops of blood from your baby's scalp. This is tested for acidity levels, which indicate if your baby is getting enough oxygen. Another way of checking this, is by simulating your baby's scalp. An increase in the fetal heart rate in response to scalp stimulation is a reassuring sign. These results help your healthcare providers to decide on the next course of action.

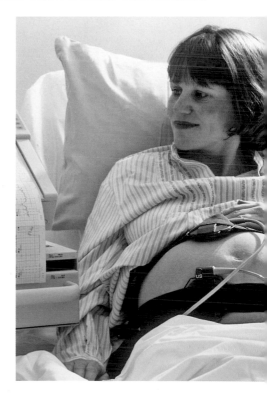

while exercising, so labour pain may be a signal to change breathing patterns, to relax muscles, or increase nourishment to help the uterus to work. In the later stages, the pain will be due to the pressure of the baby's head and body directly on your cervix but since this stage is shorter, you may find that natural endorphins and the knowledge your baby will be born soon will help to spur you on and to enable you to bear the discomfort without medications.

Medical pain control

There are a variety of ways to cope with uncomfortable sensations in labour but it's best not to rely exclusively on medical therapy for coping with contractions. For more details about analgesics, anaesthetics and tranquillisers, see Chapter 10.

It's always best to discuss your options with your doctor before labour so you can be clear about the risks and benefits of each particular treatment. Learning about the general course of labour in advance can also help you to understand the particular status of your own labour if you are considering medical therapy. Some medical treatments may be less suitable if you're close to delivery because many medications cross the placenta and can affect your baby's ability to adapt to life on his own.

Managing labour naturally

Over the centuries, women have discovered a variety of techniques and methods that can make labour more comfortable and medical intervention less likely. Some tried and tested techniques are given below. For some ways that your birth partner can help, see page 182.

♦ *Labour positions* Try out different postures to see which is the most comfortable or helps relieve backache. Changing positions can also help to guide the baby through the curvature of your

In labour, as in most situations, if you experience strong sensations without understanding them, they can lead to fear, stress and pain. Understanding what your body is up to and realizing that these sensations are totally normal can help you to interpret your contractions as 'work' and not 'pain'.

Another way your mind can help the work of your body is by focusing on a goal – in this case the arrival of your baby. You also may find that distracting yourself can help you to cope with a distressing body sensation. There are all sorts of mental distraction techniques you can employ, from breathing, massage, meditation, or imaging, to hypnosis.

While trying mental strategies to cope with potential body discomforts, don't ignore your body entirely. For instance, you may feel discomfort if your baby is descending in the wrong position, and if you change position you may help to shift him. Or your bladder may be full, and relieving it may help your baby's descent. Nausea or weakness may be an indication of low blood sugar or dehydration. Realize that labour is an amazing time and process, but one for which your body is very well equipped. Work with your body and keep things in an appropriate, positive perspective.

lower abdomen and pelvis. Suitable positions include leaning against a wall or your birth partner; sitting on a chair the wrong way round, so you're facing the chair back; kneeling forward on a pile of cushions; going on all-fours or using a birthing ball. There may be times when you find it comfortable to lie down, if so, support your body with plenty of cushions, placed under your head, beneath your bump, and underneath and between your thighs (see page 71).

♦ *Breathing* A good supply of oxygen is essential in any endeavour, and childbirth is no exception. Muscles deprived of oxygen produce lactic acid, and accumulation of this acid causes pain. Not enough oxygen going to the uterus and the placenta also can lead to distress for your baby. Breathing correctly, therefore, is an important component of successful labour.

Breathing exercises – also called patterned breathing – are often taught in childbirth classes as a tool to help to distract parents from other sensations of labour and to ensure that mother and baby get an adequate oxygen intake.

Patterned breathing doesn't work for everyone and can be confusing if you haven't practised it beforehand. If you'd like to find out more about it and how it works, ask at your childbirth class.

In early labour, slow breathing helps to promote and maintain relaxation. Taking deep, relaxing breaths at the beginning and end of contractions enhances the delivery of oxygen. When you breathe, try not to panic and hyperventilate (breathe too quickly), and don't hold your breath for prolonged periods.

In late labour, if the descent of your baby triggers the urge to push before your cervix is fully dilated, your healthcare provider may recommend panting or deep blowing, as if you're trying to keep a feather floating. This type of breathing also is helpful if you need to slow down pushing at the time of actual delivery of your baby's head. Breathing out stops your lungs from expanding and pushing down on your uterus at a time when pushing isn't appropriate.

Walking can be helpful all through labour. It's a useful distraction and keeps gravity working with labour to push your baby through your pelvis.

◆ *Massage* Kneading or stroking muscles can help to release muscle tension and promote relaxation. Relaxation, in turn, can increase blood circulation to muscles, helping to ensure that they have adequate oxygen. Between contractions, massage can provide a pleasant tactile sensation to help to lift your spirits, while during contractions massage can help to take your mind off the pain.

If you're suffering from lower back pain, you may like to ask your birth partner to gently rub the area, particularly around the sacrum (where your spine joins your pelvis). He or she should make a series of large circles using the heel of his or her hands followed by smaller circles made with the thumbs.

◆ *Relaxation techniques* Relaxation counters your body's automatic reaction to the stress response. This is an innate 'fight or flight' response, which has protected human life since time began. However, the stress response is not at all helpful in labour, because it causes the muscles to tense in preparation for action, expending energy at a high rate; and it diverts the body's blood supply to vital body organs – the heart and brain – and away from the uterus.

The mental effort required to slow down breathing and relax muscles can also serve as a distraction from painful contractions. Relaxed muscles make it much easier for your uterus to do its work so that they are also more likely to stretch as your baby passes through your pelvis.

It's important to learn relaxation techniques before the birth. Understanding what happens during labour can help you to relax, too. If you know that the powerful sensations you're experiencing are normal, this can help your mind to relax and your body to release tension.

◆ *Water* Immersion in water can provide substantial pain relief during labour and even help to progress it (see page 181). Most hospitals that use water for pain relief during labour keep it at body temperature or less – higher temperatures have been associated with fetal distress. Sometimes even a brief spell in water can advance labour so rapidly that you give birth

BIRTH POSITIONS

When it comes to giving birth, an upright position is best, as it enlists the aid of gravity to help to push your baby out. You may want to stick to one position or try a few out; do whatever makes you feel most comfortable. There's a variety of positions in which you can give birth, and you may want to assume one or more of these during labour to ease pain or help the baby's progress.

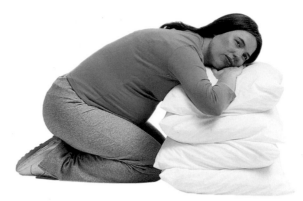

KNEE-CHEST POSITION If you have a large baby, this can help to relieve backache and rotate a backward-facing baby. It may be useful to slow down the baby's descent if he is coming too fast. Go down on your knees and rest your arms on a pile of pillows or a beanbag. If you have backache, try rocking your hips from side to side.

SQUATTING The most commonly adopted position, squatting encourages your baby to descend rapidly and may widen your pelvis by as much as 2 cm. You don't have to put as much effort into bearing down, but it can be a tiring position to hold for any length of time. Having your birth partner support you from behind or using a birthing stool can help.

LYING ON YOUR BACK Lying on your back is the position traditionally preferred by obstetricians, as it permits ease of intervention. It may also be the safest position for a highly anaesthetized mother. However, it doesn't make use of gravity, and pressure from the baby on your back may increase the risk of backache and perineal injury.

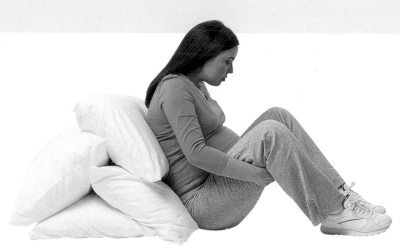

SITTING This is a good position if you're tiring, and one that can be used with continuous electronic monitoring, if your baby requires it. Sit as upright as possible with pillows supporting your back and keep your legs apart.

This position is frequently used in settings with birthing beds. It can also work well if an epidural has been used.

LYING ON YOUR SIDE If you have had an epidural, or if you're tiring, this is a good position because it can make contractions more effective and slow down the baby's descent if he's coming too quickly.

Lie on your side on the floor, resting on a beanbag or some pillows. If your upper leg gets tired, you can ask your birth partner to support it.

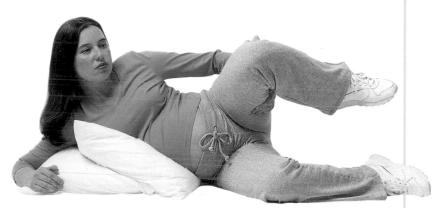

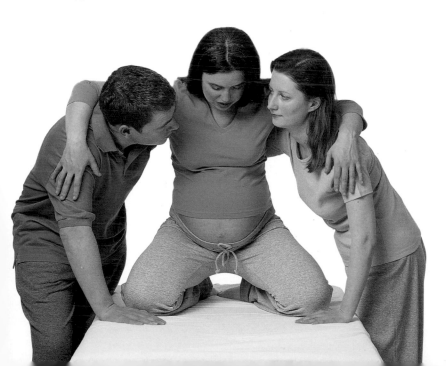

KNEELING WITH SUPPORT If your baby's in an occiput posterior position (facing backwards) this can help him to rotate. Kneel on the bed between your birth partner and healthcare provider. Put your arms round their shoulders for support as you bear down.

while you're in the water. Delivery under water doesn't appear to be a problem. Most doctors recommend bringing your baby above water immediately after birth for his first breath, as the placenta may begin to separate within seconds of delivery, and your baby will need oxygen quickly. Infants are born with an intact 'diving reflex,' which allows them to hold their breaths while submerged – they won't take their first breaths until they hit the colder air above the surface.

The second stage

Once you are through the transition period the time has come to push your baby out. The second stage usually takes an hour, but can take as little as ten minutes or as much as three hours. As with early labour, the second stage may be significantly lengthened if anaesthesia has been given.

Even after a long, exhausting labour, many women find a renewed burst of energy in the second stage, as they've achieved full dilation of the cervix and know that birth is imminent. Now you can take a much more active and mentally distracting role, which can make you feel a lot more positive.

The second stage can have another significant plus: bearing down with contractions can make discomfort seem to disappear. As long as the second stage isn't too fast and allows the perineum to stretch gradually, it can be a time of pressure, not pain. Often the extreme pressure of the baby's tight fit and the subsequent compression of nerves leads to a form of anaesthesia itself. For many women, this

THE MOMENT OF BIRTH

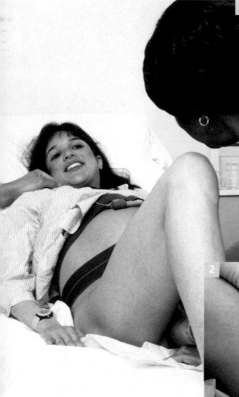

You have reached the second stage of labour and the birth is imminent.

YOUR BABY'S HEAD PRESSES AGAINST THE PELVIC FLOOR
Your caregiver can feel the head moving **1** with each contraction.

YOUR BABY'S HEAD 'CROWNS'
The widest part can be seen at the vaginal opening **2**. You will be asked to relax and pant rather than push while the head is delivered.

THE HEAD IS BORN Within one or two contractions, your baby's head will fully emerge. Your healthcare provider gently supports your baby's head while his body is delivered **3**.

THE BODY EMERGES In one or two more contractions, the rest of

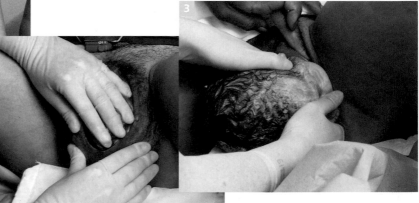

nerve compression blocks the sensation of perineal tears, surgical incisions, and repairs.

Contractions in the second stage still last for 60 to 90 seconds but may come every 2 to 4 minutes. Your position can influence their pattern – staying upright can intensify contractions; reclining and knee-chest positions may slow them down.

You'll have an overwhelming urge to push, but it's important to wait until your healthcare provider says that it's okay. You'll feel huge pressure on your rectum, and a tingling, burning feeling as your baby's head appears at the entrance to your vagina. Your emotions may veer now from exhaustion and tearfulness to excitement at the thought of meeting your baby at last.

Time to push

If you've been given the go-ahead to push, bearing down when the urge occurs will bring satisfying relief from pent-up sensations. Many women's bodies tell them before their healthcare providers do that their cervix has fully dilated and it's time to push. As your baby presses on your pelvic-floor muscles, receptors trigger an urge to bear down. The urge to push is often mistaken for the need to have a bowel movement, because the pressure of the baby on your rectum stimulates the same receptors as a bowel movement.

Usually the urge to push occurs two to four times within the course of a contraction, or you may feel one long, continuous urge. Take a deep breath, relax your pelvic muscles, and bear down with your

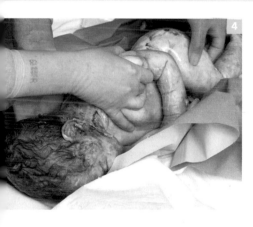

the body appears. He may be covered with vernix and have streaks of blood on his skin **4**.

YOUR BABY IS HANDED TO YOU
Once your baby has been checked, the cord is cut and he will be wrapped and given to you **5**. Lay him on your stomach so that he can be comforted by your familiar heartbeat and breathing rhythms.

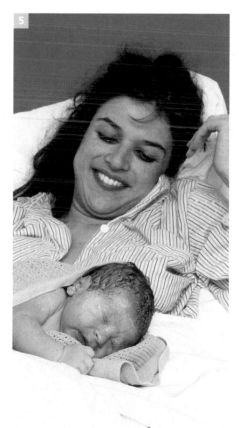

CUTTING THE CORD
Your healthcare provider may clamp and cut the cord immediately, or he or she may wait until the cord stops pulsating. Sometimes your healthcare provider may then pull gently on the cord to help you to deliver the placenta by pushing during a contraction.

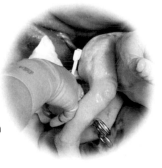

abdominal muscles. The length of the push isn't as important as timing with the contraction. Shorter pushes – for about 5 to 6 seconds – are usually fine and allow more oxygen to enter your bloodstream.

Sometimes the front lip of the cervix may not have fully dilated when the urge to push first appears. This may occur because the baby has descended too rapidly or is positioned awkwardly. Pushing against an undilated cervix can cause swelling and hinder progress. To reduce a cervical or anterior lip, as it's called, try lying on your left side, or going on all fours for a few contractions. Sometimes 'blowing' breathing can help you to avoid pushing against the lip: this is breathing as if you're blowing out a candle, and it prevents you from holding your breath, which would result in downward cervical pressure. Moving to a knee-chest position can reduce the pressure on the cervix and pelvic muscles, decreasing the urge to push.

The baby's coming

The first sign that your baby's about to be born is the distension (stretching) of your anus and perineum. With each contraction, your baby's head becomes increasingly visible at the vaginal opening. Once it has stopped slipping back, it remains at the opening, and this is called crowning.

In just a brief period of time, the perineum thins from approximately 5 cm thick to less than 1 cm.

This is totally natural, and the distension reverses within minutes after the birth. You may feel this distension as strong pressure, possibly with some mild stinging as your baby's head – or buttocks if he's breech – stretches the vaginal opening. This is the point when you may be offered an episiotomy if it looks like you're going to tear badly.

As your baby is born, slow, controlled pushing is best, as it allows the perineum to stretch gradually, helping to prevent tears. Your healthcare provider may even tell you not to push so your uterus can achieve the final expulsion with less force.

Cutting the cord

After your baby is born, his umbilical cord usually will be clamped in two places and cut in between. It's not vital to clamp and cut the cord immediately; in fact, recent evidence suggests that waiting a little before clamping the cord boosts a newborn's blood volume by a third, thus reducing the risk of anemia in a young baby, which could affect his or her brain development.

The third stage

The third stage of labour sees the complete removal of the pregnancy with the delivery of the placenta. For most deliveries, this is relatively automatic and requires little effort. As soon as your baby leaves your uterus, the uterus continues to contract, causing a massive decrease in volume, which usually shears the less flexible placenta from its walls. Further contractions push the placenta out.

Most units recommend active management of the third stage of labour to prevent heavy bleeding after delivery. Immediately after the baby is born, an injection of syntocinon or syntometrine is given into your upper leg, which encourages the uterus to stay contracted. This allows the birth attendant to help the placenta to be expelled by gently pulling on the cord. If you're lying down, he or she may massage your uterus or ask you to bear down and push.

Early breastfeeding helps to prevent problems with bleeding from the site of the placenta, as nipple stimulation releases oxytocin, the hormone that promotes uterine contractions. If you have increased bleeding, your doctor may give you syntocinon (synthetic oxytocin), via an IV, to help the uterus to contract and decrease postnatal bleeding. Once the placenta is out, it will be examined to check that fragments haven't broken off inside the uterus. Very occasionally retained placenta occurs, when the placenta remains behind in the uterus. To remove it, an obstetrician needs to feel inside the uterus and manually remove it. This usually takes place in the operating room under epidural for pain relief.

Immediately after birth

Your baby is finally born and you'll feel a range of strong emotions – relief, elation, excitement, even disbelief that you're now a mother. You may feel cold and shivery and you'll certainly be very hungry and thirsty after all that hard work.

Before you leave the birthing room, you'll be stitched if you had an episiotomy or tear. Most women hardly notice this is happening, they're so preoccupied

With nine out of 10 women it's normal that the skin and muscle between the opening to the vagina and anus (called the perineum) tears to some extent during delivery. A careful assessment after birth will be made to grade the type of tear that has occurred.

- *First degree – just skin deep so will heal naturally.*
- *Second degree – deeper tear affecting the muscle so stitches will be needed in the delivery room.*
- *Third degree – the tear has gone further down towards the anus so that the muscle controlling the bowel (called the anal sphincter) is torn.*
- *Fourth degree – the tear has extended into the anus (or rectum) itself.*

Third and fourth degree tears are more likely if this is your first vaginal delivery, your baby is large or you have a long second stage of labour. An episiotomy may help make more space for the baby to come through the vagina but does not necessarily prevent these types of tear, which need to be stitched in the operating theatre by an experienced obstetrician. For the procedure to be done properly, an epidural or spinal anaesthetic will be given and occasionally a general. A catheter will be inserted for a few hours until urine can be passed without its help. Afterwards, you will be prescribed a five-day course of antibiotics to reduce the risk of infection and laxatives to prevent constipation. Painkillers such as paracetamol and ibruprofen will be needed as the area will be sore for a few days. Pelvic floor exercises should be started to encourage healing and strengthening of the tissues.

Many hospitals offer a check-up appointment 6 – 12 weeks after birth for women who have had more extensive tears. This is make sure that the stitches have healed properly and there are no problems with how the bowels are working.

At birth, the placenta weighs about 0.5 kg (1 lb). The fetal side is smooth and covered with blood vessels. The side that was attached to your uterus is dark red and looks like raw liver.

with their babies, but you'll be given a local anaesthetic, if necessary. You'll be freshened up, and offered a fresh gown or your own nightdress. Don't be alarmed to find you start bleeding heavily. This is perfectly normal and the discharge, called lochia, will subside over the next few weeks (see page 320). In the meantime, you will need to wear maternity pads.

After spending time with you, your baby will be taken away briefly for a bath, a paediatric examination, and needed procedures. You may then be transferred to the maternity ward. Your baby will be brought back to you and a cot will be made available next to your bed.

SPECIAL DELIVERIES

BREECH

Breech babies are positioned so that their legs or bottoms are closest to the cervix. This position can make delivery difficult because the baby's head is the largest part of his body and it could get trapped if the body slips through a partly dilated cervix. Vaginal delivery is possible with breech presentation but sometimes breech babies need to be delivered by Caesarean section to avoid trauma to baby or mother.

TWINS AND MORE

The prospect of giving birth to two or more babies can be daunting to say the least. However, many women give birth to twins vaginally without any problems and the birth tends to be faster than with single babies. However, extra care has to be taken with a multiple birth, so an anaesthetist will be standing by in case you need a Caesarean. The first baby may deliver vaginally without any problem, but the second baby may be positioned awkwardly and need assistance. The second baby should arrive 10 to 20 minutes after the first. If progress is slow, you may be given syntocinon to speed up delivery, or your baby may be helped out with forceps. The placenta or placentas may follow soon after, or you may be given an injection to speed up their delivery. If you're expecting triplets or more, you'll most likely have them delivered by Caesarean.

POSTERIOR

A baby who descends into the birth canal with his head down and his back towards his mother's spine – referred to as occiput posterior (OP) – may be harder to deliver. Posterior babies present a slightly larger head diameter for passing through the narrow birth canal and posterior labours may take longer or involve greater back pain. Not infrequently, however, the baby turns in mid-labour or during the stage of pushing. If your baby doesn't turn spontaneously, your healthcare provider may be able to encourage him to rotate by strengthening your contractions with a syntocinon IV.

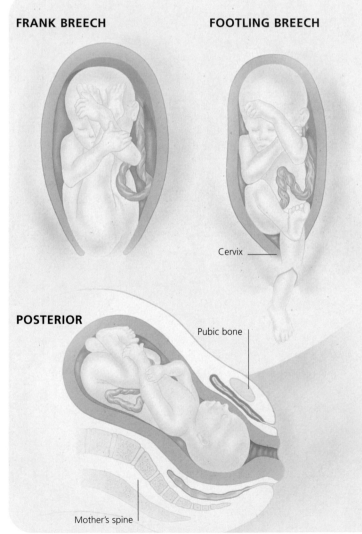

FRANK BREECH

FOOTLING BREECH

Cervix

POSTERIOR

Pubic bone

Mother's spine

Special medical interventions

Not every labour starts or progresses as it should. In these instances, medical intervention may be necessary to assist your baby's birth.

Although your healthcare provider will try to respect your wishes if you have planned for as natural a birth as possible, there may be instances when intervention is medically necessary. It may involve induction, an episiotomy, the use of forceps or vacuum extraction, or a Caesarean section.

Induction of labour

Occasionally your healthcare provider may recommend inducing your labour, usually because of some medical risk to you or your baby (see page 186). The most common reason for performing an induction is if you're overdue. It's felt that beyond one to two weeks past your due-date the placenta may cease to function well, and the baby may be at risk of decreased oxygen and malnutrition.

To get your labour started, there are a number of ways your caregiver will probably go about it. He or she may perform a membrane sweep, offer vaginal prostaglandins or rupture your membranes. If your membranes have already ruptured spontaneously or artificially, you may be given syntocinon through a drip. Often, more than one method is necessary.

Induction can be carried out in an antenatal ward if the risk is low, or in the labour ward where intensive monitoring is available if there is a risk to the mother or baby, e.g. previous Caesarean, small-for-dates baby.

Membrane sweep

This can be offered to women after the time of their due dates. Sweeping membranes can be carried out in your GP's surgery by a trained doctor or midwife. He or she introduces a gloved finger into the cervix to "sweep" or tease the membranes away from the inner edge of the cervix. There is occasional discomfort during the procedure, but no increased risk of infection or bleeding. The aim of the procedure is to bring forward the onset of labour, and it is very effective. It also reduces the likelihood that you will need other methods of induction.

Prostaglandin

Your body naturally produces many different types of prostaglandin, some of which are important in stimulating changes in the cervix and uterine contractions. Before labour, the cervix becomes softer, more compliant, and begins to shorten and open. These changes can be caused either by your

In some hospitals an intravenous (IV) line may be fitted routinely in case you need medication during labour.

body producing prostaglandin, or can be stimulated by synthetic prostaglandin.

The most common way of giving prostaglandin is into your vagina. Your healthcare provider will first ensure your baby is well by monitoring his heart rate for about 30 minutes. A vaginal examination will then be performed to establish your suitability for induction. The length, dilatation, position and softness of your cervix will be checked, and the position of the baby's head.

Synthetic prostaglandin can be administered as vaginal tablets or gels; tablets are preferred to gels. Some women start to have contractions soon after the first dose of prostaglandin, whereas other women appear to have no response for some hours. You'll be examined again either the following morning – some inductions, especially if it's your first baby, start in the evening – or three to six hours after your first dose of prostaglandin. If your cervix has changed sufficiently for your healthcare provider to rupture your membranes, that will be done at this stage. If it's not possible to rupture your membranes, you may be given a further dose of prostaglandin.

Artificial rupture of membranes

One of the most common methods of either inducing labour or speeding it along is to artificially break the bag of membranes surrounding your baby. This is called artificial rupture of membranes (ARM) or amniotomy, and is often carried out during a vaginal examination. It should be no more painful than a routine examination, and is done using a 25-cm (10-inch) long, plastic instrument with an end like a crochet hook. This is inserted through your cervix, gently catches the bag of membranes, and bursts it to let the amniotic fluid out. ARM increases the amount of prostaglandin produced locally, which will speed up labour.

Syntocinon

This is the hormone that's most widely used to induce labour once the cervix has softened and the membranes have ruptured. Syntocinon is a synthetic version of oxytocin (the hormone that initiates contractions), and is usually administered via an intravenous line (IV). The dose will be progressively increased until your contractions show a regular pattern and cervical change is underway. Syntocinon may be continued throughout labour or discontinued when labour is established. It may also be used to get labour started again if it seems to have stalled.

Syntocinon usually requires continuous monitoring, as it may be associated with fetal distress. If you do have an IV and are attached to a fetal monitor, you won't be able to move around and change position as easily.

Coping with induction

Induced labours are almost guaranteed to last longer – at least in the latent phase. Consequently, if you are induced, you should adjust your mental expectations and expect a longer labour. Some inductions take days and can still result in a normal vaginal delivery. Don't get discouraged. Prepare to distract yourself for a longer period of time while waiting for active labour.

Many women also feel that syntocinon-induced contractions are stronger – this can be the case if the contractions are too close together. When the uterine muscle contracts, its blood supply is temporarily squeezed and less oxygen gets to the muscle. Fortunately, syntocinon can usually be discontinued once active labour is in progress.

Natural alternatives to induction

Although health professionals sometimes disagree about the effectiveness of these techniques, there are a number of alternatives to medical therapy for induction. Nipple stimulation, for example, causes the release of oxytocin in the body. Speak to your healthcare provider before you try this yourself.

Other natural induction techniques include sexual activity, herbal remedies, and positioning exercises. For further information, see page 208.

Episiotomy

There are several reasons why an episiotomy (a cut to enlarge the vaginal opening) might be necessary during labour: if the perineum hasn't stretched sufficiently during the pushing stage; the baby's head is too large; it's a breech birth; the baby is in distress; forceps need to be used, and to avoid a serious tear. If your healthcare provider feels that an episiotomy is necessary, you'll be given a local anaesthetic in the perineal area unless you already have been given regional anaesthesia. Once the area is numb, the cut will be made with scissors when the head is crowning and the perineum is stretched taut. There are two types of incision that might be used: the

ALTERNATIVE CUTS

Baby's head	Baby's head
Midline	Mediolateral

midline cut is straight down towards the rectum, while the mediolateral cut is angled a little to the side, away from the rectum. Although the midline cut is easier to repair and causes less blood loss, there is a slight risk that too much pressure may cause it to tear through to the rectum. For this reason, the mediolateral cut is commonest practice.

Forceps and vacuum extraction

If your baby has entered the birth canal at an awkward angle or is in distress, or if you have a medical condition such as heart disease or are too exhausted or over-medicated to push effectively, your doctor may decide that forceps or a vacuum extractor should be used to help the baby out and shorten the second stage. Ten to 15 per cent of vaginal deliveries need forceps or vacuum extraction.

If your doctor is using forceps, you will first be given local anaesthetic or pain medication to numb the area. If you have an epidural in place, this will be 'topped up' so that it is working well. Alternatively a spinal anaesthetic may be suggested. Forceps come apart in two pieces one side at a time will be gently eased into your vagina. The 'blades' fit

around the sides of a baby's head, just as your hands would if you were to place them symmetrically along your baby's cheeks from above. While you push, your healthcare provider will gently help to pull the baby out during contractions.

If a vacuum extractor or ventouse is used, your doctor will attach the rubber or plastic cup to the back of your baby's head over the occiput. The device looks like a large bath plug. Suction is created by a pump, and the healthcare provider gently pulls on the instrument to help the baby along while you push. Although the vacuum extractor involves less risk of trauma to the mother, forceps might be preferred if speed is an issue. Your baby may well have a pronounced swelling on his head for 24 hours afterwards, but this will disappear completely.

Having your baby by Caesarean

If labour is considered a danger to mother or baby or a woman opts for an elective procedure (see page 188), a Caesarean delivery will be pre-planned. At other times, emergencies develop during labour or unexpectedly before labour, so that the baby needs to be delivered by an urgent or emergency Caesarean. With a planned Caesarean section, a date

ASSISTED DELIVERY

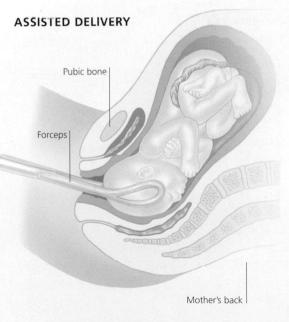

Pubic bone

Forceps

Mother's back

is set, your family can gather, regional anaesthesia can be used, and risks are generally decreased. In the case of an emergency Caesarean, there's often little time for mental preparation and you may need to be put to sleep with general anaesthesia.

What happens during a Caesarean

Prior to an elective procedure, you will be told not to eat or drink for six hours. Some hospitals now allow sips of water up to two hours beforehand. This helps to avoid anaesthetic complications. You may be admitted to the hospital at least two hours before the surgery. Once in hospital, your health and pregnancy history will be taken and an intravenous drip (IV) will be started in your arm, to keep you hydrated and able to receive necessary medications. You will be offered prophylactic antiobiotics before the surgeon makes an incision as this reduces the risk of endometritis, and urinary tract and wound infections (occurring in eight per cent of women).

Depending on your medical condition and the reason for the Caesarean, you'll be given either a general or a regional anaesthetic. A general anaesthetic is an anaesthetic gas mixed with oxygen that is given through a tube in your throat via your mouth. It puts you to sleep and you won't remember anything. Regional anaesthetics block pain from the waist down (see page 179). If you have a regional anaesthetic, you'll be awake and alert and able to see and, perhaps, to hold or touch your baby. It's preferable for you to meet the anaesthetist before your surgery so that you can discuss all the options.

Before surgery, a catheter will be placed in your bladder to drain urine during and for several hours following surgery and a small area of your lower abdomen, where the incision will be made will be shaved. Your surgeon should talk to you about the type of incision before the surgery (see page 232).

Depending on the hospital's policy and if you are awake, one or two support people may accompany you into the operating room. If so, they should: sit or stand by your head to communicate with you; follow the staff's instructions; remain in one spot; and refrain from touching anything.

Your abdomen will be prepared with an antiseptic wash and sterile drapes. An incision will be made with a scalpel through the skin in the lower abdomen. The muscles of the abdomen aren't usually cut but are separated in the midline and pushed aside. The bladder may be pushed down to protect it from instruments. Another incision will be made in the uterus. You may hear a whooshing noise as the amniotic fluid is sucked out.

Once your uterus is open, your baby will be lifted out through the incision. Frequently at this time, the top of the uterus is squeezed – just as you would do when pushing – and you'll feel pressure and a tugging sensation. The baby will be handed to another member of the team, who will give her a physical examination as well as some basic tests, including the Apgar score (see page 287). If you have general anaesthesia or there is some concern about the baby, a paediatrician will be present. You may be able to see your baby immediately or after she has been assessed physically.

After the surgeon has removed the placenta, your uterus and the layers of the abdominal wall will then be sewn closed. These sutures are absorbable and won't need to be removed. Your skin will then be closed with either sutures or staples. Once this is done, you will probably be united with your baby before you leave the surgical suite.

Once surgery is completed, and you and your baby are ready to be moved, you will be taken to a recovery room where you will be observed by trained staff until you are deemed to be in a satisfactory condition. Here, you should be able to hold, bond with, and breastfeed your baby.

You will be offered pain medication during your stay in hospital – an average of three to four days) but you may be allowed home sooner (after 24 hours) and your incision attended to there if you are recovering well and there are no complications. For information about recovery, see page 324.

Having a Caesarean makes you more vulnerable to having a pulmonary embolism or deep vein thrombosis, so tell your doctor immediately if you experience an unexpected cough, shortness of breath or a painful swollen calf. If you are considered to be at higher risk, you will need to have a daily blood thinning injection (Heparin) for five to seven days.

An urgent (emergency) Caesarean

This may be necessary if your baby is at risk of trauma from the birth process because he is premature or in distress. Or, you may develop a serious medical condition, such as pre-eclampsia (see page 253), and require a rapid delivery.

DID YOU KNOW...

YOU CAN HELP TO AVOID AN UNNECESSARY CAESAREAN Research shows that in 2010 over 24 per cent of deliveries in the United Kingdom were by Caesarean. Once you've gone into labour you can help to avoid a Caesarean in several ways: don't arrive at the hospital too early; walk and change position frequently; labour in an upright position; practise relaxation techniques and natural pain relief; try to rest between contractions.

Although the surgical process involved is much the same as for a planned one, the circumstances can make an emergency Caesarean birth more stressful. The staff may seem more rushed, your birth partner may be asked to leave the room, and you may be given general anaesthesia. If the baby is in an awkward position or if it's necessary to work fast, a larger incision may be necessary.

Try to trust in the skill of your doctor and believe that the outcome – the safe delivery of your healthy baby – is more important than the birth process.

Pain relief options for Caesareans

Caesarean deliveries are safest if they can be performed with regional anaesthesia – an epidural or spinal (see page 179). Less medicine is passed to the baby, the mother can be awake to greet her newborn, and family members can also be present. Sometimes, however, general anaesthesia is necessary for the mother's or baby's safety.

Usually, general anaesthesia is a combination of IV medication and anaesthetic gas administration. During the surgical procedure, general anaesthesia can require the use of a respirator to protect the mother from developing serious pneumonia and from aspiration (inhaling food particles and stomach acid into her lungs). General anaesthesia is faster and may be a necessity if it's an emergency Some mothers may require general anaesthesia for certain

UTERINE CAESAREAN INCISIONS

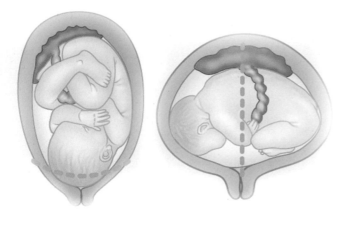

Low transverse incision   Vertical incision

medical conditions such as back problems, which may rule out regional anaesthesia.

Alternative incisions

During a Caesarean, the doctor will make two separate incisions: one through the skin and abdominal wall and the other, beneath this, through the uterine wall. The scar that you see on the outside doesn't necessarily mirror the incision made on the uterus beneath it. There is a very low risk, about 2 per cent, of fetal lacerations.

The skin incision that is most often used is the 'bikini' incision, made across the lower abdomen, just above the pubic hairline. This is preferable because it leaves a small, unnoticeable scar. It is also associated with a shorter operating time and reduced postoperative complications.

Rare circumstances – if you have had previous surgery or currently have large fibroids –

may require a vertical skin incision from the pubic area to the umbilicus (belly button).

The most common uterine incision is the low transverse (side-to-side) incision, which is made across the lower part of the uterus (see left opposite). As this is the segment of the uterus that stretches rather than contracts, incisions made here have less risk of reopening or rupturing in future labours. Many women who have this incision have a successful vaginal delivery with their next pregnancy.

A vertical uterine incision allows more room to avoid birth trauma to mother and baby if the baby's in an awkward position, if it's a multiple pregnancy, or if the lower uterine segment isn't stretched enough to allow delivery through a transverse incision. If you require a vertical incision and it extends into the upper portion of the uterus, you will need to have a Caesarean for future deliveries as there's a higher risk – greater than 2 per cent – of scar separation in future labours.

MORE **ABOUT**   repeat caesareans

There is no scientific evidence to say what the maximum number of Caesarean sections it is safe to have. However, after two, the risk of complications increases.

- *Repeated Caesarean operations tend to result in internal scar tissue, called adhesions, forming. This can make repeated surgery difficult. Part of your bowel or bladder can get stuck to the front of the uterus or under the abdominal wall scar so these organs can get injured during the birth.*

- *The placenta can grow too deeply into the wall of the uterus where it has been opened at a previous Caesarean delivery. This results in a condition called placenta accreta (see page 276).*

- *Placenta previa (where the placenta lies over the cervix) is more likely so the uterus bleeds more heavily at the time of birth.*

Doctors will warn you that the risk of excessive bleeding at delivery increases with the more Caesarean section births you have. Blood transfusion may be necessary although many hospitals use a machine called a Cell Salvage device that can collect the blood you lose and infuse it back to you through an intravenous line. Occasionally blood loss can be so heavy that a hysterectomy is carried out.

Your baby's experience of birth

Birth is not only a lengthy and physically demanding process for you, but it involves considerable changes for your baby as he adapts to life outside the uterus.

Your baby is well prepared for his journey to the outside world. For instance, because the plates of his skull aren't fixed, his skull is able to 'mould' to the shape of the birth canal as he travels through it. Your baby's skull will then recover its normal shape within 24 to 48 hours of delivery. It also appears that the neural connections that would lead a baby to interpret birth sensations as 'pain', may not have developed at the time of labour.

Adapting to life

The pressure on your baby's body as he squeezes through the narrow birth canal is actually helpful in preparing him to live outside the uterus. Pressure on his head causes the release of thyroid and adrenal hormones that help him to regulate his temperature after birth.

The compression of a baby's chest while in the birth canal helps to expel fluid and mucus from his lungs. This pressure also prevents him from breathing and inhaling fluid and blood as he passes through the birth canal. This helps to prepare him to take his first breath upon emerging.

Once outside your body, your baby's chest is able to expand and the pressure on his head is released, both of which promote the instinctive response to hypoxaemia, which is inhalation. This is the impetus to breathe.

Your baby's first breath

To provide his own oxygen supply after the cord is clamped and cut, major changes have to take place in your baby's heart and lungs. While he was in your uterus, his oxygen was supplied from your blood vessels in the placenta and not by his breathing. As his heart had to pump blood along the umbilical cord as well as around his body, the blood was largely diverted from his lungs.

The first time that your baby breathes, it initiates major changes in his body. As his lungs fill with air, the tiny air sacs in the lungs begin to expand. The oxygen causes the blood vessels in the lungs to relax, and this initiates an increase in the flow of blood. The openings in his heart that permitted diversion of blood from his fetal lungs, close shortly after birth. Your baby's umbilical cord stretches and, as this occurs, arteries close down, otherwise your baby would lose blood when the placenta separates.

Your baby's first cry

Although not all babies cry when they are born, the shock of birth usually produces some reaction from a newborn. Your baby may cry for several minutes after delivery, or may give a startled shriek and then settle down. If, however, he is sedated by pain-relief medication you were given, he may not cry until some time after the birth.

DID YOU KNOW...

YOUR BABY INSTINCTIVELY LOOKS FOR YOUR NIPPLE Your baby's ability to find your nipple immediately after birth is remarkable. Research has shown that a baby connects the smell of the fluid on his hands with the smell of his mother's nipples. If placed on his mother's tummy, he makes crawling movements to try to reach the breast. He also may use his touch and sight to try and find the breast. This is why the first hour can be crucial for successful breastfeeding.

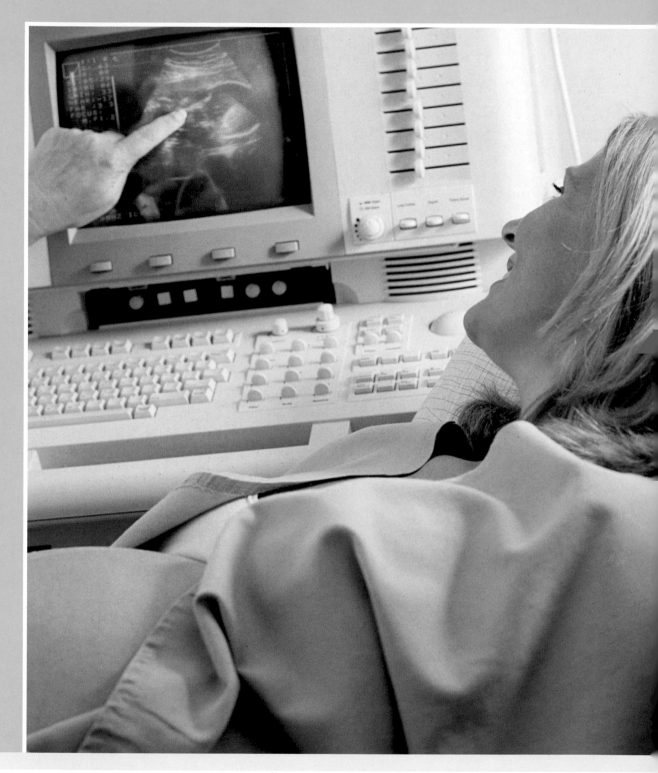

PART III

Antenatal Directory

Antenatal tests

During your pregnancy, your healthcare provider may recommend a variety of tests that are intended to confirm that your baby is developing normally. The decision whether to have these tests or not is yours – you do not have to agree to any procedure you are not comfortable with. Understanding the procedures involved, why the tests have been offered, and what they will tell you about your baby, will enable you to make an informed decision.

Screening tests

These procedures consist of ultrasound or blood samples to check for abnormalities in the baby and/or disease in the mother. These tests do not give a definite 'yes' or 'no' answer and, occasionally, further tests are needed. They can give 'false positives' indicating there is a problem with the baby when everything is in fact fine, or 'false negatives' when a problem is missed. Their attraction for many women is that unlike diagnostic tests they're noninvasive and therefore pose no threat to the baby.

Ultrasound

This technology makes use of sound waves and their echoes to create a picture of the uterus and developing baby. Ultrasound examinations are painfree, and cause no harm in the short or long term to you or your baby.

Ultrasound scans be performed either transvaginally, using a probe that inserts into the vagina, or trans-abdominally, using a transducer that is moved across the mother's abdomen. The technology of scannng is evolving rapidly, and 3D technology is now widely available. 3D means that a life-like picture of your baby can be built up from images taken in each of the three planes of vision of the scanner. These images are covered by computer to a full picture. The term 4D refers to a moving 3D image. These scans take no longer than conventional 2D scans because all the pictures are taken simultaneously.

Doppler ultrasound scanning traces the blood flow between the placenta and your baby through the umbilical cord. Using colour Doppler, the

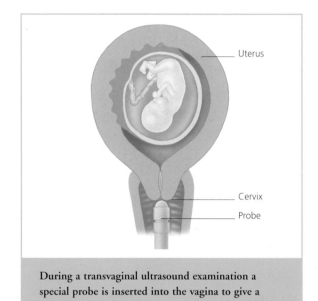

During a transvaginal ultrasound examination a special probe is inserted into the vagina to give a clear picture of the baby.

sonographer can identify the different blood vessels in your baby and take measurements from them (particularly those in the umbilical cord and brain) to check your baby's well-being.

Scans performed before 8 to 10 weeks of pregnancy are usually done vaginally because this gives a clearer picture, being much closer to the baby at this stage of pregnancy. Occasionally, you may need a transvaginal ultrasound later in pregnancy to examine the cervix. Although it's understandable to worry, there is no evidence that the probe can harm you or your baby.

Scans later in pregnancy are usually done transabdominally since the baby is clearly visible in the abdomen by then. Gel is spread over the abdominal skin and the transducer is moved on the gel. The sound waves travel through liquid such as the amniotic fluid but are reflected (bounced back) by more solid structures such as the heart, brain and uterine wall. The quality of the pictures depends on several variables:

- *The quality of the scanning machine;*
- *The training and skills of the person doing the scan;*
- *The length of time for which you are scanned;*
- *The way your baby is lying (sometimes the scanner can't see the heart clearly so you may be asked to go for a walk to alter the baby's position before scanning is resumed);*
- *Whether you are very overweight, or there is a lot of scar tissue.*

In pregnancy, ultrasound scans are used for several types of reasons depending on the stage. Early in pregnancy, a scan can help confirm the dates and make sure the pregnancy is in the uterus, not the tube (ectopic pregnancy) and that the baby is viable (i.e. you have not miscarried). Scans can be used to help in diagnosis of a problem, for example, if you have twins, or as a screening procedure to see whether you have a normal or higher risk of an abnormality such as Down's syndrome or congenital heart disease. Scans also can help show whether the placenta is in the correct place, whether the baby is growing well, and can determine the sex of your baby. Finally, scanning is used to aid other procedures such as amniocentesis and CVS.

Although scanning is a useful aid, it can supply only a certain amount of information and may pick up anomalies that rectify themselves or miss small problems. They must be interpreted along with all the other data available.

An an NHS patient, you will be routinely offered at least two scans during your pregancy.

Early/dating scan

This is usually carried out between 11-13 weeks of pregnancy. All women who book before this stage in pregnancy are counselled and offered screening for Down's syndrome (see page 241) at this appointment as well. The scan helps:

- *Locate the pregnancy* – Is it in the uterus?

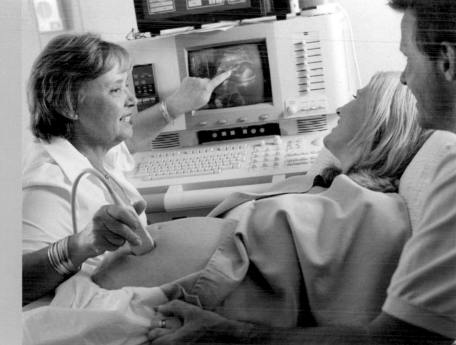

Transabdominal ultrasound is a painless procedure which is most commonly used after the first trimester to check on the well-being of your baby.

- *Establish an accurate due date* The length of the baby is measured from the head to the bottom, called the crown-rump measurement. This gives a very accurate indication of your dates if you are under 14 weeks pregnant and will be used to confirm your estimated date of delivery.
- *Check the number of babies* If you have twins (or more), the appearance of the membrane separating the babies and the position of the placenta can show whether the babies share one placenta or have one each.
- *Check the uterus and ovaries* The size and shape of the uterus and appearance of the cervix are assessed, and if you have fibroids (common benign overgrowths of the muscle wall of the uterus), they can be measured. Sometimes a small ovarian cyst is seen, which formed when the egg was released. These corpus luteum cysts disperse during pregnancy. Occasionally larger ovarian cysts are noticed, unrelated to the pregnancy.
- *Assess the risk of Down's syndrome* by measuring the baby's nuchal translucency (NT) (see below) and sometimes nasal bone length (the presence of the nasal bone in this scan is an early and positive marker for a low risk of Down's). The NT measurement is used in combination with a blood test (the Combined or Integrated Test, see different screening tests, page 241) routinely used to test for Down's.

Nuchal translucency (NT)
The nuchal translucency is a fluid filled area behind the baby's neck that can be accurately measured at the time of the dating scan. If it is thicker than average, your baby has an increased risk for Down's syndrome or a heart problem.

Anomaly scan
This is performed at around 18 to 20 weeks and is much more detailed than the early scan. It checks:
- *Fetal anatomy* This looks at all the baby's organs including the brain and spinal cord, heart, chest cavity, stomach, face, kidneys and bladder, and arms and legs. Even the number of toes and fingers can be counted. If the scan

suggests an abnormality, you may be referred to a specialist doctor called a Fetal Medicine Consultant for further scanning and assessment. Occasionally an MRI (magnetic resonance imaging) scan is needed to evaluate it further.
- *Gestational age*
- *Growth rate* The baby's head, abdomen (waist) and thigh bone (femur) are measured and plotted on a graph to assess the baby's size.
- *Amount of amniotic fluid*
- *Location of the placenta* The position, size and function of the placenta is checked. If the placenta is low-lying, near or across the cervix, you will be rescanned later in pregnancy. If, later on, the placenta or its blood vessels are seen to cover the cervix, you will need to have a Caesarian. The placenta can be investigated further using colour Doppler scanning to trace the blood flow through the uterine arteries to screen mothers for per-eclampsia. Umbilical artery Dopplers can be used to evaluate placental blood flow and assess why a baby is small on scan measurements.
- *The baby's gender* After 16 weeks it is often easy to see if you have a boy or a girl. Don't depend completely on this though!

Further ultrasounds
A number of ultrasound examinations may be needed if any of the following arise:
- *Multiple pregnancy.*
- *Problems with the baby's growth rate (too small or too large).*
- *Too little or too much amniotic fluid.*
- *High risk for premature labour.*
- *Diabetes, high blood pressure, or other medical problems that may affect the baby's growth.*
- *If you're pregnant and bleeding.*
- *If you have a low-lying placenta.*
- *If you are 41 weeks pregnant or more.*

Maternal blood tests
Early in pregnancy, usually at your first (booking) antenatal check, your blood will be tested to

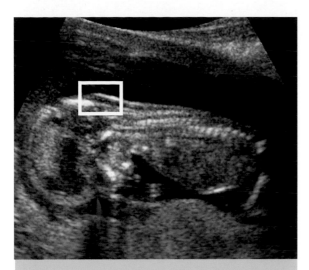

During a nuchal translucency scan, ultrasound is used to visualise the fluid-filled area at the back of the neck so it can be measured in order to assess the risk of Down's syndrome.

screen for anaemia, to check your blood group and Rhesus factor status, and to assess your immunity or previous exposure to certain infections. Currently all women are tested for rubella, Hepatitis B, syphilis and HIV. You will have pre-test counselling for all these checks. Later in pregnancy you may have blood testing to assess your risk of Down's syndrome.

Blood group and rhesus (Rh) status

It's necessary for your doctor to know your blood group in case you need a transfusion during pregnancy or labour. Your rhesus status is important because of a pregnancy condition called rhesus incompatability.

If a mother is rhesus negative and her baby is rhesus positive, the mother's body can develop antibodies to the baby's blood when the two bloods mix, for example during delivery. Although this is unlikely to have an effect on a first pregnancy, it could cause a problem in a subsequent pregnancy with a second rhesus positive baby, as the antibodies that have formed in the mother's body can attack and destroy the

baby's blood cells. This leads to haemolytic disease of the newborn and blood conditions ranging from mild jaundice to severe anaemia.

Fortunately, however, these conditions are now rare. Rh-negative mothers are given injections of Rh immunoglobulin (anti-D) at 28 weeks of pregnancy, as well as after delivery. They prevent the mother from making antibodies that can cross the placenta and attack her baby's red blood cells. Anti-D can also be given if the mother experiences vaginal bleeding after the 12th week of pregnancy and after chorionic villus sampling (CVS), amniocentesis, or external version (see page 205). A woman who is Rh negative should receive the injection, unless she knows for certain that the father is Rh negative, too, in which case the baby will also be Rh negative.

Full blood count

This blood test checks the levels of each type of blood cell: red blood cells, white blood cells and platelets. Your red blood cell level is particularly important (see page 90), as a low level is associated with anaemia.

Towards the end of pregnancy, a few women experience a drop in platelet levels. Although rare, it is possible that a very low platelet count can affect the clotting mechanisms of the blood and so put a woman at high risk of heavy bleeding during delivery. A low count may also prevent a spinal epidural from being performed. For these reasons, your platelet count will be checked at your booking appointment and at least once again during the last few weeks of your pregnancy. If your platelet count is low, your doctor will monitor your levels carefully.

Pregnant women commonly have high white blood cell counts but an extra-high white blood cell count may indicate infection, so your doctor may monitor this if infection is suspected, for example, if your membranes rupture early.

Rubella (German measles)

A routine test can indicate whether you are immune (see page 89). Most women are immune to this virus, either from having had rubella as a child or from a previous vaccination.

If you are not immune and you come into contact with somebody who has, or is suspected of having, rubella, tell your doctor immediately, as this infection can lead to serious pregnancy complications (see page 258).

Hepatitis B
This viral liver infection is usually caught from blood (even just a few drops) used in transfusions or contaminated needles used by tatooists, acupuncturists or drug addicts, or having unprotected sex with an infected person. Hepatitis B is the most common liver infection in the world. Although its incidence in the UK is relatively low, the Department of Health is looking at introducing a vaccination programme for all babies. Currently, only babies born to infected mothers are vaccinated. If you carry this virus, it could infect your baby at delivery. To reduce this risk, your baby will be given a vaccine immediately after she is born.

Hepatitis C is an unpreventable viral disease that can result in serious liver damage; there is a small risk it will pass to your baby if you are infected. Tests for hepatitis C aren't usually offered routinely as part of antenatal care. If you think you might be at risk, talk to your caregiver who can arrange a test. If you're infected, you'll be referred to a specialist, and your baby can be tested after it's born.

Syphilis
Although syphilis is very uncommon these days, there is still a chance that you may have been unknowingly infected in the past and have never shown any symptoms, which is why a routine blood test to check for syphilis is given during early pregnancy. The organism that causes syphilis can be transmitted to your baby from early in pregnancy and can result in facial abnormalities and mental retardation. Fortunately, once identified, syphilis can be treated early in pregnancy with antibiotics – usually penicillin – which will not only prevent your baby from being affected but will also cure you of this disease.

HIV
All pregnant women in the United Kingdom are now routinely offered a blood test for HIV, as it is possible to be infected without realising it. Doctors now have many ways of preventing HIV from being transmitted to an unborn baby, so the

---

BLOOD TESTS FOR INHERITED CONDITIONS

If you or your partner have a history of an inherited disease in the family you may be offered a blood test to help to diagnose whether your unborn baby is at risk (see page 246).

A blood test may also be recommended if there is a better-than-average chance that you and your partner could be carrying a defective gene for a particular disorder, even though there is no known history of the condition in your immediate family. For example, Jewish couples whose families originate from Eastern Europe, should be offered testing for Tay-Sachs and Canavan's diseases, Cystic Fibrosis and Familial Dysautonomia.

Afro-Caribbeans who are at a higher-than-average risk of sickle cell disease may be offered testing for the condition. People whose families originate from the Mediterranean may be offered a test for thalassaemia – a hereditary form of anaemia.

Blood tests are also used to identify diseases that can be passed on from only one carrier parent, such as haemophilia, or from an affected parent, as in the case of Huntington's disease.

Your healthcare provider will be able to advise you about genetic testing, and may refer you to a genetic counsellor.

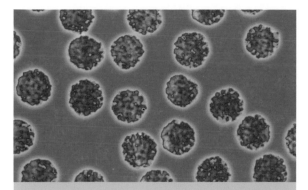

The hepatitis B virus (show above) is the cause of serum hepatitis, or hepatitis B, which is usually transmitted through blood or unprotected sex.

outlook for babies of HIV-positive mothers is better than ever (see page 268).

Glucose tolerance test

A form of diabetes – known as gestational diabetes – is a complication of pregnancy. Gestational diabetes is detected in different ways. In some practices you may be given a sugary drink at your first visit and have a blood sample taken two hours later, which is sent for laboratory testing. In other clinics, you may have a blood sugar test every three months or you may be tested only if you fall into one of the risk groups or are found to have sugar in your urine. The commonest time to have a test is between 26 and 28 weeks.

Screening for Down's syndrome

The risk of a baby having Down's syndrome can be estimated by a combination of NT screening (see page 238) and blood tests, which form part of normal antenatal care. These tests pick up 80–90 per cent of women whose babies are at risk. The actual diagnosis can only be made by chorionic villus sampling or amniocentesis, which look at the baby's chromosomes.

The different screening tests

There are specific substances in the maternal blood which have come from the baby and the placenta, which are higher or lower in pregnancies with Down's syndrome. These are alpha-fetoprotein (AFP), human chorionic gonadotrophin (hCG), a placental substance (PAPP-A), oestriol and inhibin A. The following tests are available:

- *The combined test* (NT, hCG and PAPP-A), performed from 11 to 14 weeks.
- *The quadruple test* (hCG, AFP, estriol and inhibin A) is done between 15 to 23 weeks if NT wasn't measured.
- *The integrated test* (an ultrasound scan to check NT and a blood test for hCG and PAPP-A done between 11 and 13+ weeks followed some weeks later by a blood test for AFP, estriol, inhibin A and hCG).

Raised AFP levels in the mother's blood can indicate a neural tube defect, such as spina bifida (see page 375), or fetal abdominal wall problems, although these types of problems are usually picked up by an anomaly ultrasound.

This type of screening, however, is not necessarily suitable for multiple pregnancies, as blood levels of these substances are naturally much higher in these circumstances, making the test invalid. It can depend of whether the twins are identical (having the same DNA) or not.

Diagnostic tests

Depending on your age, your medical, obstetrical and family history and other factors, you may want to or be advised to undergo one or more tests designed to detect certain genetic diseases or conditions by evaluating the chromosomes of your developing baby. Abnormalities in the number or structure of chromosomes can lead to problems in the baby. The most common chromosomal abnormality in live-born babies is Down's syndrome, which is associated with severe learning difficulties. Tests can detect abnormalities by yielding a karyotype, an enlarged picture of the individual chromosomes.

In addition, the DNA obtained from these procedures can be used to test for certain hereditary diseases from which you may be at risk

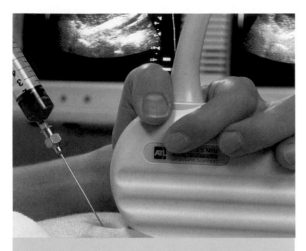

During transabdominal CVS, ultrasound is used to determine the placenta's position, and to guide the needle through the abdomen and the uterine wall to the edge of the placenta, without harming the baby.

based on your family history or your ethnic background; for example, Tay-Sachs, cystic fibrosis or sickle cell disease. However, unless a couple is known to be specifically at risk for one of these rare genetic disorders, this specialised testing won't be routinely done.

Traditionally, women aged 35 or older – or who will be at their due date – are offered one of these diagnostic tests to check for abnormalities. Thirty-five is the target age, because a woman's risk of having a baby with a chromosomal abnormality increases significantly after she reaches that age (and if the baby's father is also considered older, see page 94). It's also the age at which the risk of miscarriage from the procedure itself is roughly equal to the chance that the baby has a chromosomal abnormality.

However, while the risk of a chromosomal abnormality is much less for women under the age of 35, most babies with Down's syndrome are born to women under this age, because far more women under 35 are having babies than women over the age of 35.

What if you are advised that you have an increased risk of a chromosomal problem but you find the risk of miscarriage associated with the test unacceptable, or you have decided that you wouldn't wish to terminate a pregnancy even in the case of an abnormality? Can you refuse? You can – you have the right to decide whether or not to agree to any procedures that are offered – but you need to bear in mind that even if pregnancy termination isn't something you would consider, prior knowledge of an abnormality can give you more time to make preparations for a child that may have special needs.

If you are under the age of 35 and want to have your baby tested for chromosomal abnormalities, this is completely reasonable, as long as you understand the risks and benefits of the testing.

Chorionic villus sampling (CVS)

Tiny, finger-like pieces of tissue known as chorionic villi make up the placenta. They develop from cells arising out of the fertilised egg, so they have the same chromosomes and genetic make-up

NON-INVASIVE PRENATAL DIAGNOSIS (NIPD)

From as early as 8 weeks of pregnancy, small amounts of your baby's DNA can be detected floating in your blood stream. Recent scientific advances mean it is now possible to isolate this fetal DNA by a simple blood test from the mother. This technology, known as NIPD, can be used to accurately check the baby's sex, blood group and diagnose if the baby has Down's syndrome with 99% accuracy. Currently, only available in certain high risk circumstances it is likely that this test will eventually replace standard screening for Down's syndrome and a number of other chromosomal or genetic conditions in the baby.

as the developing baby. A sample of chorionic villi will enable your healthcare provider to see whether or not the chromosomes are normal in number and structure. DNA from the chorionic villi can also be used to test for some genetic diseases, if the baby is thought to be at risk.

The main advantage CVS has over amniocentesis is that the results are available earlier in the pregnancy. This means that if the test reveals an abnormality in the baby, and if pregnancy termination is an option, it can be done earlier, which is easier for the mother, both physically and emotionally.

How it's performed
CVS is typically done from 11 weeks of pregnancy onwards and can be performed in one of two ways – either by withdrawing placental tissue, which contains chorionic villi, through a hollow needle inserted through the maternal abdominal wall (transabdominal CVS) – or by inserting a device through the cervix to take a 'bite' of placental tissue (transcervical CVS). Ultrasound is used to guide the doctor to the right location and to avoid injury to the baby as the procedure is performed. The tissue is then processed in a laboratory and a karyotype (a picture of the chromosomes) is prepared. The decision on whether to perform CVS through the abdomen or the cervix depends on where the placenta is located within the uterus and the uterus' general shape and position.

Risks and side effects
Regardless of whether the CVS is performed through the cervix or the abdomen, neither method is riskier than the other, although having an invasive test always slightly raises the risk of miscarriage (1:100 to 1:1000). Studies show that the experience of the person performing the procedure is important in reducing this risk. Babies tested by CVS before nine weeks have an increased risk for limb and facial defects, which is why the test is always performed after 11 weeks.

Some vaginal bleeding may occur after CVS and should not be a cause for concern, although you should report it to your midwife if it lasts for three or more days. There is also a very slight risk of infection, so you should also report if you have a fever in the days following the procedure.

Results
CVS results should be available in seven days, but it can take two to three weeks for a full report. Occasionally (1 in 100 cases), results are

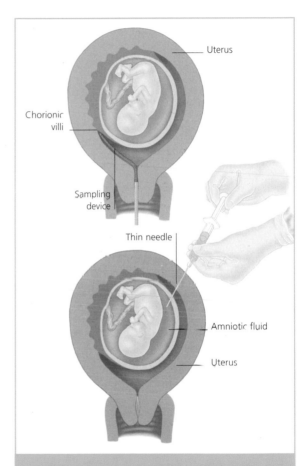

CVS (top) and Amniocentesis (bottom) are both diagnostic tests that can be carried out if an abnormality is suspected. Which one to choose is a matter of discussion between you and your caregiver. There is no statistical difference between the two when it comes to miscarriage. With both tests ultrasound is used to guide the doctor to the right location in the uterus and to avoid injury to the baby.

inconclusive and an amniocentesis is then needed to confirm the genetic makeup of the baby.

Amniocentesis

This test involves withdrawing amniotic fluid from the uterus, which contains cells from the baby that can be used to obtain information about the baby's chromosomes.

An amniocentesis to test for genetic abnormalities is usually done at 15 to 20 weeks. It primarily tests to see that 23 chromosome pairs are present and that their structures are normal. It doesn't routinely test for all possible genetic diseases or structural abnormalities. It may also be used to test for specific genetic disorders for which the baby is known to be a high risk – for example, if both parents are known to be carriers of cystic fibrosis, or Tay-Sachs disease, or if one parent is a carrier for a genetic disease that can be passed by just one parent, such as Huntington's disease. Amniocentesis will be offered if you had a high-risk result from the Down's syndrome screening, or if your ultrasound examination was abnormal, indicating, for example, poor fetal growth or suspected structural abnormalities.

Further amniocentesis

You may be offered amniocentesis later in pregnancy to test for:

◆ *Infections* Some pregnant women may be at risk of developing such infections as toxoplasmosis, cytomegalovirus (CMV), or parvovirus. The amniotic fluid can be tested for evidence of such problems in women who are considered to be at risk.
◆ *Abnormalities* If any abnormalities were picked up at the anomaly scan (see page 238), these may raise suspicions that your baby has a chromosomal disorder.
◆ *Premature labour* An infection within the amniotic fluid may be a cause of premature labour. If this is suspected, the amniotic fluid can be sent to a lab for tests to look for any such infection. If an infection is present, your doctor may suggest the immediate delivery of your baby to minimise any harm to either you or the baby.

How it's performed

The procedure is usually carried out by a specialist obstetrician. The ultrasound scan is used to identify a 'pocket' of amniotic fluid away from the baby. A thin needle is inserted through your abdomen and the wall of the uterus, into the amniotic sac. About 15 to 20 cc (1 to 2 tablespoons) of amniotic fluid is withdrawn, after which the needle is removed.

Some women think that the needle is inserted through the navel, but it isn't. The exact point of insertion depends on where the baby, the placenta, and the amniotic sac are located within the uterus.

Many women have heard that an amniocentesis needle is exceptionally long, and they fear that such a long needle causes pain. But the needle's length, which enables it to reach the amniotic sac, doesn't make it painful. It's the thickness of a needle that determines how uncomfortable it is. An amniocentesis needle is very thin, so any discomfort should be minimal.

The procedure only lasts about 1 to 2 minutes, although it may feel longer. It's mildly uncomfortable but not terribly painful. Most women report that it isn't as bad as they expected it to be. Generally a slight, brief cramping sensation is felt as the needle goes into the uterus, followed by a strange pulling sensation as the fluid is withdrawn through the needle. While some doctors choose to give local anaesthesia, others feel that the discomfort caused by the injection of the anaesthetic agent isn't worth the benefit. After all, the anaesthesia only numbs the skin, and doesn't numb the uterus where any discomfort will be felt. Afterwards, your doctor may advise that you rest for one to two days and avoid strenuous activity and sex during this period.

Risks and side effects

There is a small risk of miscarriage (1:100 to 1:1000) with this test. After the procedure some women experience cramping for several hours.

The best treatment for this is rest. You may experience a little leakage of amniotic fluid through the vagina – no more than a teaspoonful. A small leakage that then stops is usually all right, but if you experience a gush of fluid, call your doctor immediately. You may also experience spotting which lasts a few days.

Many parents worry that having an amniocentesis will harm the baby, but the chance of this happening is extremely rare, given the use of ultrasound guidance.

Results

The amniotic fluid cells taken during the amniocentesis must be incubated and cultured, which takes some time. Results are usually available in one to two weeks. Under certain circumstances, some laboratories will perform a preliminary, rapid test called a Fluorescent in Situ Hybridisation (FISH) which takes 24 to 48 hours for a result. A FISH isn't a final result, and only tests for certain common chromosomal abnormalities. FISH is most commonly used if there is a high suspicion of a chromosomal abnormality like Down's syndrome, trisomy 18 or trisomy 13.

Fetal blood sampling

Also known as percutaneous umbilical blood sampling (PUBS) or cordocentesis, fetal blood sampling is a procedure in which fetal blood is withdrawn from the umbilical cord. Usually performed after week 18 of pregnancy, the test lets your doctor obtain blood for rapid chromosomal diagnosis when a fast result is critical. It is also sometimes carried out in order to diagnose some fetal infections, to detect evidence of fetal anaemia, or to diagnose and treat a condition called hydrops, in which fluid accumulates abnormally in the baby.

Some babies develop anaemia, which can be treated within the uterus with a blood transfusion. The transfusion is done during a fetal blood sampling and blood is actually transfused into the umbilical cord. Conditions that may lead to

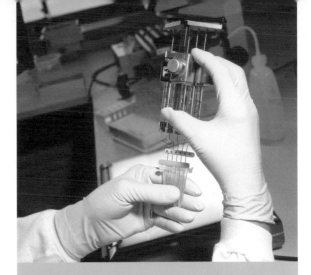

Fetal blood is taken from the unborn baby's cord during percutaneous umbilical blood sampling (PUBS) for testing in the laboratory (see above). The blood can be used to diagnose a number of different conditions.

anaemia include certain infections, such as parvovirus, genetic diseases (see page 240), or some blood group incompatibilities (see page 90). However the commonest reason is when the mother has anti-D antibodies in her blood stream that have crossed over the placenta to destroy the baby's red blood cells (see page 239)

How it's performed

The procedure, which is carried out by an experienced maternal-fetal medicine specialist, is performed under ultrasound guidance. It's similar to an amniocentesis, except that the needle is directed into the umbilical cord rather than into the amniotic fluid.

Risks and side effects

The risk of loss of the baby is higher than amniocentesis. Other risk factors include infection and rupture of the membranes.

Results

It usually takes three days for the results to come through. Although there is no definitive research at present on the test's reliability, the results are thought to be highly accurate.

Genetic counselling

You could be referred for genetic counselling before, during, or following a pregnancy if you may be at increased risk of having a baby with an abnormality. Ideally, genetic counselling should take place before conception when testing and decision making is less rushed.

Why you may want counselling

The purpose of genetic counselling is to:

◆ Determine the probability of your baby having a congenital (present at birth) abnormality or genetic disorder.

◆ Explain the effects of the disorder and the amount of risk to the baby.

◆ Outline any treatments available.

◆ Highlight what antenatal tests are available to detect the problem.

◆ Explain possible courses of action.

◆ Help you reach a decision appropriate for you.

Many fetal abnormalities can be diagnosed antenatally. However, antenatal tests are entirely optional and can be declined. If a mother chooses to have an antenatal test and is told there's a possible problem, or if the baby is found to have a serious abnormality – either during pregnancy or after delivery – the implications can be discussed at a genetic counselling session with a doctor, midwife, or genetic counsellor.

Many people mistakenly believe that all types of congenital abnormalities happen more often to babies born to older mothers. In fact, most abnormalities aren't related to the mother's age, and, as most babies are born to women under the age of 40, these babies represent the largest population with congenital abnormalities. However, older mothers do have a greater risk of having babies with chromosomal problems.

Why you might be referred

Couples who are at a higher-than-average risk of having a baby with an inherited disease or congenital abnormality should be referred for genetic counselling before pregnancy or in the early stages of pregnancy. Such people:

◆ *Have had children with abnormalities* Counselling may discuss if and how this affects the chances of having another baby with the same problem.

◆ *Are from particular ethnic groups* Some genetic disorders are more common in certain racial or cultural groups. For example, people of Ashkenazi Jewish origins are at above average risk of carrying a gene for a degenerating neurological disorder called Tay-Sachs disease. Afro-Caribbeans, on the other hand, are at higher-than-average risk of carrying the gene for sickle cell disease, and people of Asian or Mediterranean descent are at increased risk of carrying the gene for thalassaemia.

◆ *Are known carriers* If either of the parents carry an abnormal gene or an unusual chromosome is found – via testing because of ethnic origin, family history, repeated miscarriage, or a general screening programme – then the healthcare provider should recommend genetic counselling to determine what significance this has for children and other family members.

◆ *Are married cousins* If the expectant parents are first cousins, they will share one in eight of their genes – second cousins share 1 in 32. Therefore there's an above-average risk of both having the same abnormal gene, so the chances of the baby having a recessively inherited genetic condition are also higher than average. It is important to remember, however, that most marriages between cousins produce normal, healthy children.

◆ *Have had repeated miscarriages* A mother can be referred for chromosome testing if she's had repeated miscarriages, as an unusual chromosome pattern in one parent can be the cause. Testing isn't usually offered until there have been two or three losses, because miscarriage is common and doesn't usually indicate a problem in either parent.

- *Have had harmful exposure* If the mother suspects that shortly before or during her pregnancy she could have been exposed to something hazardous, such as X-rays, chemicals or certain medications, which could have harmed the unborn baby.

- *Have had a potential problem found on an antenatal test* If an ultrasound scan or other antenatal test detects an abnormality.

What happens during a session

You will be asked questions by a geneticist, specialist nurse or genetic counsellor about your relatives, in order to construct a family tree to find out if any disorders seem to 'run in the family' and to assess the chances of your baby inheriting such a condition. To get more detailed information, both partners and other family members may be asked to give a blood sample or a saliva sample for gene or chromosome testing.

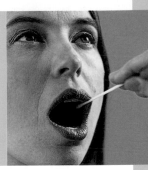

A saliva sample may be used for gene or chromosome testing when assessing the risks of an inherited disease. The inside of the cheek is rubbed with a cotton swab which is then sent to a laboratory for analysis.

If your baby is thought to be at high risk of having a genetic or chromosomal abnormality, amniocentesis (see page 244) or chorionic villus sampling (see page 242) will be offered, or if the mother is over 20 weeks pregnant, fetal blood sampling (see page 245) may be offered.

If, once all the information and test results are available, the unborn baby is found to have a disorder, you will be told how the disorder will affect him, what treatments are available, and whether a termination of pregnancy is an option. You won't be told what to do. All the tests are voluntary, and whatever course of action you decide upon is acceptable. The pros and cons of different options will be put forward, and you will be given any further information you may require, but you will have to make all decisions.

How diseases are inherited

A baby has two genes for each characteristic: one from the mother and one from the father (see page 17). It's likely that the parents and the child will carry some abnormal genes – most people do – but the abnormal genes probably won't cause problems. An abnormal gene is only likely to cause problems if it's dominant, if it's recessive and the baby has inherited two copies of the affected gene, or if it's X-linked and the baby is a boy (see page 248). The figures given are average risks for the different types of inheritance. Bear in mind, that just as one couple can have six boys or six girls in a row, so a couple could have many children with a problem, for which the risk is one in two or one in four, or they could have many normal, problem-free children.

MICROARRAY CGH TEST

Comparative genomic hybridisation uses the latest technology to check for small changes or alterations in the chromosomes such as additions or loss of normal chromosome material. This is a more sensitive test than just checking the number of chromosomes present in each cell. A tiny amount of DNA is placed on a small 'chip'. If the DNA contains any of the abnormalities coded on the chip, a chemical reaction occurs that causes the chip to change colour in the area on the chip corresponding to the abnormality. A special scanner can pick up the colour change and identify the abnormality. Although it can be helpful in explaining why an abnormality has arisen in a baby, further research is needed to fully understand all the test results. You may be offered it at amniocentesis or after birth if there are concerns for your baby.

DOMINANT GENES

Examples of diseases: Huntington's disease, achondroplasia and myotonic dystrophy.

If a person carries an abnormal dominant gene, he or she will probably know already because the person will have the problem – unless the effects aren't apparent until later in life. If such a gene is carried, every egg or sperm produced has a 50:50 chance of containing this abnormal gene.

Chances of baby inheriting problem: Each child has a one-in-two chance of being affected.

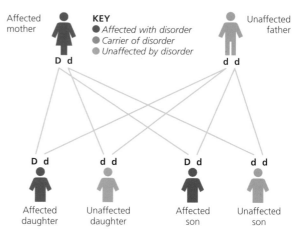

D = Abnormal, dominant gene   d = Normal gene

RECESSIVE GENES

Examples of diseases: cystic fibrosis, thalassaemia and sickle cell disease.

An abnormal recessive gene won't affect the mother's or father's health provided that the matching gene is normal. However, if a baby inherits two copies of the abnormal gene, one from each parent, he'll be affected. If he inherits one copy, he'll be a healthy carrier of the problem – like his parent.

Chances of baby inheriting problem: Each child has a one-in-four chance of being affected. Each unaffected child has a two-in-three chance of being a carrier.

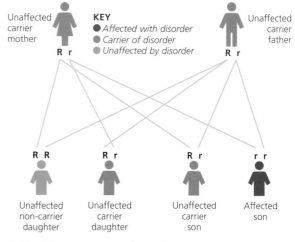

R = Normal gene   r = Abnormal, recessive gene

X-LINKED GENES

Examples of diseases: haemophilia, Duchenne muscular dystrophy and colour blindness.

If a woman carries an abnormal gene on an X chromosome, she probably won't have a problem, as her other X is likely to carry a normal version of the gene. A man carrying an abnormal gene on his X chromosome will suffer from the disorder, as he won't have another X chromosome with a normal version of the gene.

Chances of baby inheriting problem: If the mother is a carrier, a daughter has a one-in-two chance of being a carrier. Her sons have a one-in-two chance of being affected. If the father is affected, all daughters will be carriers, sons will not be affected.

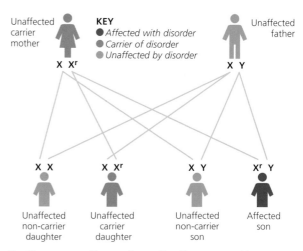

X = Chromosome with normal gene   Y = Chromosome without gene
X^r = Chromosome with abnormal gene

New mutations

Sometimes a baby is born with a dominant or X-linked problem, which neither parent has – a new mutation. Mutations arise from a mistake in the copying of a gene during the egg or sperm production process. If you have a baby with a new mutation, although your future children won't be at high risk of having the problem, the affected child could pass on the gene to his children.

Chromosomal problems

It's extremely important for a baby to inherit the correct number (46) of chromosomes – an additional chromosome means thousands of extra genes; an absent one, thousands of missing genes.

Trisomies

If a baby inherits an extra copy of a chromosome, he'll have three copies instead of the normal two. Most trisomies cause a pregnancy to miscarry, but some allow a baby to develop. The most common of these is Down's syndrome, also called trisomy 21 because the baby has three copies of chromosome 21. Edward's syndrome (trisomy 18) and Patau syndrome (trisomy 13) are rarer and more serious disorders. The risk of having a baby with Down's syndrome increases with a woman's age: at 20 it's about 1 in 1,500, at 30 it's 1 in 900, and at 40 it's increased to about 1 in 100.

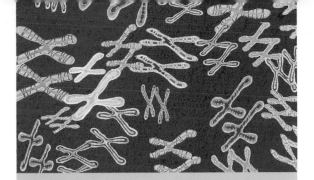

The male sex chromosomes are seen here as bright yellow (centre left) with the larger X chromosome below the small Y chromosome. The Y chromosome is responsible for masculine characteristics.

Extra sex chromosomes

Studies show that at least one baby in 1,000 has an extra sex chromosome. Such babies are usually normal in appearance and behaviour, and many progress through life without being diagnosed as having an extra chromosome. However, some of these children may have problems – for example, males with an extra X chromosome are infertile. If tests show that your baby has extra chromosome, you will be offered genetic counselling.

Translocations

About one person in 500 has one or more chromosomes on which pieces have been swapped with another or have broken off. A balanced translocation will cause no problems, since all the genes are present, but in a different location. If there is an unbalanced translocation (with extra or missing genetic information) a miscarriage will usually occur – if the baby is born he could suffer major physical and intellectual problems. People with balanced translocations are at increased risk of producing eggs or sperm with unbalanced translocations.

Fragile X Disease

Here, one of the genes on the X chromosome is faulty. As the normal form of the gene makes a protein necessary for brain development, the chief symptom is mental retardation. It affects 1 in 3,600 men and 1 in 4,000 to 6,000 women of all races and ethnic groups.

> **MULTIFACTORIAL OR POLYGENIC DISORDERS**
>
> Many abnormalities, such as spina bifida (see page 375) or heart defects (see page 374), aren't usually caused by an abnormal gene or chromosome but arise from a combined effect of many different genes and the environment. When a baby is born with one of these disorders, the risk of recurrence that the parents are given is based on observations of what has happened to other couples in the past who have had similarly affected children.

Complicated labours

Every woman's experience of labour is different, and every baby's experience of birth is unique. Some babies take their time to be born; others pop out without any fuss. Then there are the babies who arrive late, and those who arrive early. Occasionally, problems occur which affect the progress of labour.

Premature labour

Not all labours occur at term (between 37 and 41 weeks after your last menstrual period). If regular contractions start before 37 weeks and occur at a rate of six or more in an hour and don't settle with rest, you may be having premature labour. Because the baby may not be mature enough to cope on her own if she's delivered too early, you should be examined as soon as possible.

Just as with term labour, no one knows exactly what causes premature labour but there appear to be many possible causes or contributing factors. Among these are:

◆ Uterine infection, which can trigger the release of prostaglandins, that may induce labour.
◆ Problems with or inadequacy of the placenta which may cause the baby to release substances that bring on early labour.
◆ Uterine anomalies such as large fibroids, which decrease the ability of the uterus to stretch and accommodate the growing baby.
◆ Expecting more than one baby.
◆ Polyhydramnios (excessive amniotic fluid) (see page 262).
◆ History of prior premature labour.

Premature contractions may feel as strong as labour at term, possibly because they're unexpected. Some women experience them as persistent or rhythmic low back pain or pelvic pressure; others feel them as menstrual-like cramps or groin pulling. Increasing vaginal discharge may be a sign that the cervix is dilating, especially if it's blood-tinged.

Management
If you suspect you may be having premature contractions, plenty of fluids and bed rest can sometimes relieve the symptoms. Resting also allows you to attend to your body. In particular, keep a hand on your lower abdomen, over your uterus. If you feel repeated episodes of tightening, and they persist when you're resting, call the hospital and ask to be seen as soon as possible.

Slow labour

There are several types of labour in which progress is slow or nonexistent. These include:

Delayed first stage labour
A diagnosis of delay in the first stage of labour needs to take in all aspects of progress and is not just a set time. Relevant factors that impact on the diagnosis include;

◆ For first labours, cervical dilatation of less than 2 cm in 4 hours, or slowing in progress for second/subsequent labours.
◆ Changes in strength, duration and frequency of uterine contractions.

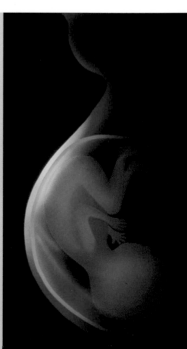

The baby can be seen in this artwork in the head-down position in the uterus, ready for birth.

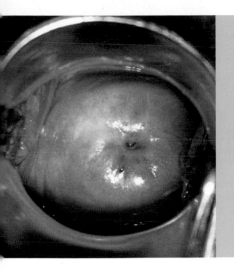

During pregnancy the opening of the cervix (centre left) remains tightly closed. Hormones and an increased blood supply gives the cervix a deep pink colour.

♦ Delay in descent and rotation of the fetal head. A prolonged first stage may be treated with sedation and rest. Sometimes this will distinguish true from false labour. Alternatively, you may encouraged to walk around, which can help position the baby properly. Don't tire yourself out, however; you will need to save some energy for active phase labour and pushing.

Protracted active phase

The active phase of labour begins when the progressive dilation in the cervix proceeds at one or more centimetres per hour. This usually occurs when you've dilated to between 3 and 5 cm. Once active phase labour occurs, complete dilation is usually reached within 4 to 8 hours. Contractions are more intense during this phase as they work to fully dilate the cervix and guide the baby farther into the pelvis – usually 1 cm deeper per hour.

Protracted active phase occurs when progress stalls and it takes over an hour to dilate 1 cm. This can happen if the baby is in the wrong position, or after an epidural has been inserted. It is a very common occurrence in first labours. You may be given syntocinon, a synthetic form of oxytocin, to help to stimulate contractions. If labour is still not progressing, the baby's head may be too large to fit through the pelvis – known as cephalopelvic disproportion (CPD) – and a Caesarean will be necessary.

Back labour

Many women feel their contractions most strongly in their backs. This is usually because the baby isn't in the most common position for labour but in the occiput posterior position, in which she faces away from her mother's spine and the occiput (back of head) presses against the spine. Back labour can be relieved by getting into the knee-chest position, pelvic rocks, walking, or keeping upright to encourage the baby to descend – babies often turn when they descend. Back massage and occasionally acupressure, and water therapy can also help. For information on all these, see Chapter 12.

Fast labour

Occasionally, the cervix dilates very rapidly, so that it becomes fully dilated within a very short time. This 'precipitate' labour – taking three hours or less from start to finish – doesn't usually cause any problems for the baby. Very occasionally, however, a rapid labour can deprive the baby of oxygen, or result in tearing or other damage to the cervix, vagina, or perineum. Medication may be given to slow labour down so that the baby can be delivered safely without damage to the mother.

Vaginal breech labour

A vaginal breech labour is always considered a trial of labour and is allowed to proceed only as long as it progresses normally. Some doctors will not use syntocinon if progress slows, because this could be an indicator that the baby is too large for the vaginal route. Any deviation from normal labour will mean that your doctor will recommend a Caesarean. Once the cervix is fully dilated, it is common practice to wait for the baby's bottom to be visible at the entrance of the vagina before pushing is encouraged. If vaginal breech birth goes ahead, the legs and body are usually allowed to deliver naturally. The birth attendant then helps to deliver the shoulders and head – occasionally an episiotomy and forceps are needed.

Pregnancy complications

Many women suffer minor health problems during pregnancy, but more serious complications occasionally arise. When these occur, treatment is usually required, so it is important to report any unusual symptoms to your healthcare provider immediately.

Blood disorders
Anaemia

A common condition in pregnancy, anaemia occurs when there aren't enough blood cells circulating in the mother's blood. Many pregnant women develop some degree of anaemia at some point, but in mild cases it doesn't cause any problems. And, because your body diverts its resources in favour of your baby, he is unlikely to be lacking in iron. But, if anaemia occurs as a result of hereditary abnormalities in haemoglobin, this can threaten the health of both of you.

The most common anaemia of pregnancy is dilutional anaemia. The amount of blood circulating around the body increases by as much as 50 per cent to sustain the growing baby. This dramatic rise is mainly achieved by an increase in the serum component of blood. Unless red cells increase at the same rate, they will be diluted.

Iron deficiency is the other major cause of anaemia in pregnancy. Because you need to produce enough red blood cells for both you and your baby, you need more iron during pregnancy to maintain blood volume. Most women don't have enough stored iron and it's difficult to ingest sufficient amounts. Consequently, a large number of women become anaemic in pregnancy. Unless nutritional intake of iron is supplemented during pregnancy, a woman will be deficient in iron stores at the time of birth, placing her at risk if postnatal bleeding occurs.

Anaemia also can be caused by a folic acid or vitamin B_{12} deficiency so your midwife or doctor may arrange a blood test to check your blood levels as well as test your blood ferritin (iron) level.

Symptoms
- Fatigue, loss of energy
- Pallor
- Decreased ability to fight illness
- Dizziness, fainting, shortness of breath

Treatment
During pregnancy, iron deficiency anaemia is treated with an iron supplement. In addition, iron-rich foods – molasses, red meat, kidney beans, spinach, fish, chicken and pork – should form a major part of your diet. To increase iron absorption, vitamin C is needed, so take your iron pill with orange, tomato or vegetable juice.

Rarely, a woman unable to absorb adequate iron by mouth may require an intravenous infusion of a liquid iron preparation to boost her own levels especially if labour and delivery are near. A B_{12} deficiency is treated by injections.

Deep vein thrombosis (DVT)
This is a condition which occurs when a blood clot blocks a vein in one of the legs – usually the calf vein or a vein in the upper leg or groin area.

Symptoms
- Pain, tenderness and swelling of the calf, upper leg or groin
- Swollen area feels warm

Treatment
If you suspect you may have DVT, you need to go straight to the hospital. This condition shouldn't be ignored, because if left untreated, the clot can travel to the lungs causing a pulmonary embolus, which can be life-threatening. A special blood test is available which can confirm the diagnosis. An

ultrasound scan called a Doppler is also available that will quickly tell doctors if a DVT is present. Treatment usually consists of blood-thinning injections or medication.

It's easy to confuse DVT with the common and harmless condition of superficial thrombophlebitis. Sometimes the small surface veins in the lower legs become red and sore in pregnancy, especially if you're overweight. In this case, only soothing cream and support tights are required.

Gestational diabetes

Unique to pregnancy, in this type of diabetes the body fails to make enough insulin to cope with the increased blood sugar levels. The placenta produces a hormone, human placental lactogen, which acts against insulin and can therefore expose a tendency to diabetes. For women with gestational diabetes, the main complication is that the baby can become very large. Delivery often has to occur by 39–40 weeks gestation to ensure the baby's well-being.

You're at risk of gestational diabetes if you've had it before, if you're over 35, overweight, Asian, if your previous baby was over 4 kg (8 lb 13 oz), if you have a parent or sibling with diabetes, a previous baby with an abnormality or a previous stillbirth. The diagnosis is based on testing the sugar levels in your blood when fasting and after eating a fixed amount of sugar.

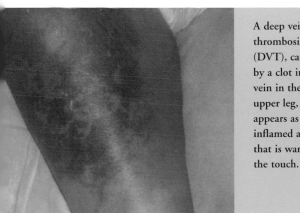

A deep vein thrombosis (DVT), caused by a clot in a vein in the upper leg, appears as an inflamed area that is warm to the touch.

Symptoms

- Sugar in urine
- Excessive thirst
- Excessive urination
- Fatigue

Treatment

Most women with gestational diabetes can control their sugar levels by following a relatively sugar-free diet. For some women, however, watching their diet is insufficient and they will need to start oral medications or at least twice-daily insulin injections to control their blood sugar. If you are one, this is managed with the hospital diabetic team, who will teach you how to check your sugar levels and how to give yourself injections.

High blood pressure (hypertension)

If blood pressure (BP) is raised before pregnancy, this is known as essential or chronic hypertension. PIH or pregnancy-induced hypertension occurs when a woman's blood pressure is elevated only during pregnancy and occurs in 16–18 per cent of all pregnancies, and is defined as a BP greater than 140/90. It normally develops after 20 weeks, and becomes more common the nearer the delivery date. It is more common in first pregnancies.

Mild high blood pressure may cause no problems. Severe high blood pressure may lead to kidney failure or stroke. The major risk is to the 1 in 4 women with PIH who go on to develop pre-eclampsia (see below).

Symptoms

There are usually no symptoms until some organs, such as the kidney and eyes, are affected by the decreased blood supply that can accompany hypertension. Because untreated hypertension can eventually lead to serious complications, blood pressure checks are routine at antenatal visits.

Pre-eclampsia

A syndrome that occurs only in pregnancy, pre-eclampsia is characterised by high blood pressure, protein in the urine and increased swelling of the legs and feet. Pre-eclampsia affects 8–10 per cent of pregnancies, and 85 per cent of these are first-time pregnancies. Mothers who are over 40; teenage mothers; and mothers who are over-weight, have diabetes, a history of blood-pressure problems or previous pre-eclampsia, or kidney or rheumatology disorders; or who are expecting twins or more also are at higher risk.

Many women with pre-eclampsia feel perfectly well and only realise they have this condition because they are told their blood pressure is high. If the following symptoms develop the condition becomes more serious.

Symptoms
- Sudden excessive lower leg, hand or facial oedema (swelling) or excessive weight gain
- Persistent headaches
- Blurred vision, flashing lights or spots before your eyes
- Upper abdominal pain on right side of the body, just below ribcage

Treatment
The cause of pre-eclampsia remains unknown, and consequently no treatment has been consistently shown to prevent or treat it. Birth is the only cure, with induced delivery for women who are close to their due dates or who are severely affected. If it is still early in the pregnancy or if pre-eclampsia is mild, blood-pressure tablets can help to reduce blood pressure. Low-dose aspirin – 81 mg daily – may reduce your risk of developing it. Attend all your check-ups, so any problems can be detected early. Try not to get stressed, as this can raise blood pressure. Cut down on sodium and fat; eat more calcium-rich foods, fruit and vegetables, and drink plenty of water. You may be asked to monitor your blood pressure so you can spot any dramatic change.

Eclampsia
Pre-eclampsia can develop into eclampsia, a rare but very serious condition.

Symptoms
- Seizures

Treatment
Eclampsia is a medical emergency, and oxygen and drugs will be given to the mother to prevent any further seizures occurring. Urgent delivery of the baby is usually required to enable proper treatment of the mother.

HELLP syndrome
A life-threatening condition, HELLP syndrome is a unique variant of pre-eclampsia. It stands for its characteristics: H is for haemolysis (the breaking down of red blood cells); EL for elevated liver enzymes; and LP for low platelet count. HELLP syndrome occurs in tandem with pre-eclampsia, but because some of its symptoms can occur before those of pre-eclampsia they can be mistaken for other conditions. As a result, the right treatment may not be given, leaving both mother and baby in a very vulnerable state. In the United Kingdom, 8 to 10 per cent of all pregnant women develop pre-eclampsia. Between 2 and 12 per cent of these go on to suffer from HELLP syndrome. Older white women with more than one child are most at risk of getting HELLP.

Symptoms
- Headache
- Nausea, vomiting
- Abdominal soreness and pain in the right upper section – from liver distention

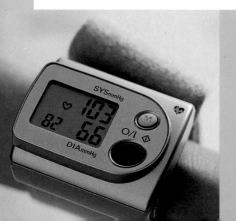

A simple home blood pressure monitor can be used to keep a check if you are thought to be at risk for pre-eclampsia.

These symptoms may or may not be present:

- Severe headache
- Visual disturbances
- Bleeding
- Swelling
- High blood pressure
- Protein in the urine

Treatment

The only effective treatment is delivery. The quicker pre-eclampsia is detected and managed, the better the outcome for mother and baby.

Obstetric cholestasis

Also called OC or cholestasis of pregnancy, this is a poorly understood, multi-factorial condition originating in the liver. Overall, 0.7 per cent of pregnancies are affected, but if you are from an Asian background, your risk is twice that.

Deranged liver function leads to a build-up of bile salts in the bloodstream and causes intense itching, and consequent sleep deprivation. Although there is no harm to the mother and the condition disappears after birth, there are some risks to the baby. You may go into labour early, and there is a small risk of the baby dying before birth (intrauterine death) if bile salts are very high.

Symptoms

- Itching, which may be all over but most commonly on the palms and the soles
- Abnormal liver enzymes on blood testing

Treatment

Doctors may prescribe a drug called ursodeoxycholic acid or ursadiol to improve the liver abnormalities. Antihistamine medication and cooling creams can help the itching. Vitamin K supplements may be given to the mother and postnatal vitamin K to the baby. Early delivery may be advised, although the evidence for this is not very good. The timing of the risk of stillbirth is not known or predictable.

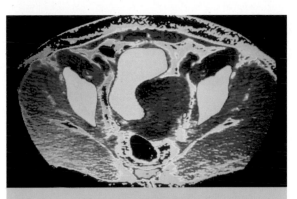

A large fibroid, a benign tumour, can been seen (round black area) in the uterus (yellow), on this colour-enhanced CT scan.

Uterine and tubal problems
Fibroids

Benign growths on the wall of the uterus, fibroids are more common in older women, and usually don't affect pregnancy. Pregnancy hormones can make fibroids grow larger, and occasionally they may cause problems, such as preventing the baby from growing properly. A fibroid's position may sometimes make a vaginal delivery impossible.

Symptoms

- Pain
- Abdominal tenderness
- Slight fever

Treatment

If fibroids are causing discomfort, pain-relieving medications are usually the only treatment during pregnancy. They usually shrink in the weeks after delivery. If they continue to be a problem, they may be surgically removed some months after delivery. It's considered unsafe to remove fibroids at the time of a Caesarean section, because of the risk of severe blood loss and the possible need for hysterectomy to control bleeding.

Ectopic pregnancy

This is a serious condition that occurs when a pregnancy develops outside the uterus, normally in a Fallopian tube. It can mimic a miscarriage, because the symptoms and signs can be very similar, in that abdominal pain and vaginal bleeding occur, though normally any bleeding is light. Pain in early pregnancy should always be investigated by ultrasound to exclude an ectopic pregnancy. Blood tests are often required to monitor the levels of human chorionic gonadotropin (hCG) in the blood before this type of pregnancy can be diagnosed.

Symptoms

◆ Severe abdominal pain that may also be accompanied by shoulder or rectal pain.

Treatment

Laparoscopy (key-hole surgery), usually will be used to remove the pregnancy. A drug called Methotrexate is now being used to treat some ectopic pregnancies in a number of hospitals.

Hydatidiform mole or molar pregnancy

This is a rare type of pregnancy complication affecting around 1 in 2000 pregnancies. The cells in pregnancy called trophoblasts, which normally form the placenta, grow out of control and stop the fertilised egg from developing normally. The uterus becomes full of very abnormal tissue, which produces high levels of HCG hormone. The diagnosis can be confirmed by ultrasound.

Symptoms

◆ Brownish discharge
◆ Severe morning sickness
◆ An unusually large uterus
◆ Absence of a fetal heartbeat.

Treatment

A D&C (dilation and curettage) will be carried out to remove abnormal tissue from the uterus, as in rare cases it can spread to other parts of the body. Close monitoring of HCG hormone levels will be necessary for several months to ensure that all the tissue has gone away. Attempts to conceive again should be delayed for a year until all traces of the pregnancy hormone have disappeared.

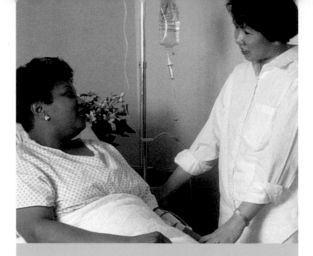

Dehydration, caused by hyperemesis gravidarum, may require a stay in hospital so that rehydrating fluids can be given through a venous line.

Anal fissure

Occasionally pregnancy or a difficult delivery can lead to a tear in the anal mucosa (lining of the anus). Bowel movements can reopen this tear, resulting in bleeding and intense pain; continual opening prevents healing and can result in scar tissue. Anal fissures are usually linked to bowel problems; constipation or frequent stools can cause straining and exacerbate the problem. Anal fissures also can be caused by syphilis, tuberculosis, Crohn's disease and tumours.

Anal fissures are generally diagnosed with a proctoscopy, which examines the anal canal and can rule out haemorrhoids (painful swellings at the anus caused by enlarged veins and genital warts). They can usually be prevented by keeping bowel movements regular and soft through eating plenty of fibre and taking stool softeners.

Symptoms

◆ Pain during and after a bowel movement
◆ Bright red bleeding
◆ Constipation

Treatment

Anal fissures can be acute or chronic, and it's important to get them treated as early as possible or complications can set in. Treatment depends on the severity of the condition. Acute or recent fissures are usually treated with a bulk-forming laxative, and a local anaesthetic cream. In severe cases, a surgical procedure may be necessary. After treatment, it's important to follow a high-fibre diet, eat regularly and drink plenty of fluids.

Hyperemesis gravidarum

Rarely, morning sickness can develop into this more extreme condition. Approximately 1 in 200 women in early pregnancy need to be admitted to hospital because they're vomiting excessively and need to be rehydrated by intravenous drip. If left untreated, hyperemesis gravidarum can result in low levels of potassium in the bloodstream and prevent the liver from functioning properly.

Symptoms
- Excessive nausea and vomiting
- Weight loss
- Dehydration
- Dark yellow urine
- Passing small quantities of urine

Treatment

Fortunately, treatment by admission to the hospital, stopping all oral intake and giving rehydrating fluids via a venous line (a drip) is usually very successful. Food is then slowly reintroduced and you will be discharged after a matter of a few days.

Infections
Cytomegalovirus (CMV)

A member of the herpes virus family, CMV is a common congenital infection, which is spread by contact with saliva, urine and faeces. About 1 per cent of newborns are infected every year. The vast majority aren't affected by the virus but about 8000 babies a year develop lasting disabilities such as learning difficulties, deafness and blindness. A woman who contracts CMV for the first time during pregnancy has a 30 to 40 per cent risk of passing it to her baby. Women who contract CMV at least 6 months before getting pregnant,

appear to have little risk of developing complications. A lab test can determine whether a woman has had the infection before, while a culture can be grown from a urine specimen to detect active infection. If CMV is diagnosed, the baby can be tested for the infection by amniocentesis. In newborns, the virus can be identified in body fluids within 3 weeks of birth.

Symptoms
- Sore throat
- Fever
- Body aches
- Fatigue

Treatment

No preventive treatment for congenital CMV exists, but an hyperimmune gamma globulin may be offered to a women with an acute CMV infection to reduce the risk of her passing it to her unborn child. An antiviral drug, ganciclovir, may help babies with the infection. The risk of contracting CMV can be reduced through careful hygiene, such as thorough hand-washing after contact with the saliva and urine of a young child.

Toxoplasmosis

Although quite rare in the United Kingdom, this infection can seriously affect the fetus. It can be

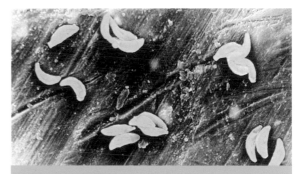

Toxoplasmosis organisms can be seen here as yellow, crescent-shaped parasite cells. If a pregnant woman becomes infected, it can affect her unborn baby.

caught through contact with cat litter and lambs, and by eating undercooked meat and unwashed vegetables. If a pregnant woman becomes infected, the chance that she will transmit the infection to her baby, and the possible effects it may have depend largely on when she contracts it. If it's during the first trimester, the chance that the baby will become infected is less than 2 per cent, although the effect it has on the baby's development is greater. If the infection isn't contracted until later in pregnancy, the chance that the baby will become infected is higher, but the effects of the infection are much less severe. There may be some general symptoms (see below), but it is possible to have the infection without knowing.

Not all doctors routinely screen for toxoplasmosis in early pregnancy. It often depends on your own particular risk factors, such as whether you own a cat or handle lambs.

Symptoms
- Feeling generally unwell
- Slight fever
- Swollen glands
- Rash

Treatment
If blood tests show that you have developed toxoplasmosis either immediately prior to conception or during pregnancy, you should see a maternal-fetal medicine specialist or your own doctor to discuss the possible implications. You may need to be given certain antibiotics to decrease the chances of transmitting the infection to the baby, and possibly have an amniocentesis (see page 244) in the second trimester to determine if the baby has contracted the infection. Even if your unborn baby is infected, treatment with appropriate antibiotics gives an excellent chance that he will be fine.

Listeriosis
Caused by listeria, a bacteria found in unwashed raw vegetables, unpasteurised milk and cheese, and raw and undercooked meat, poultry, fish and shellfish, listeriosis can cause serious illness in pregnancy, which can lead to premature birth, miscarriage, still birth, or infection of the baby. Listeriosis is relatively rare and hard to detect; symptoms can appear any time between 12 hours and 30 days after contaminated food is eaten, and may be ignored, as they are similar to those of flu, or mistaken for normal pregnancy side effects.

Symptoms
- Headache
- Fever
- Muscle aches
- Nausea and diarrhoea

Treatment
Antibiotics are needed to treat and cure listeriosis.

Rubella (German measles)
A relatively mild infection normally, but in pregnancy rubella can have very serious implications; it can cause birth defects ranging from deafness to encephalitis (inflammation of the brain), heart defects and learning difficulties. Fortunately, most women are immune. As part of your antenatal care, a blood test (see page 89) will check your immunity.

Women are advised to have their immunity assessed before getting pregnant and if not immune, be vaccinated against the disease and then wait three months before trying to conceive. If you received the vaccine before being aware you were pregnant (you won't be immunised during pregnancy), the chances of it harming the baby are very low. A detailed ultrasound may be carried out at 18 weeks to check your baby's progress.

Symptoms
- Rash first appearing on the face and spreading to other parts of body
- Fever
- Swollen glands

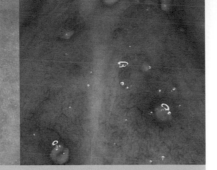

A rash is a symptom of both rubella (left) and chickenpox (right). Although most adults are immune to these diseases, they can cause serious complications if a woman becomes infected with them during pregnancy.

Treatment

If you contract rubella during pregnancy, the risk to your baby depends on when you caught it. If it was in the first month, there's a one-in-two chance the baby will be affected. By the third month, the risk drops to one in ten. Unfortunately, nothing can be done during the pregnancy to protect your baby. Your healthcare provider will explain your options and what tests are available.

Chickenpox and shingles

Both infections are caused by the varicella-zoster virus; chickenpox is the illness you get the first time you catch the virus, while shingles is a reactivation of it. Most adults in the United Kingdom have had chickenpox as a child, so have immunity to it, and won't get it again even if they are in contact with an infected person (though its best to avoid this). There's only a very small risk to a baby if the mother becomes infected early on in pregnancy (before 10 weeks). In 1 in every 100 cases, damage can occur to the eyes, limbs and brain of the baby, known as congenital varicella syndrome. Chickenpox just before delivery means the baby can be born with chickenpox, resulting in severe neonatal complications,

Symptoms
Take 10 days to three weeks from catching the virus:
- Itchy blister-type rash
- Fever
- Malaise
- Fatigue

Treatment

If you are pregnant, aren't immune to chickenpox and have been in contact with a case, let your doctor know as soon as possible. You will need a blood test to confirm you do not have antibodies to the virus so that you can be given an injection of immunoglobulin (called VZIG) to try to protect you from getting ill. Untreated, the disease can lead to a severe pneumonia in adults. If you do catch it, you also can be given antiviral drugs to treat the infection.

Yeast infections

As mucus production increases in pregnancy, a greater vaginal discharge is usual. As long as the discharge is thin and white – although it may be yellow when dry – it's probably normal. However, hormonal changes in pregnancy can encourage microorganisms in the vagina to overgrow, resulting in yeast infections caused by a fungus called candida albicans. Candida is very common – 25 per cent of women have it in their vaginas.

Symptoms
- Thick, curd-like, white discharge
- Burning sensation while urinating
- Redness and itching of the vulva

Treatment

While candida won't affect your pregnancy, if the infection isn't treated, your baby can contract oral yeast (thrush) while passing through your vagina at birth. Candida can be treated by vaginal creams, ointments, suppositories and oral medication. Many of these are available over the counter, but before using any medication, check with your healthcare provider. To alleviate symptoms and prevent candida from occurring, avoid feminine hygiene sprays and scented bath products, cut down on carbohydrates and sugar, wear cotton underwear and cotton gusset tights, and avoid tight-fitting garments. Always wipe from front to back after going to the toilet. Eating live yogurt (containing lactobacillus acidophilus) each day can help to reduce the risk.

Urinary tract infections (UTIs)

UTIs include infections of the bladder and the kidneys, the ureters (the tubes that lead from the kidneys to the bladder), and the urethra (the tube that carries urine from the bladder to outside of the body). UTIs are very common in pregnancy. Infection can be mild to severe, ranging from bacteria in the urine to kidney infection. As UTIs can be present and not lead to any symptoms, urine specimens are routinely tested throughout pregnancy. If bacteria are found, antibiotics can stop a mild infection from affecting the kidneys.

Symptoms

- An urgent need to urinate
- A sharp pain or burning sensation on urination
- Very little urine is eliminated, and it may be tinged with blood, be cloudy or smell bad
- The need to urinate returns minutes later
- Soreness may occur in the lower abdomen, in the back or in the sides
- Back pain, chills, fever, nausea and vomiting if infection spreads to kidneys

Treatment

Untreated UTIs can trigger contractions and possibly premature birth. You should contact your doctor, as antibiotics are usually necessary. To help to prevent a recurrence, drink plenty of water to help to flush bacteria from your system. Empty your bladder frequently and, as you do so, lean forwards on the toilet to make sure that the bladder is completely emptied – stagnant urine is the perfect breeding ground for bacteria. Fresh cranberry juice can help, too, as it makes urine more acidic and so less agreeable to bacteria.

Group B streptococcus (GBS)

This normally harmless bacteria is found in the vagina of one in ten healthy women. It can be transmitted to the baby during delivery and may

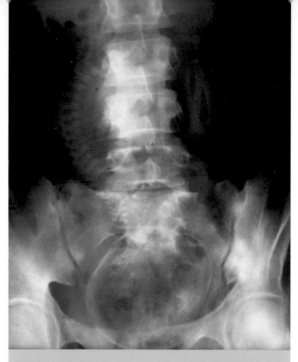

Pressure from the baby, seen here on this colour-enhanced X-ray in the head-down position in the pelvis, sometimes causes the symphysis pubis joint (below the baby's head) to separate.

cause serious illness (see page 363). For this reason, women who are found to be GBS carriers should be treated with antibiotics during labour.

Joint problems

Carpal tunnel syndrome

The carpal tunnel, in front of the wrist, houses the tendons and nerves that run to the fingers. If the hand and fingers swell in pregnancy, in common with other tissues, the carpal tunnel swells, too, putting pressure on a nerve resulting in the sensation of pins and needles spreading down into all the fingers except the little finger. The symptoms of carpal tunnel syndrome tend to be worse at night, but usually ease during the day as the joints are used and become more supple.

Symptoms

- Pain in the wrist
- Pins and needles extending from wrist down into hand
- Stiffness of fingers and joints of hand

Treatment

Sleeping with your hands raised on a pillow can prevent fluid from building up. On waking, dropping your hands over the side of the bed and giving them a vigorous shake can help to disperse fluid and ease any stiffness. Wearing splints on the wrists can help, also. This condition should disappear in the days following delivery.

Symphysis pubis dysfunction

The pelvic girdle is made up of three bones – one at the back and two at the front – joined by ligaments. The bones meet to form three 'fixed' joints, one at the front, called the symphysis pubis, and one at each side of the base of the spine. In pregnancy, the hormone relaxin loosens all the pelvic ligaments to allow the baby easier passage at birth. However, these ligaments can loosen too much, making the pelvis move, especially when weight is put on it. The weight of the baby makes this worse and sometimes the symphysis pubis joint actually separates slightly. The result is mild to severe pain in the pubic area called symphysis pubis dysfunction (SPD). This condition can develop at any time from the first trimester onward. It can also occur if you've been immobile for a long time or if you are overactive or after an activity such as swimming breaststroke or lifting something incorrectly.

Symptoms

- Pain, usually in the pubis and/or the lower back, but can be in the groin, inner thighs, hips and buttocks
- Pain is made worse when weight is on one leg
- A sensation of the pelvis separating
- Difficulty when walking

Treatment

Unfortunately, SPD is untreatable during pregnancy as it's due to the effect of hormones. The condition should improve, however, as your body returns to its pre-pregnancy state. In the meantime great care should be taken not to make SPD worse. Avoid putting weight on one leg as

much as possible – sit down to get dressed, get into the car by putting your buttocks on the seat first, and then lifting your legs into the car. Avoid breaststroke when swimming and keep your knees together when turning over in bed. If the pain is severe, ask your healthcare provider about painkillers and arrange to see a physiotherapist, who may advise a pelvic support belt.

Special care needs to be taken during labour and birth. Your legs need to be kept as close together as possible. Good birth positions are on all fours, kneeling up against the back of the bed, or side-lying with the top leg supported.

Problems with baby

Sometimes a baby seems to be growing too slowly or too rapidly. Both can cause problems. How well a baby grows can be affected by a number of factors. For example, if you smoke, your baby will generally be smaller than average, while if you have diabetes you are likely to have a larger baby. If abnormal growth is suspected, ultrasound can accurately measure your baby's size and growth for your dates. It also can be used to look for the amount of fluid around the baby; both too little and too much are problemmatical.

Finally, there may be problems with the cord at delivery or the baby become distressed.

Baby too small

A very small baby may move less often, will practise its breathing less and may be less active. In conjunction with a heart-rate trace from the baby, these features comprise the biophysical profile (BPP). A normal BPP suggests that the baby is currently healthy.

Another very useful test when trying to decide whether a poorly growing or small baby is healthy is the umbilical artery Doppler estimation. This is also an ultrasound scan and can tell how fast the blood moves along the umbilical cord. When the speed is reduced it suggests that the placenta isn't functioning well.

When making a decision about delivery, how mature your baby is, how ill he is suspected to be, and your health are factors that will be considered. Some very ill babies will need to be delivered by Caesarean. If your baby is ill and needs to be delivered prematurely, you may be given steroid injections to help his lungs mature.

Baby too big

Taller or heavier mothers tend to have larger babies than shorter or lighter mothers. But there are some serious conditions that cause a baby to become over-large. The most common is diabetes.

Many mothers worry about whether they'll be capable of delivering a large baby. Ultrasound isn't always very accurate in the measurement of large babies, and, in assessment of a baby's weight, there's about a 10 per cent error. If your baby is big and you are near the end of your pregnancy you may be offered an induction of labour, to try to deliver your baby before he becomes even bigger. If your baby is large for your dates but you still have some time to go before the birth, it's best to discuss a plan with your doctor.

Polyhydramnios (hydramnios)

About 2 per cent of pregnant women have too much amniotic fluid, a condition known as polyhydramnios. Most cases are mild and are a result of a gradual build-up of fluid during the second half of pregnancy. About half the time, polyhydramnios goes away and women will deliver healthy babies with no problems. Rarely, polyhydramnios can be a warning sign that there's a birth defect or that a medical problem such as gestational diabetes has developed.

Polyhydramnios may also occur in conditions that cause fetal anaemia or certain viral infections. If polyhydramnios is severe, it may make the uterus contract and trigger premature labour.

Symptoms
- Larger than normal uterus
- Abdominal discomfort
- Indigestion
- Swelling in the legs
- Breathlessness

Treatment
Polyhydramnios is normally diagnosed with ultrasound. If the condition is advanced, amniocentesis may be performed to remove excess fluid. If membranes rupture, there's a risk of cord prolapse (the cord is delivered before the baby), so you should contact your caregiver immediately.

Oligohydramnios

This is a condition in which there's too little amniotic fluid in the uterus. Most women with this condition will have a normal pregnancy, but occasionally it can signal or result in problems. Fluid will decrease if the placenta is functioning poorly. In early pregnancy there is a slight risk of the baby developing talipes (club foot) because there isn't enough room for normal growth. Later in pregnancy it can be a sign of fetal distress. Rarely it accompanies some form of fetal defect, such as problems with the kidneys or bladder. If oligohydramnios lasts for several weeks of

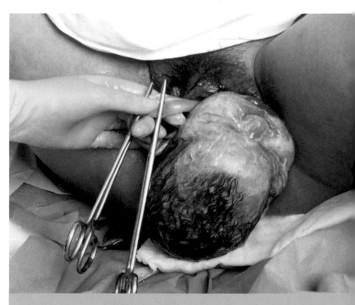

Sometimes the umbilical cord becomes wrapped around the baby's neck and immediate delivery is necessary. When this occurs, the cord is clamped and then cut as soon as the head is born.

pregnancy, it can lead to pulmonary hypoplasia (underdevelopment of the fetal lungs).

Symptoms
- The uterus may be smaller than average
- Less frequent fetal movement
- Slowed growth

Treatment
Reduced amniotic fluid around your baby s normally picked on an ultrasound scan. Further tests will be done to assess the baby's growth or well-being. Any concerns may lead to your baby being delivered earlier than expected so that labour may need to be induced. Caesarean section is also more likely as there is less fluid to cushion the baby during labour, resulting in fetal heart rate abnormalities.

Knotted cord
Sometimes the umbilical cord becomes knotted or tangled in the uterus, even wrapping around the baby's neck or other part of the his body. A cord around the neck is common, appearing in up to 30 per cent of all births. It usually doesn't prove a problem, but if the cord gets compressed, it can cause drops or decelerations in the fetal heart rate. Again, this usually is not a problem but if the heart rate remains low, delivery may need to be expedited.

Symptoms
- Decrease in fetal activity
- Variable deceleration in the fetal heart tracing

Treatment
An immediate delivery, usually by Caesarean.

Cord prolapse
Rarely, the baby's umbilical cord can fall into the birth canal ahead of the baby's head or other parts of the baby's body. A prolapsed cord can be very harmful to the baby. When the cord is squeezed, the baby's supply of blood and oxygen is cut off, which can have very serious consequences.

Prolapse is more likely to happen: if polyhydramnios is present; during delivery of the second baby of twins; if the baby is breech or in a transverse lie; or if the membranes rupture, either naturally or during a vaginal examination before the baby descends into the pelvis.

Symptoms
- Decreased fetal heart rate

Treatment
If the cord is still pulsating and can be seen or felt in the vagina, the doctor will support the part of the baby delivering first to take pressure off the cord. To assist with this you may have to get on your knees and bend forward. The doctor will keep a hand in the vagina until the baby is delivered the fastest way possible – by Caesarean or possibly with forceps or vacuum extractor.

Fetal distress
Used to describe any situation in which the unborn baby is thought to be in jeopardy – usually through decreased oxygen flow – distress can be caused by a variety of problems including: maternal illness such as hyper- or hypotension or heart disease; a placenta that is no longer functioning well or has separated prematurely from the uterus; umbilical cord compression or entanglement; fetal infection or malformation and prolonged or excessive labour contractions.

Symptoms
- A change in fetal movements
- Absence of fetal movement
- Fetal heartbeat changes

Treatment
Immediate delivery is usually recommended. If vaginal delivery is not imminent, then an emergency Caesarean is likely to be performed. The mother may first be given medication to slow contractions, which will increase oxygen to the baby, and to dilate her blood vessels, which will improve blood flow to the baby.

Pre-existing medical conditions

If you had a medical condition before you became pregnant, it may affect the way your pregnancy is managed. Your healthcare provider will want to ensure that your treatment is safe for you and your baby. Sometimes special precautions are necessary, and you may require more frequent antenatal checks.

Respiratory diseases
Asthma
This is the most common respiratory disease encountered in pregnant women, occurring in between 1 and 4 per cent of all pregnancies. The effect of pregnancy on asthma is highly variable, causing symptoms to worsen in 22 per cent, improve in 29 per cent, and remain unchanged in the remainder of cases. In general, asthma tends to improve from 36 weeks, and it is highly unusual to suffer a severe asthma attack during labour. In well-controlled asthma, there is little or no effect on the pregnancy.

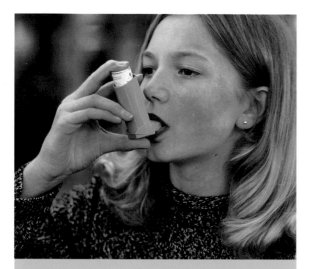

There is no evidence to suggest that the use of asthma inhaler pumps can cause any harm to your baby during pregnancy.

Management
If you have asthma, it can worsen in pregnancy if you don't continue to use your usual medication. You can continue to use an asthma inhaler pump, and even if steroid tablets are needed to control asthma, they won't do any harm. Long-term use of steroids can very occasionally cause high blood pressure or raised sugar levels, but both of these can be treated.

Immune disorders
Anti-phospholipid syndrome (APS)
Also known as lupus, APS is an autoimmune disorder in which antibodies that harm the body are made. The antibodies make the blood sticky and can cause small or large blood clots. This syndrome may also accompany another disorder called systemic lupus erythematosus (SLE) and it's then called secondary anti-phospholipid syndrome. APS is a serious condition as it can cause miscarriage, pre-eclampsia, blood clots, as well as stillbirth.

Management
APS can be treated with low-dose aspirin – 75 mg daily – and, for some women, daily injections of heparin. If you have this condition, you will need to be treated by an obstetrician who will closely monitor your pregnancy and the growth of your baby. It is important to discuss your condition with your healthcare provider as soon as pregnancy is confirmed, as with the correct treatment the chance of a successful pregnancy is high, whereas without treatment, over 70 per cent of pregnancies will miscarry.

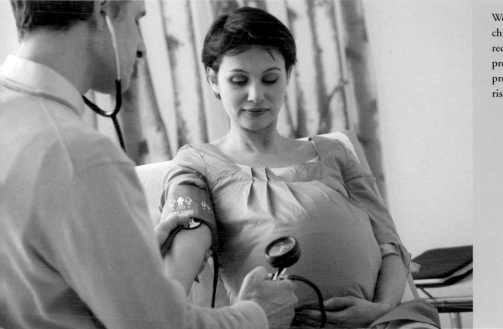

Women who suffer from chronic hypertension require frequent blood pressure checks during pregnancy because of the risk of pre-eclampsia.

Circulation/blood disorders
Chronic hypertension

If you already had high blood pressure before you got pregnant, the condition is described as chronic hypertension. This is more common in women over the age of 40, Afro-Caribbean women, and those with mothers or sisters with high blood pressure. Certain medical conditions can make hypertension more likely, such as diabetes, renal disease and being overweight.

The main risk of hypertension in pregnancy is the increased risk of developing pre-eclampsia (see page 253). In women with pre-existing hypertension, the risk of developing pre-eclampsia is around 20 per cent. In general, unless pre-eclampsia develops, the risks of hypertension to the mother and baby are small.

Management
As your pregnancy will be considered high-risk, you will be referred to a hospital specialist to monitor your pregancy. You are likely to have more checks and tests than usual. It's important to discuss your medication with your doctor as early on as possible, as certain blood-pressure drugs

aren't safe in pregnancy. Your blood pressure is likely to decrease in the first three months. As the pregnancy progresses it's not unusual to need to increase the medication or even add in a second or even third type of drug.

With hypertension, it's important to have expert medical supervision and to take good care of yourself, which means following a low-salt diet, getting plenty of rest and doing relaxation exercises such as yoga. This way you're increasing your chances of a healthy pregnancy.

Heart disease

Most women have healthy hearts. Although no longer common today in the UK, in the past, the most common form of heart disease was due to an infection called rheumatic fever, which can damage the heart valves. Some women may have experienced it as children if they were brought up in a developing country.

If you or your partner were born with a heart defect you should mention this to your caregiver at your first antenatal visit. It may be that the only precaution that is required is to give you antibiotics during childbirth to prevent you getting an infection in your heart. On the other hand, if you have a complex abnormality, it may be that pregnancy will have some danger. A detailed scan of your baby's heart can usually show if she has inherited a similar problem.

You can be referred for genetic counselling prior to conception.

Management

If you've had rheumatic heart disease, you'll probably have a replacement heart valve. If so, the main problem with pregnancy is the management of your anticoagulation. You will probably be on warfarin to stop a clot forming in your heart around the new valve. Warfarin is a very useful drug but shouldn't be used between weeks 6 and 14 of pregnancy, so your cardiologists will change to a form of heparin. This is another anticoagulant that can only be given by daily injection but doesn't cross the placenta. Some doctors continue the heparin until delivery; others prefer to put women back onto warfarin from 14 to 36 weeks and then change back to heparin again until delivery.

Sickle cell disease

An inherited abnormality of the red blood cells, sickle cell disease occurs predominantly in Afro-Caribbean people and developed as a natural protection against malaria. If you inherit sickle cell from just one parent, it has little effect upon your health but protects you to a certain extent from malaria. If you inherit sickle cell from both parents, you can become unwell with the disease.

Sickle cell disease causes problems with joint pains and anaemia, which start from childhood. Pregnancy can be a special problem as it puts extra stress on the body and can precipitate sickle crisis. Common complications include joint pains, breathlessness, chest pain and chest infection for the mother, and growth restriction and premature delivery for your baby.

Management

Your healthcare providers will work together with you to monitor your pregnancy closely and decide when blood transfusions are useful. You will continue to be treated with folic acid and penicillin throughout the pregnancy, and you're likely to be induced at 38 weeks' gestation.

Sexually transmitted diseases
Bacterial vaginosis (BV)

While BV is classified as a sexually transmitted disease (STD), you don't have to be sexually active to get this vaginal infection. You may be tested for BV at your first antenatal visit. If BV is left untreated there may be an increased risk of premature delivery. The main symptoms are a watery white or grey discharge, which has a highly unpleasant or fishy smell. However, it's possible to have BV and not experience any symptoms.

Management

BV is usually treated with antibiotics, but it can also be treated with vaginal creams.

Chlamydia

This is a bacterium that is generally transmitted by sexual intercourse. The symptoms in men can be minimal which means that they may not be aware that they're infected – although infected men may suffer pain when passing urine. In women, the symptoms can be nonexistent, although some women have a vaginal discharge and may experience pain on passing urine. Sometimes women experience severe pelvic pain and become unwell with acute pelvic inflammatory disease. The severity of the symptoms doesn't appear to be related to the risk of the long-term effect of infertility.

Management

If you have had chlamydia in the past, and both you and your partner have been treated so that there's no risk of reinfection, the only concern in pregnancy is how the infection may affect your Fallopian tubes. If your Fallopian tubes have been damaged, you may suffer an increased risk of an ectopic pregnancy. If you have progressed beyond 12 weeks of pregnancy, or you have had a scan showing the pregnancy is situated in your uterus and is not ectopic, the previous infection will have no detrimental effect on the pregnancy.

If you have untreated chlamydia in pregnancy there's a slight increase of premature birth and a small risk that your baby may become infected during delivery. If she's infected he may develop a sticky, infected eye, and then, between one and three weeks after delivery, she may develop a chest infection. Chlamydia in pregnancy should be treated with erythromycin not tetracycline, as the latter can affect your baby's tooth and bone development.

Hepatitis B

This viral liver infection is carried in blood and body secretions and is most commonly transmitted by having sex with an infected person, infection during childbirth, or using contaminated needles. If you've been infected you're likely to carry the virus forever and remain infectious to others. In the long term, hepatitis B can cause liver damage. In some parts of the world, such as West Africa and Southeast Asia, hepatitis B is widespread as the virus can be passed from mothers to their unborn baby.

Management

If you are a hepatitis B carrier, you should be referred to a liver specialist for monitoring during pregnancy. Your partner should be tested as well, as he can be immunised against this virus if he hasn't already caught it. Hepatitis B can be transmitted to your baby at the time of birth, but this can be prevented from developing by giving your baby a course of vaccinations, starting immediately after the birth. This will protect your baby when breastfeeding.

Herpes simplex virus (HSV)

There are two types of herpes simplex virus: type 1 typically affects the lips and causes cold sores, and type 2 affects the genitalia. Both types can be transmitted by close contact such as kissing or sexual intercourse. In both types you will suffer

from small painful ulcers on the skin, which can occur at any time but typically are preceded by a tingling feeling. If your partner has an active HSV lesion on his penis, he should wear a condom during intercourse so you don't become infected. This is especially important during pregnancy.

Management

If you have genital herpes it can be transmitted to your baby during childbirth. This is usually only a problem if you have your first ever attack during childbirth. If you already have HSV, your body will have developed antibodies, which will be transmitted to your baby before she's born and therefore give her protection until she's three months old. If your baby is affected by HSV during childbirth she could develop a brain infection known as encephalitis. This presents as lethargy and poor feeding but can develop into a life-threatening illness.

To protect your baby, most doctors recommend a Caesarean if you have your first ever attack of HSV in labour and the membranes haven't ruptured. If you have a recurrent attack, which is much more common, the advice is less certain, but most doctors will still recommend a Caesarean. The risk of your baby becoming unwell is less than 1 in 100. Some doctors

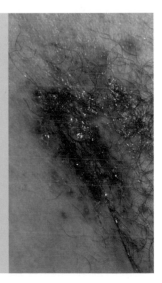

Type 2 herpes simplex virus affects the genitalia and the area around the groin. It can be seen here as an inflamed area with crusting yellow scabs.

recommend prophylactic oral Aciclovir – an antiviral medicine – from 36 weeks gestation to keep you from having an outbreak around the time of delivery.

Human immunodeficiency virus (HIV)/AIDS

Unprotected intercourse is the most common form of transmission of HIV/AIDS, but it can also be transmitted by the use of contaminated needles, through a blood transfusion with infected blood, and during childbirth.

Management

If you have HIV – commonly known as being HIV positive – and you are not on treatment, there's a 15 to 25 per cent risk that your baby will become infected. With appropriate treatment, this risk can be reduced to 1 to 2 per cent. Treatment consists of anti-retroviral medication, Caesarean delivery in some situations, and refraining from breastfeeding. In some circumstances, for example, if you're on HAART regime and your viral load is undetectable, vaginal delivery may be just as safe for your baby. If you're on treatment before you get pregnant, your doctor may suggest changing your regime. If you're put on just one drug during pregnancy – usually zidovudine – you can usually stop treatment after delivery.

Pregnant women should be offered screening for HIV early in pregnancy because appropriate antenatal intervention can reduce maternal-to-child transmission of the infection. They also should be screened for other genital infections as early as possible, and again later in pregnancy. Women diagnosed as HIV positive during pregnancy should be managed by a multi-disciplinary team.

Understandably, confidentiality may be an important issue for women with HIV, so if are affected, you will need to decide who you want involved in discussions about your care. Your usual healthcare provider will need to know about your treatment as he or she will be concerned with your and your baby's long-term care.

Syphilis

You'll be offered testing for this disease at your first antenatal visit; however, the good news is that the instances of syphilis in pregnancy are currently lower than ever.

Treatment

A course of antibiotic treatment given in the first trimester is usually successful in preventing any harm to the baby.

Trichomonias vaginalis

While this STD isn't too serious, it can increase the risk of premature delivery so it is very important to have treatment. It's also often associated with other sexually transmitted diseases, particulary syphilis and HIV. The main symptoms are a greenish, frothy vaginal discharge with a fishy smell, and itching.

Management

An oral medication is usually given, which is safe for use in pregnancy.

Neurological disorders
Epilepsy

If you have epilepsy, the chances are that you'll enjoy an uncomplicated pregnancy. Seizures (fits) rarely harm a baby but are best avoided. Morning sickness can make it difficult to take your usual medication so you need to contact your doctor if you are can't keep anything down.

Management

Ideally, see your doctor prior to conception so that your medication can be reduced, if possible, and altered to the best combination for pregnancy. There's an increased risk of having a baby with an abnormality (such as spina bifida or cleft palate) and this can be reduced by taking an increased dose of folic acid (4 mg daily) for three months before you get pregnant and continuing until the baby is born. If you're already pregnant, it's important to see your doctor as early as possible to check you are on the best anti-epileptic drugs

(AEDs). If your seizures get more frequent, you may need a higher dose. You will be offered extra scans to check that your baby is developing normally. Remember to take your AEDs during labour and delivery at the right time to prevent a seizure occurring during the birth. Some AEDs affect your ability to absorb vitamin K, so you may be prescribed vitamin tablets from 36 weeks of pregnancy. Your baby should have the vitamin K injection after delivery (see page 286).

Multiple sclerosis

A degenerative neurological condition of unknown origin, multiple sclerosis (MS) consists of relapses and periods of remission. There is no evidence that pregnancy affects the long-term prognosis of MS, although relapse after delivery isn't uncommon.

Management

While MS doesn't appear to affect pregnancy, regular antenatal care is important. You can be more prone to anaemia and infections such as UTIs (see page 260). Keep yourself as healthy as possible by getting plenty of rest and avoid stress and overheating. If you're on medication, check with your healthcare provider that it's safe to take in pregnancy, as some MS medications aren't.

Infections

Chronic fatigue syndrome

Also known as myalgic encephalopathy (ME), this is a chronic debilitating illness that appears to start after a viral infection, although the nature of the infection and the cause of the chronic fatigue are unknown. If you have ME, you will need to discuss any medication you are taking – including herbal and homeopathic – with your healthcare provider in case it could have a detrimental effect on your pregnancy.

Management

Some women with ME find that their symptoms improve during the pregnancy, possibly as a result of the hormonal changes; but they tend to suffer a relapse after delivery. The delivery itself can be daunting. You need to plan well and consider an epidural to reduce the stress and tiredness that a long painful labour can bring. There's no reason why you shouldn't try for a normal delivery, but you may need help in the second stage if you're too exhausted to push.

The important thing to consider with ME is ensuring that you have sufficient support during the pregnancy, which you are likely to find very tiring, and especially after delivery. Don't hesitate to accept offers of help from your partner, mother, sisters and friends.

Other chronic conditions
Diabetes

This is a tendency to have high blood sugar levels. This condition can also develop during pregnancy (gestational diabetes, see page 253). Whether your

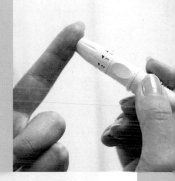

A home testing kit can be used to measure your glucose levels. A drop of blood is drawn from your finger, using a small lancing device (right). The blood drop is applied to the target area of the electrode and the monitor displays your glucose result (bottom).

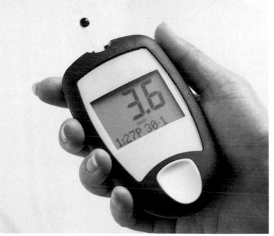

diabetes is controlled with tablets or with insulin injections, the risks for your baby are similar. The main risks for the baby – apart from the increased risk of abnormalities – are macrosomia (growing too large) and stillbirth. The main risks for you are hyperglycaemia (sugar going too high) and hypoglycaemia (sugar going too low), which is common if you're suffering morning sickness. You're also at increased risk of pre-eclampsia. Because of the risk of stillbirth, many obstetricians will recommend delivery by 38–39 weeks and will suggest that if you haven't delivered by then you should be induced.

Management
It's vital that you control your sugar levels prior to and in the first few months after conception, as this will decrease the chance of your baby developing an abnormality. Once you're pregnant, tablets normally will be switched to insulin injections. The aim during pregnancy is to control your sugar levels as tightly as possible, achieving a 2-hour post-meal sugar level of less than 7 mmol/L. Increasing the number of daily injections from two to four often achieves this. The amount of insulin you need increases every week as the placenta grows, up until about 34 weeks.

It's important to have a healthy, balanced, stable diet to help you to predict how much insulin you will need. Don't worry if you need to increase your dose of insulin, it doesn't mean you're eating too much; insulin requirements will increase as your pregnancy progresses.

Kidney failure
Many women have problems with their kidneys. Most are relatively minor problems such as urinary infections and cystitis (see page 260), but more serious problems such as kidney failure can occur. If you have kidney failure, the way it affects your pregnancy will largely depend on the severity of your condition.

Management
Women with kidney failure should discuss the implications of pregnancy with their renal physician and a maternal-fetal medicine specialist. The chance of a successful pregnancy depends on how well your kidneys are working. If you have had a transplant and your new kidney is working well then you have an excellent chance of having a healthy baby. Most drugs used to prevent rejection are safe for use in pregnancy; your healthcare provider should be able to advise you about any medication you are taking.

If you're awaiting transplant and you're on dialysis the results aren't as good. Many women on dialysis don't even manage to get pregnant, and those who do have difficult pregnancies, with most babies born very premature. Women with moderate kidney damage are at risk of pre-eclampsia and should discuss these risks with their healthcare provider to try to minimize the risks associated with this condition.

Thyroid disease
The thyroid gland can be overactive or underactive – both extremes are bad for your health and may affect your pregnancy. If your thyroid isn't working properly you are likely to be on medication to regain the balance. Although this shouldn't affect your pregnancy, your healthcare provider will monitor you closely until after your postnatal check.

Management
Hypothyroidism (an underactive thyroid) can be easily treated with replacement thyroxine. You should have your levels checked every three months during the pregnancy, but you're unlikely to need to have your dose changed.

If you have hyperthyroidism (an overactive thyroid) you may need treatment with carbimazole or propylthiouracil. Both these drugs control the activity of the thyroid. If you're first diagnosed in pregnancy you may need a large dose to start with, but this is usually reduced after a few months. Both drugs cross the placenta, and in

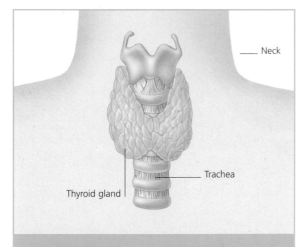

The thyroid gland is situated in the neck, and is responsible for the production of a hormone called thyroxin, which regulates your metabolism.

rare cases cause the baby to have a swollen thyroid gland and to become hypothyroid. Using the lowest effective dose reduces this risk.

If you have thyroid disease it's important to have your levels checked six weeks after delivery, as your thyroid can become inflamed at this stage – a condition known as postnatal thyroiditis – and your medication may need altering.

Rheumatoid arthritis (RA)

Many women with RA find the pain and swelling in their joints improves during pregnancy, particularly by the second trimester.

Management

Talk to your doctor about which medication is safe to take in pregnancy. Non-steroidal anti-inflammatory drugs like ibuprofen are not normally advisable after early pregnancy. Corticosteroids can safely be used in low or moderate doses throughout pregnancy. Hydroychloroquine and sulphasalazine can be continued, too. Methotrexate should be stopped at least three months prior to falling pregnant as it can cause birth defects. Newer drugs, such as anti-

TNF agents, can need specialist advice as their effects on pregnancy are unknown.

If your arthritis affects your hips or mobility, discuss with your healthcare provider how best to cope in labour.

Cancer

There is no indication that pregnancy directly affects the course of cancer, but it does add a complication, as the treatment you need may not be good for your baby. If the cancer is discovered after you are already pregnant you may have to consider whether to continue with the pregnancy. This will depend on the type of cancer, how advanced it is, and the effects the best treatment will have on you and your baby.

Management

During pregnancy your healthcare provider will need to find a balance between the treatment that's best for you and the safety of your baby. Chemotherapy during the first trimester increases the risk of birth defects. During the second and third trimesters, chemotherapy may lower your baby's birth weight, but the degree of risk for other complications varies depending on the medication used. Radiotherapy may or may not affect your baby, depending on the location of the cancer, the strength of the exposure and how advanced your pregnancy is. The most vulnerable period for your baby is between 8 and 15 weeks. Surgery is usually possible during pregnancy and does not often cause a risk to your baby. However, if inflammation or infection occur in the abdomen, this increases the risk of premature labour.

Medical emergencies

Most pregnancies are straightforward and proceed without any problems. Just occasionally, situations do occur that could put the mother and baby at risk. Fortunately, most of these, if detected early enough, can be successfully treated. If you've had an accident, don't feel well or something doesn't seem quite right, call your healthcare provider right away for advice.

Abdominal pain

The odd ache and mild transient discomfort is to be expected during pregnancy, but any persistent abdominal pain that causes discomfort or seems in any way out of the ordinary needs to be urgently evaluated by medical staff.

Sharp lower abdominal pains just to one side or both sides of the uterus, may just be stretching of the ligaments (round ligament pain) but could signal ectopic pregnancy, miscarriage, placental abruption or premature labour. Constant abdominal pain associated with hardening or tense feelings in the uterus is of particular concern and needs urgent treatment.

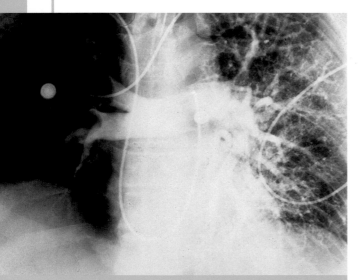

A pulmonary embolus – blood clot on the lung – (shown in an X-ray above) is a serious condition that needs urgent medical treatment.

In the first few weeks, the first sign of an ectopic pregnancy is often lower abdominal pain, cramping or a dull ache, which may just be one-sided or all around the abdomen. Shoulder pain and pain around the rectum, particularly on opening the bowels, often feature as well. Vaginal bleeding is common but normally not very heavy. Urgent hospital treatment is needed, because the internal bleeding can be very dangerous.

Later on in pregnancy, upper abdominal pain in the area of the liver (right side, just below the rib cage) could be a sign of serious pre-eclampsia and needs immediate medical assessment. It can also be a sign of gallstones or indigestion, which are obviously much less serious. However, this type of pain should never be ignored.

Groin pain or lower backache can be the sign of a kidney infection and needs to be treated urgently with strong antibiotics. A high fever or rigor (shivering attack) may accompany the pain, which indicates that treatment in hospital with intravenous antibiotics is needed.

Chest pain

A pain in the chest should never be ignored. It could indicate a pulmonary embolus (a blood clot in the lung) or pleurisy. Both conditions need urgent treatment.

Chills and fever

If you have a fever over 37.8°C (100°F) without other symptoms you should consult the doctor the same day. If your fever is over 38.9°C (102°F), or you have other symptoms such as a sore throat or shortness of breath or cough, you need immediate treatment, as you may have swine flu (see below) or an infection that requires antibiotics and rest. If the fever remains high for a prolonged length of time, the baby's development could be hindered.

Swine flu

This is a new strain of influenza so-named because it is thought to have originated in pigs (though this is not certain). Pregnant women are at particular risk because their immune systems are naturally suppressed; they are more likely to catch it, and if they do, they are more likely to develop complications. That being said, most pregnant women will only have mild symptoms and the risk of complications is very small.

Symptoms are similar to regular flu – a fever or high temperature (over 38°C/100.4°F) and two or more of the following: unusual tiredness, headache, runny nose, sore throat, shortness of breath or cough, loss of appetite, aching muscles, diarrhoea or vomiting. Recovery generally takes about a week but women who are in their second and third trimester are more likely to suffer possible complications including pneumonia (an infection of the lungs), difficulty breathing, and dehydration, and these can lead to premature labour or miscarriage.

You can reduce your risk of infection by being vaccinated (see below), practising good hygiene habits and avoiding unnecessary travel and crowds where possible. If a family member or other close contact has swine flu, your doctor may prescribe you antiviral medication (usually Relenza) as a preventative measure.

If you think that you (or someone close to you) may have swine flu, call your doctor for an assessment immediately. If your doctor confirms swine flu over the phone, you will be prescribed antiviral medication to take as soon as possible and advised how and where to pick it up. Do not attend the surgery. You will usually be given a course of antiviral drugs, which should be taken as soon as possible. Relenza, which is inhaled using a disk-shaped inhaler, is recommended for pregnant women because it easily reaches the throat and lungs, where it is needed, and does not reach significant levels in the blood or placenta. It should not affect your pregnancy or your growing baby. However, Tamiflu should be offered to you if you have a condition such as asthma or chronic obstructive pulmonary disease, have difficulty taking an inhaled antiviral, or develop a severe or complicated disease due to influenza (where you will probably be treated in hospital).

You can also take paracetamol to reduce fever and other symptoms.

Pregnant women are advised to have the swine flu vaccination, Pandemrix, whatever the stage of their pregnancy. There is no evidence that this vaccine, which is inactivated, will cause any harm to pregnant women or their unborn babies.

Excessive lower leg puffiness (oedema) or excessive weight gain

These symptoms shouldn't be overlooked as they can be associated with pre-eclampsia.

Excessive vomiting and/or diarrhoea

Contact your doctor if you keep being sick or have diarrhoea. There's a risk of dehydration if you can't keep anything down, while excessive diarrhoea depletes you of body fluids, which is dangerous. You may need to go to the hospital and have an IV to replace lost fluids. If the vomiting is accompanied by fever, or the diarrhoea contains blood or mucus, call your doctor immediately.

Fall or car accident

Falls aren't always harmful, as the baby is well protected inside the uterus, surrounded by amniotic fluid, but if you do fall over, call your healthcare provider as soon as you can and explain what happened. If you experience contractions, leaking fluid, or any bleeding, call your healthcare provider right away.

Headaches, flashing lights in front of the eyes or double vision

These are all indications of pre-eclampsia and dangerously high blood pressure and require urgent hospital treatment.

Heavy vaginal bleeding

A small amount of painless vaginal bleeding in the early weeks of pregnancy is common (see page 20). So, too, are spotting and staining in the early months (see page 275). However, bleeding that occurs after the first trimester or is heavy, should be evaluated by your healthcare provider. Any bleeding associated with pain could indicate a miscarriage (see page 278) or ectopic pregnancy (see page 255), so you should contact your doctor urgently. Very heavy vaginal bleeding or bleeding associated with severe pain needs immediate attention, and you should go straight to the accident and emergency department.

Itching all over

This may be a sign of obstetric cholestasis (see page 255) especially if there is jaundice (yellow skin and dark urine). There's no danger to the mother, but there is an increased risk to the baby. For this reason, doctors advise close monitoring of the baby if cholestasis is diagnosed, and normally an early delivery is recommended.

Leaking of fluid from the vagina

This should be reported immediately, because this could be a leakage of amniotic fluid and indicate that the membranes have ruptured. This could be a sign of premature labour and leaves the baby exposed to infection.

Painful or burning urination, with fever, chills and backache

You may have a urinary tract infection, a condition that should be treated with antibiotics.

Seizures (fits)

If a pregnant woman known to have epilepsy has a prolonged seizure, immediate hospital assessment is recommended. However, an unexpected seizure could be a result of eclampsia, which is a medical emergency and requires oxygen and drugs to prevent any further seizures occurring. Call the emergency services without delay as urgent delivery of the baby is usually required to enable proper treatment of the mother.

Slowing or absence of fetal movements

Feeling the baby move usually occurs at around 16 to 20 weeks of pregnancy. After 28 weeks you should be aware of at least ten movements every day. If your baby seems to have been less active over the last 24 hours, or there have been fewer than ten movements over a period of 12 hours during the day, call your doctor and go straight to the hospital for evaluation. Your baby's heartbeat will be recorded for 20 to 30 minutes on a fetal monitor to ensure that all is well. Reduced fetal movements can be a sign that the baby is under stress, so should never be ignored. On the other hand, the vast majority of babies start to move vigorously as soon as fetal monitoring begins, and there is nothing wrong.

Swollen or painful leg

A painfully swollen leg that's warm to the touch may be a deep vein thrombosis (DVT). Call your healthcare provider immediately if you suspect you may have this condition (see page 252). It can be confused with the common and harmless condition of superficial thrombophlebitis – that affects the small surface veins in the lower legs which become rather red and sore in pregnancy, especially if you are overweight. Ultrasound will distinguish between the two conditions.

Thirst and infrequent urination

If you experience a sudden increase in thirst accompanied by little or no urination, this could be a sign of dehydration or kidney failure, both potentially dangerous conditions for mother and baby. Contact your doctor, who will then arrange for you to be evaluated.

Bleeding in pregnancy

Approximately one-in-four women will experience vaginal bleeding during their pregnancies. The bleeding can vary from spotting or staining to a substantial blood loss that requires urgent hospital treatment. While it's important to treat any bleeding in pregnancy seriously, remember that in at least 90 per cent of cases no harm is going to come to the pregnancy.

Early bleeding (before 12 weeks)

Bleeding or spotting in the first few weeks of pregnancy is particularly common but doesn't necessarily mean that there's a problem. A good indicator is the amount of pain associated with the bleeding. Painless vaginal bleeding is much less of a concern than bleeding that is associated with cramping lower abdominal pain and/or backache over several hours. If you have vaginal bleeding, your healthcare provider will carry out various investigations. You may have a pelvic examination, an ultrasound, or a blood test in order to measure levels of the pregnancy hormones human chorionic gonadotropin (hCG) and progesterone. As the pregnancy progresses, hCG levels increase, so you may have to have more than one test. Often no cause for the bleeding can be found and the pregnancy continues without any problems. A small number of women go on to experience slight bleeding on and off throughout their pregnancies for no obvious reason.

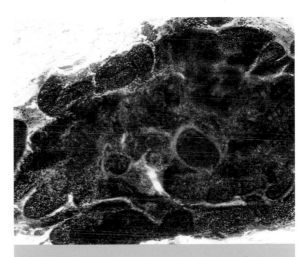

Cervical ectropion occurs when a layer of cells normally found on the inner lining of the cervix appear on the outside. Above can be seen abnormal cell growth caused by cervical ectropion.

Implantation bleed

Occasionally a small amount of vaginal bleeding occurs for 24 to 48 hours as the fertilized egg implants itself into the wall of the uterus around ten days after conception. This is a natural process and is of no concern.

Hormonal bleeding

Some women experience a light period-like bleed at around four and eight weeks of pregnancy, just at the time that their period would have occurred. This is why some women don't realize that they are pregnant.

Cervical ectropion

Spotting during early pregnancy may be caused by a cervical ectropion, which occurs when the cells on the inner lining of the cervix extend onto its surface and become inflamed. Bleeding can occur after sexual intercourse because the cervix is softer and more delicate during pregnancy. Unless an infection is suspected, a cervical ectropion won't affect your pregnancy.

Later bleeding

Vaginal bleeding in pregnancy between 12 to 24 weeks is much less common than in the first three months. Miscarriage at this stage in pregnancy is considerably less likely. Later miscarriages – after 20 weeks – may be a result of an infection or an abnormality in the uterus, such as an incompetent cervix (see page 279), or in the placenta.

Bleeding after 24 weeks of pregnancy should always be reported to your healthcare provider. Often there's no cause for concern if the bleeding is light, particularly if it has occurred after sexual intercourse or an internal examination. However, admission to the hospital for observation for 24 hours is normal if a woman reports vaginal bleeding, especially if any pain is associated with the bleeding.

Any woman who has a Rhesus negative blood group after twelve weeks of pregnancy should receive anti-D immunoglobulin in the event of bleeding, to protect against forming antibodies against the fetal blood.

The following conditions should be investigated if bleeding occurs later in pregnancy:

Marginal placental bleed

Painless bleeding can occur as a result of a rupture in one of the small blood vessels at the edge of the placenta. Usually the bleeding settles quickly, although a small blood clot can form near the cervix and lead to a brownish vaginal loss for a few days afterwards. Sometimes it can be painful, as the blood irritates the uterus and causes mild contractions. There is no undue cause for concern, and rest and observation are usually prescribed.

Placenta praevia

When the placenta lies low in the uterus, it can partly or completely cover the cervix. Many women are told that they have placenta praevia (a low-lying placenta) when they attend a routine 20 weeks' scan, but during the last few weeks of pregnancy the placenta tends to move up so that it no longer blocks the cervix. However, in 1 per cent of pregnancies, the placenta remains covering

In placenta praevia, the placenta lies low in the uterus and may partially, or completely, cover the cervix (see right). There is a risk to both the mother and baby from excessive bleeding.

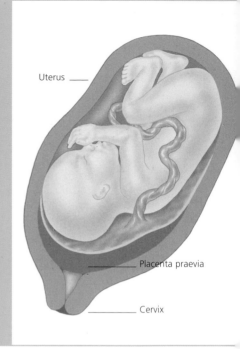

Uterus

Placenta praevia

Cervix

the cervix. In this position the placenta is less well attached to the uterine wall and is more likely to bleed from one or more of the huge number of blood vessels that cross the placental surface. Fortunately, although it can be heavy, the bleeding often stops of its own accord. You'll be advised to rest in hospital from 34 weeks until the baby is born so that you can be treated quickly should you bleed again.

Placenta praevia is more likely to occur in women who have had more than one child or a Caesarean delivery, or who are carrying twins or triplets. Bleeding is usually painless but can be extremely heavy. It may start lightly enough as an early warning but suddenly become very heavy, requiring emergency treatment for the mother, including a blood transfusion.

Vasa praevia

A related condition to the above, blood vessels in the umbilical cord may run through the membranes covering the cervix and when the membranes rupture and the waters break, the vessels too may tear resulting in vaginal bleeding.

As a result of this rare condition (about 1 in 3000 to 6000 births), a baby can lose and great deal of blood and may even die. It is difficult to diagnose but may be spotted on an ultrasound scan.

Placental accreta

A very rare complication of pregnancy, where the placenta grows into the deeper layers of the uterine wall and becomes firmly attached. The most common variant is accreta, where the placenta becomes directly attached to the uterine wall. Occasionally, however, the placenta extends deeper into the uterine muscle – this is known as placental increta. In the third, very rare variant, the placenta extends through the entire wall of the uterus – this is known as percreta.

The condition most commonly occurs in women who have had a previous Caesarean, or have scarring from uterine surgery. Placenta praevia may also be a cause.

Often there are no symptoms until the third stage of labour, when the placenta doesn't separate from the uterine wall. Rarely, the condition causes rupture or partial rupture of the uterus. Treatment involves surgical removal of the placenta. Very rarely, if the bleeding cannot be controlled, a hysterectomy is required.

Placental abruption

This is when the placenta separates or shears away from the wall of the uterus. Usually the bleeding is associated with severe abdominal cramps but not always if the placenta only separates a small amount. The amount of bleeding experienced is variable but can be heavy with clots.

A particularly dangerous form of abruption is called a concealed abruption. This rare condition occurs when the placenta separates in the middle portion, causing a large blood clot to build up between the placental surface and the wall of the uterus. Usually the mother experiences severe pain and feels very faint. No bleeding is seen because all the blood loss is captured behind the back of the placenta. Urgent medical treatment is essential and immediate delivery of the baby is necessary.

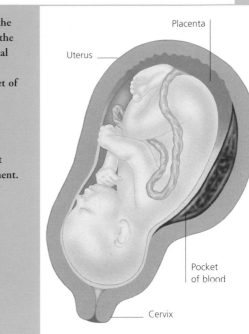

Separation of the placenta from the uterus, placental abruption, can lead to a pocket of blood forming between the placenta and uterus, which requires urgent medical treatment.

Placenta

Uterus

Pocket of blood

Cervix

Uterine rupture

Very occasionally a rupture or tear occurs in the uterus during pregnancy. Sometimes, the uterus may rupture during labour. Usually the cause is a weakness in the uterine wall caused by a scar from a previous Caesarean or a previously repaired uterine rupture. Abnormalities to the placenta, such as placenta praevia, or placental accreta, can also increase the risk of uterine rupture. Being induced during a VBAC labour with certain medications also increases the risk of rupture.

The first sign of a rupture is usually a searing pain in the abdomen, accompanied by a feeling of something 'tearing' inside, and some vaginal bleeding. If the rupture occurs during a trial of labour after a previous Caesarean section, contractions will probably slow down or cease. The fetal heart rate monitor will demonstrate abnormalities indicating the baby is compromised.

When a rupture occurs, an immediate Caesarean is required, followed by surgical repair of the uterus. Rarely, a hysterectomy is necessary.

After a rupture you will be closely monitored and antibiotics will be given to prevent infection.

Miscarriage

Sometimes a pregnancy ends in miscarriage. There are a lot of reasons why this may happen – in the early weeks it is often the body's way of rejecting a fetus that could never develop healthily. Occasionally it is caused by a problem that occurs during pregnancy, or because of a pre-existing medical condition. Recurrent miscarriages need to be investigated, as treatment may be required.

Loss of a baby before 24 weeks (before the baby is able to survive outside the uterus) is known as a miscarriage or a spontaneous abortion. Most miscarriages occur before 12 weeks, when doctors tend to refer to the miscarriage as being an 'early or first trimester' miscarriage. Early miscarriage is very common, affecting about one in five pregnancies. The figure is probably even higher than this because a woman may not even be aware that she's pregnant before she miscarries with what seems like an extra-heavy period. If you smoke, are an older mother, have had previous miscarriages, or have fibroids, lupus or diabetes, you face an increased risk of miscarriage.

At least half of all miscarriages in the first trimester are caused by chromosomal abnormalities that prevent the fetus from developing into a healthy baby. Infections, uncontrolled diabetes, thyroid problems, uterine abnormalities, or a woman's production of certain antibodies also can cause an early miscarriage.

Vaginal bleeding, accompanied by lower backache or cramping abdominal pains, similar to period cramps, which may be constant or occur intermittently, may be a sign of a threatened miscarriage. Despite these symptoms it's still possible that the pregnancy isn't going to miscarry.

But, once the uterus starts to expel the pregnancy, then it's inevitable that a miscarriage will follow. The cervix opens and pieces of liver-like tissue are passed. In this case, vaginal bleeding and pain may be quite severe.

Ultrasound is normally used to establish whether a pregnancy is continuing normally. A pelvic examination is also helpful because a closed cervix indicates the pregnancy may be all right.

A complete miscarriage

When the uterus has expelled the pregnancy entirely, a miscarriage is complete. The bleeding and pain subside and an ultrasound scan will show that the uterus is completely empty.

Incomplete miscarriage

When the uterus doesn't completely expel all of the pregnancy and pieces of tissue are retained a miscarriage is described as incomplete. It's usually obvious on ultrasound, but doctors may make the diagnosis if bleeding is very heavy or if tissue can be seen in the cervix on examination.

At this stage you'll probably be offered a minor procedure under anaesthetic to clean out the uterus, known as an ERPC (evacuation of retained products of conception). This involves dilating (widening) the cervix and scraping tissue away from the endometrium (the lining of the uterus).

Alternatively, the tissue may be left to expel itself naturally over the next few days, as long as you're not bleeding too heavily and you're well enough to cope with this.

Missed miscarriage or blighted ovum

Occasionally a miscarriage occurs without any symptoms, or with very minor signs such as a small amount of brownish vaginal discharge. This type of miscarriage is usually detected by ultrasound, because an empty sac can be seen inside the uterus, meaning that the fetus has never formed – this is called a blighted ovum. To be absolutely sure, your doctor may wish to re-scan you in seven to ten days to check that a baby is not going to develop in the sac. Occasionally a fetus can be seen inside the sac

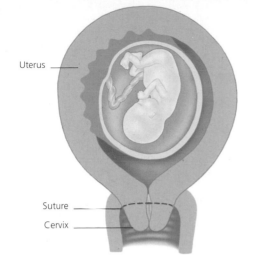

Uterus

Suture

Cervix

If cervical incompetence has been diagnosed, a stitch (see above) may be inserted to reinforce the cervical muscle. Inserting a stitch is most successful if it is performed early in pregnancy.

but the heart has stopped beating, indicating that the fetus has clearly died at a very early stage. You will then be offered an ERPC to remove the remains of the pregnancy, or you may be given the option of waiting to see if your body will naturally expel the pregnancy over the next few days.

Incompetent cervix

Believed to be responsible for 20 to 25 per cent of all second trimester miscarriages, an incompetent cervix is one that opens under pressure of the growing uterus and baby. It can be caused by a genetic weakness of the cervix; extreme stretching of or severe lacerations to the cervix during one or more previous deliveries; a cone biopsy for cervical cancer; or cervical surgery or laser therapy. It is usually diagnosed when a woman has previously miscarried in the second trimester or when ultrasound or a vaginal examination shows the cervix shortening and opening during pregnancy.

Once the condition is diagnosed, a procedure known as a cervical cerclage will be carried out – the opening of the cervix is stitched or sutured to keep it closed. The procedure is performed through the vagina under local anaesthetic or epidural at around 12 to 16 weeks of pregnancy. The stitches or sutures are usually removed a few weeks before the estimated date of delivery; in some cases they remain in place until labour has begun. With a stitch the chances of carrying a baby to term are excellent.

COPING WITH MISCARRIAGE

It can feel devastating to lose a much-longed-for pregnancy. To grieve is natural, as is feeling sad and depressed. Often hospitals treat the situation as routine, which can be very distressing.

It can be hard to accept that miscarriage is very common and that it is usually nature's way of dealing with pregnancies where defects have arisen in the very early stages of the baby's development. Never feel guilty that somehow you were to blame; this is a natural

process and not a situation that you have caused. The happy fact is that next time you have an excellent chance of a successful pregnancy.

Remember to continue taking folic acid and keep up a well-balanced nutritious diet. There is no reason to wait before conceiving again, although many couples do take a rest before trying for their next pregnancy.

A small number of women experience repeated miscarriages. If you've had three or more

miscarriages in a row, ask your healthcare provider to arrange for you to be referred for some extra tests. Some women carry antibodies in their blood that prevent a pregnancy from implanting properly, and treatment can be given in early pregnancy to help.

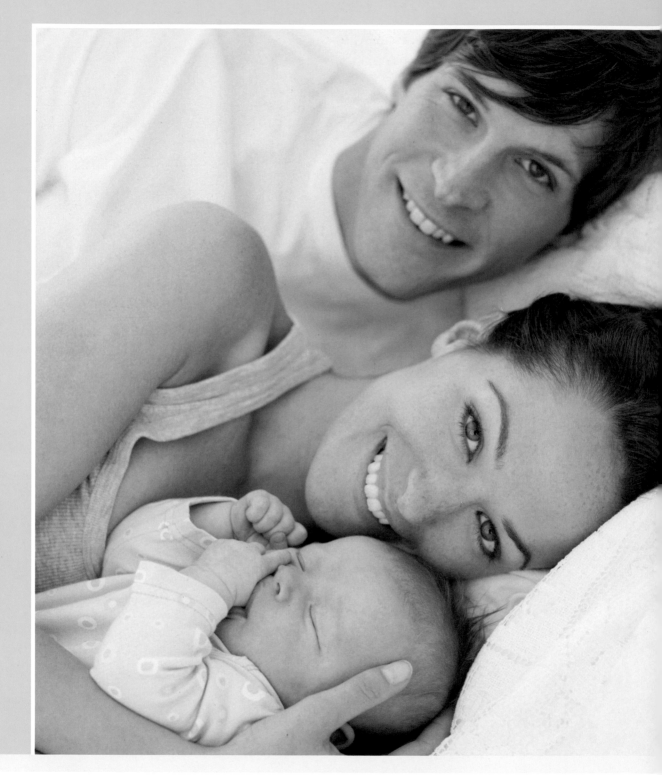

PART IV NOW YOU'RE A FAMILY

13

CHAPTER

Your marvellous newborn

After all the months of waiting, your baby is finally

here, and that moment when you hold her for the

very first time is certain to exceed any expectations

you might have had. You'll very soon get to know

her, what she looks like and what she can do – and

understand what she needs to thrive.

What your baby looks like

Throughout your pregnancy, you're bound to have wondered what your baby will look like. Will she have a lot of hair and what colour will it be? Will she be long and lean or petite and plump? Will she look like you? Well, now you can check her out from head to toe.

As you hold your beautiful baby and begin to examine her all over, she might not look quite like the little cherub you imagined. Exactly how your newborn will look depends on how she was positioned in your uterus, her genetic make-up and what sort of delivery she had. Caesarean babies, for example, who haven't had to squeeze down the birth canal, may have more normal-shaped skulls and less

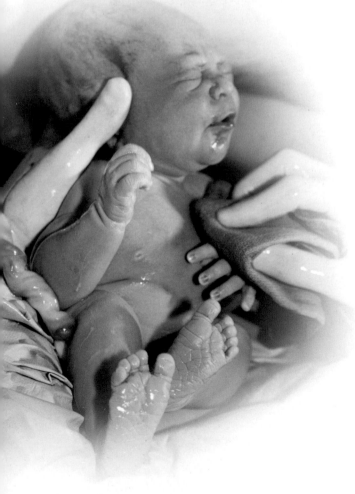

squashed faces than babies who have had a vaginal birth. It's not unusual for a mother to feel a little let-down by her baby's appearance immediately after the birth, and if this is the case, don't worry. In a very short time, all those newborn features will fade, and she'll look as beautiful as you could wish. In the meantime, here are some of the things you may notice about your baby.

Typical newborn characteristics

All newborns share certain features that can be a surprise to some parents. Make sure you take the opportunity to ask your healthcare providers any questions you have about your baby's appearance. Draw on their professional knowledge, too, to acquire the skills to take care of her basic needs.

An elongated, swollen and bruised head

Your baby's skull bones are soft at birth to allow her head to pass through the birth canal. As she's squeezed and pushed out into the world, her head bones are moulded, which can leave her head with a conical, pointed shape. Even some babies who are delivered by Caesarean have a degree of head moulding, because they have spent the last few weeks upside down, wedged tight in their mother's uterus. Either way, the moulding doesn't last long and you'll notice that your baby's head starts to become rounder within a few days.

Your baby may have a soft tissue swelling on her head known as a caput. This can be caused by her head pressing against the dilating cervix during contractions or by the suction of a vacuum delivery (see page 229). This harmless swelling should disappear in a matter of days. Also, your baby's head may look bruised, especially if she was delivered by forceps or had a fetal scalp electrode (see page 217) attached during labour. This bruising generally gets better within a week or so.

Fontanelles

You also may notice a soft, pulsating spot on the top of your baby's head. This is called the anterior fontanelle, and is one of two your baby has on her head. They're simply gaps where the bones of your baby's skull haven't yet fused, and they are there to allow her head to grow quickly during her first year. They act also as a cushion, protecting her head from injury. By the time your baby is about 2 years old, the fontanelles will have closed.

Although these soft fontanelles look like they're very vulnerable, they're actually covered by tough, fibrous tissue, so you won't hurt your baby if you touch the area gently. You can comb the hair over the soft spot without any problem.

A squashed face

Looking straight at your baby's face, you may notice that her nose looks a little flattened, maybe even pushed to the side. Your baby's eyes may look bloodshot and her eyelids puffy. She may even have some trouble opening up one eye or the other at first. Again, these are caused by your baby's position in the uterus and the tight trip down the birth canal. All these effects should improve quickly over a day or two. If your baby is reluctant to open her eyes at first, don't try to force them open. If you like, you can encourage your baby to open her eyes naturally simply by lifting her above you with her head higher than yours.

While you look at her eyes, notice the colour. Many babies are born with dark blue eyes, because melanin, the body's natural pigment, is not present in the irises at birth. The colour of babies' eyes often alters as the pigmentation increases, and any changes are usually complete by 12 months of age.

Some babies are born with a common condition called 'sticky eye'. If your baby has this, you'll probably notice it as a yellow discharge around the eyelids. Although this isn't serious, your doctor will want to rule out conjunctivitis (see page 365).

Vernix and hair

At birth, most babies are covered with blood and mucus, as well as a protective layer of thick, white grease, called vernix. This develops during the last trimester of pregnancy and protects a baby's skin from becoming waterlogged. Babies born prematurely have a lot of vernix on their skin, while overdue babies have virtually none at all. In some hospitals the vernix is washed off, while in others it's left to wear off naturally, usually within a few days.

Many babies – and particularly those who are born a bit early – have a layer of fine, downy hair over their skin called lanugo. Nobody knows for certain why lanugo is there, but it's thought that it might help to keep the vernix in place and regulate your baby's body temperature. Most of this hair will fall out by itself during the first few months.

Your baby may have been born with a thick head of hair or almost no hair at all. If she has hair, much of this will be replaced by new growth over the next few months, and her hair colour and texture may change quite a lot from what you see at birth.

Blue hands and feet and long nails

Your newborn's hands and feet may have a bluish tinge during the first few days. This phenomenon, known as acrocyanosis and caused by poor circulation, is normal and will improve as she gets older. The rest of her body should be nice and pink.

Your baby's fingernails may be long, especially if she was born late, but they are very delicate, and it's best not to cut them at this stage. You can file them gently or your healthcare provider may put scratch-mitts on your baby's hands if it's thought that she might scratch herself.

Swollen breasts

You may notice that your baby's breasts are slightly swollen. In some newborns it's even possible to see a milky white discharge. This is perfectly normal in both boys and girls. Both the swelling and the discharge are caused by pregnancy hormones remaining in your baby's body. The swelling and discharge will disappear in a few days.

Swollen genitals

If your baby is a boy, you may notice that his scrotum (the sack that surrounds his testicles) is somewhat swollen. This swelling, known as a hydrocele, is caused by fluid surrounding the testicles and usually goes down within a few months. If it doesn't, then speak to your healthcare provider, as surgery may be required. Also, some baby boys are born with a condition known as undescended testes, which means that their testes have not yet moved outside the body. If your baby has this condition, your healthcare provider will keep a check on it (see page 378).

If your baby is a girl, she may have slightly swollen genitals and a white vaginal discharge. When she is between a few days and a couple of weeks old, she also may have a very small amount of vaginal bleeding. Both the discharge and the bleeding are caused by pregnancy hormones remaining in her body and will cease as the hormone levels drop.

The umbilical cord

Shortly after the birth, the umbilical cord is clamped and then cut (see page 224). However, a small stump will remain, which will have a clamp on it to prevent bleeding. Within a few hours, the cord will dry out and go from being soft and spongy to dry and black. The cord will fall off by itself, usually within one to two weeks. Before this you should treat the cord gently, particularly when washing your baby (see page 312).

Dry skin and spots

Once your baby has had her first bath, her skin may appear dry and cracked. This is a result of the time that she's spent immersed in liquid. Dry skin is often more noticeable in babies born a bit after their due dates, because all the vernix will have worn off, leaving the skin unprotected. Any dry patches should get better within a few weeks. In the meantime, it's fine to apply a very mild moisturiser to any dry patches on her arms and legs. Make sure this doesn't contain any added perfumes, as these might irritate her delicate skin.

During the first few days, your baby is likely to have a rash or two. There are several common rashes among newborns, for example:

♦ *Erythema toxicum* This consists of red, blotchy spots with white heads in the middle and appears mostly on a baby's trunk. Its causes are unknown.

♦ *Milia* Also known as 'milk rash', this appears as whitish-yellow dots on a baby's face, especially on the nose, and, less commonly, on the roof of her mouth. This is caused by enlarged oily glands in your baby's skin.

♦ *Pustular melanosis* This usually starts as small, white dots that then break and become scaly, brown rings. Its causes are unknown.

All of these rashes are harmless and will disappear by themselves during the first couple of weeks.

However, you should always get a rash checked by your baby's healthcare provider. Very occasionally, rashes are an early sign of an infection that will require treatment.

IDENTIFYING YOUR BABY'S BIRTHMARKS

These are very common and are usually harmless. But your baby's healthcare provider may want to check them as your baby grows.

STORK MARKS These collections of dilated blood vessels appear as a red mark on the back of a baby's neck. Stork marks may not go away but are soon covered by hair.

SALMON PATCHES These are similar to stork marks but appear on the forehead **1**, over the eyelids or under the nose. Unlike stork marks, salmon patches fade with time.

STRAWBERRY MARKS These raised, red marks **2** are collections of blood capillaries. They may grow during the first year, but almost all fade by age of 9 if left untreated.

MONGOLIAN SPOTS These are common on dark-skinned babies and appear as bruise-like, flat, bluish-gray patches around a baby's bottom **3**, shoulders, back and arms. They are caused by clusters of pigment cells in the skin and usually fade within a year.

PORT WINE STAINS These red or purple marks, usually on the face, head or neck, are rare. They don't fade but may be treatable with laser therapy or plastic surgery.

CAFÉ-AU-LAIT PATCHES Small, flat, brown or coffee-coloured oval patches are very common. They are usually permanent.

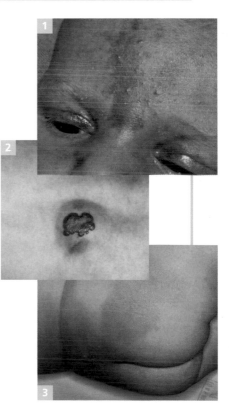

Your baby's postnatal care

After you and your baby have spent some time getting to know each other, your baby will probably be taken to the nursery for a bath, a physical examination and some routine procedures. If you have the birth at home these will be carried out by your healthcare provider.

You may be able to stay in the same room for the labour, delivery and recovery, or based on your delivery needs, your baby may be born in a separate labour and delivery suite, after which you'll be transferred to another, more comfortable room. Following a hospital birth, most women go home within 24 hours, depending on how they feel. Some women, with plenty of help at home, are discharged home after two hours! After a Caesarean the usual stay is three to four days. Your length of stay in hospital will be negotiated with hospital staff. Your own and your baby's health and wellbeing as well as the level of support available following discharge will be the primary factors to be considered. In hospital you will be in a small maternity postnatal ward or single room, and your baby will be with you at all times. Well mothers and babies should not be separated. There may be a separate room for bathing and feeding your baby.

MEDICAL ATTENTION FOR YOUR BABY

Your baby will receive a considerable amount of medical care immediately after his birth and during his first few days to make sure that all is well.

A FULL PHYSICAL EXAMINATION
At 1 and 5 minute intervals after the birth, hospital staff will perform the Apgar test (see box, opposite). Then at some stage within the first few days your baby's features, spine, anus, fingers and toes will be checked, he'll be weighed, and his head size and length may be measured **1**. His hips will be checked for proper movement and placement **2**.

VITAMIN K INJECTION Babies receive an injection or drops of Vitamin K shortly after birth. This is because newborns often have low levels of this vitamin, which is necessary for the process of normal blood clotting. Further doses are given in subsequent weeks.

BLOOD SPOT SCREENING
After the first 24 hours, a blood sample will be taken taken from your baby's heel. This is used to check for congenital hypo-thyroidism, sickle cell disorders, cystic fibrosis, MCADD and phenylketonuria – all rare but serious conditions. In some areas babies are also screened for other conditions so enquire about which ones your baby is given.

HEPATITIS B INJECTION Before being discharged from hospital, some babies receive the hepatitis B vaccine to prevent an infection of the liver. This is given if a baby's mother, or another member of the close family, is a carrier. If given, the

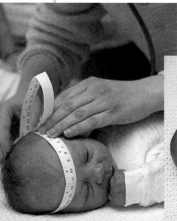

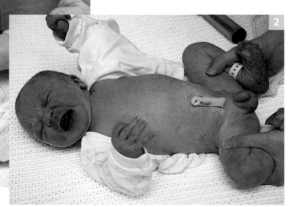

Once you return home, you'll receive regular home visits from a midwife.

Learning to care for your baby

If you haven't already attended parenting classes (see page 172), your hospital stay can be a useful time to learn how to take care of your baby with the help and support of expert staff. They will be able to show you how to change a nappy, give him a bath and take care of the cord, as well as answer any queries you have about feeding. Many hospitals organize short classes, in which you can learn about caring for your baby. These classes also give you the chance to meet other new parents going through exactly the same experience as you. This should help you to be as relaxed as possible about looking after your baby on your own. Of course, worries and concerns may crop up once you're home, but your baby's healthcare provider will be happy to speak with you or see the baby, if necessary. For information about what you'll need on the journey home, see page 206.

If you're not having your baby in a hospital, speak to your healthcare provider to find out about classes you can attend in your area.

course is completed in three doses by the time the baby's a year old.

BODILY FUNCTIONS After your baby's birth it's a good idea to keep track of how much and how often he is feeding, as well as noting the frequency and appearance of his stools and urine.

WEIGHT Your baby will probably be weighed regularly in his first few days. Don't be alarmed if his weight drops at first; it's normal for babies to lose up to 10 per cent of their birth weight in the first few days. He should begin to gain weight again by the time he's 1 week old.

HEARING All babies are screened for hearing problems in the first few weeks after birth.

MORE **ABOUT**   the Apgar score

This test was developed by Dr Virginia Apgar to allow a quick assessment of a newborn's health. The word 'Apgar' stands also for the signs that the doctors and nurses are looking at. For each of these, your baby will be given a score of 0, 1 or 2. Babies rarely receive a total score of 10, but a score above 6 is usually fine. If your baby receives a low score, don't worry – it simply means he needs some temporary medical help and close monitoring. It's not an indicator of his future health.

SIGN	POINTS		
	0	1	2
Appearance	Pale or blue	Body pink, extremities blue	Pink
Pulse	Not detectable	Below 100	Over 100
Grimace (reflexes)	No response to stimulation	Grimace	Lusty cry, cough, or sneeze
Activity (muscle tone)	Flaccid (no or weak activity)	Some movement of extremities	A lot of activity
Respiration	None	Slow, irregular	Good, crying

What your baby can do

Your baby might seem helpless at birth, but, in fact, she has capabilities and a personality. Over the following weeks and months, she'll be adding to her store of knowledge very rapidly, as this is what she is programmed to do.

From the moment your baby is born, her senses are flooded with information, activating her brain into a surge of development. Neurons (nerve cells) start to work overtime, creating thousands of connections with other cells. The brain's structure is stimulated and physically changed by the types of messages it receives. If your baby's brain doesn't receive enough information, development in one area may be arrested or impaired – for example, if a squint is left uncorrected for too long, the brain will learn to look through one eye, and that habit can't be corrected, even with glasses. On the other hand, if you talk, sing, and play with your baby from very early on, you will be actively encouraging the neural pathways to form.

You can't get your baby to do something before the appropriate brain pathways have been established, but she will get there in her own time and at her own developmental rate. In fact, your baby's brain will more than double in size during the first year after birth, and to maintain this tremendous growth, her brain will use 60 per cent of the energy she gets from food. But, because this process takes some time, your baby will already have some bodily functions in place and certain reflexes that help her to survive (see below).

Breathe, feed and digest

Perhaps the most miraculous skill your baby acquires is the art of breathing independently. While she was in the uterus, her lungs weren't needed, as the placenta provided her with oxygen from her mother's blood. The moment she's born, she has to switch to using her lungs to obtain vital oxygen for life. As she takes a breath, contact with the outside air results in the lungs expanding and blood passing directly to the lungs, instead of to the placenta. Your baby may follow her first breath with a bout of coughing to clear her airways, but as soon as she begins to breathe normally, she will probably cry.

Your newborn may hiccup quite a lot at first, but these bouts of hiccups won't upset her. They are caused by the sudden, irregular contractions of the immature diaphragm, which hasn't quite got breathing in and breathing out into steady rhythm. As the muscles involved become stronger, your baby will hiccup less.

Your newborn is also perfectly equipped to feed and digest food. Put a newborn baby to her mother's breast and she'll probably take to it right away, because of her strongly developed sucking reflex.

Tune in to her environment

At birth, all of your baby's senses are intact and ready to be used. She can already see, albeit fuzzily; she can hear, she can taste, she can smell and she can sense touch.

Your baby's sight

Immediately after birth, you may notice your baby staring at you. She can see you quite well, but focuses best at 20 to 25 cm (8 to 12 inches) away from something. Interestingly, this is the approximate distance between you and your baby's face when you're holding her at your breast. Your baby will enjoying watching you and will track your movement for short periods. Sometimes you might notice her eyes crossing, which is normal and is a result of her lack of control over her eye muscles. As she gets used to seeing, this should disappear within a few weeks – if not, speak to your doctor.

Your baby's hearing

Babies hear very well when they're born, too. You may notice your baby turning towards you when you speak, and she'll have a definite preference for the voices she heard while she was still in the uterus. You may notice that your baby seems to brighten when she hears your voice – this is a useful natural reaction, as you are vital to her survival.

Your baby won't like loud voices or noises, which will startle her and may even make her cry. If she's crying or fretful, white noise – the low-pitched sound of the washing machine or the dishwasher, for example – may have a miraculous calming effect. This is probably because they remind your baby of the type of noises she heard while in the uterus. Likewise, if you sang a particular song to your baby while you were pregnant, singing it again after the birth may bring about a delighted reaction.

Your baby's sense of taste

Babies seem to be able to distinguish certain flavours from birth, and many experts believe that they, in fact, have a more delicate sense of taste than adults. Research has shown that if a baby is given bottles containing water with subtly different degrees of sweetness, she'll spend more time sucking on the bottle that contains the sweetest water.

Your baby's sense of smell

Newborns have surprisingly pronounced smell preferences. A baby can distinguish her own mother's breast milk from another mother's, and responds better to her own mother's milk. She may

HOW TO bond with your baby

A baby is usually very aware of her surroundings from birth, which is why the time you spend together in the first few hours and days will be important for you both. Immediately after the birth, hold her close to you and look into her face. Babies have an inborn ability to distinguish people from other objects, and your baby will want to look at your face rather than anything else. Look into her eyes and smile to encourage this attachment.

Communicate your strong feelings for your baby through close physical contact. During her initial alert period after the birth, hold her naked against your skin so that she becomes familiar with how you feel and smell. Also talk to her in a quiet soothing voice – she'll recognize your voice from before she was born. As she gets older your baby will try to copy the noises you

make to her and will want to imitate your facial expressions. Through bonding in this way, your baby will begin to get to know you, learn to rely on you and trust you. Make sure your partner has plenty of contact with her, too, so that your baby can develop an attachment to both of you. The early stages of your relationship with your baby can have an impact on her future, and knowing that she can depend on you will give her the courage to venture out and explore as she gets older and becomes independent.

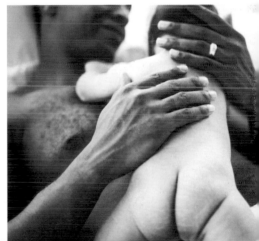

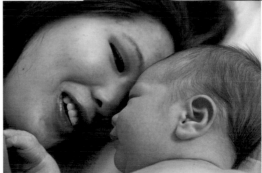

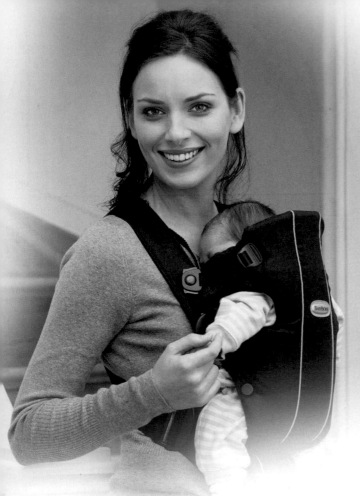

If your baby is fretful, carrying her in a baby carrier so that she is held close to your body will soothe her.

in the same way we do, if not more. Even in the uterus, a baby will move away from external pressure during examinations.

Your baby's personality

Your baby has her own individual personality from the moment she's born. She has her likes and dislikes and reacts in her own unique way to you and her environment.

One of the most exciting aspects of parenting is getting to know your baby's patterns of behaviour in a way that no one else can. As a newborn, your baby has very limited ways of communicating with you. But through observation, you'll gradually learn the details of your baby's personality, and the more you interact and play with her, the easier it will be for you to know what she wants.

Getting to know your baby

Some babies like to be rocked, while others enjoy being still. Some babies like to be swaddled tightly, while others prefer to have their hands and legs free. Some babies quickly become uncomfortable in a wet nappy, others don't seem to mind it at all. Babies' behaviour patterns are influenced by their temperaments. You'll soon get to know your baby's temperament, but in the early days you may find yourself trying several strategies for caring for her (see page 306) to find out what suits her best.

Understanding your baby's temperament

If your baby cries a lot, it may mean that she's highly sensitive to stimulation. Sensitive babies sometimes have trouble settling into a regular sleeping pattern or feeding schedule. If your baby has this type of temperament, she may respond best to peace and quiet, rather than bright lights and lots of stimulation. Introduce her to new people and situations slowly to give her plenty of time to adjust.

even use smell to help her to find the breast. Babies also seem to show preferences for certain smells, being repelled by those she finds unpleasant, and attracted by others that she finds pleasant.

Your baby's sense of touch

All babies love the feeling of being cuddled and held close, which usually calms and reassures them. Your baby will be soothed by the sound of your beating heart and the secure, warm pressure of your body. It's been found that premature babies, in particular, thrive on skin-to-skin contact, or 'kangaroo care' as it's also called. Research has shown that removing a preterm baby from her incubator and placing her against her mother's skin for just a short spell every day frequently leads to quicker weight gain and more rapid development.

It used to be thought that babies were developmentally too immature to feel pain, but a relatively recent discovery is that they experience it

YOUR BABY'S REFLEXES

Your baby is born with a number of important ingrained behaviours. These are automatic responses that are thought to help babies with basic needs. Many of these early reflexes will slowly disappear over the first 6 months,

THE SUCKING REFLEX This is your baby's natural instinct to suck on whatever is put in her mouth. She'll suck readily on your nipple, on the teat of a bottle or on your finger. This reflex is crucial for survival, and a strong suck is a sign of a healthy baby. Your baby may also suck her fingers or thumb to soothe herself.

THE ROOTING REFLEX This occurs if you stroke the side of your baby's cheek: she'll turn towards the side seeking the breast (or the bottle) **1**

This reflex helps a baby find food. It can help to tickle your baby's lips when encouraging her to feed.

THE GRASPING REFLEX If you place your finger in your baby's hand. she'll grasp it tightly, and this grasp can be so strong that you could almost lift her up by her arms **2**. When you try to remove your finger, her grip will get tighter.

THE STARTLE REFLEX Also known as the Moro reflex, this occurs when your baby hears a loud noise or is moved suddenly. During the startle, your baby's hands will suddenly go out to her sides with her fingers spread **3**. Then she'll bring her arms back into her chest with clenched fists, and probably end this with a crying episode.

THE WALKING REFLEX Also called the stepping reflex, this occurs if you hold your baby upright under her arms and let her feet touch a

flat surface. She'll naturally make stepping movements and try to move forwards **4**.

DIVING REFLEX Although you should never leave your baby to swim under water, if you place your newborn under water for a short while, she'll swim happily without any problem. This is because her lungs automatically seal off once she hits the water.

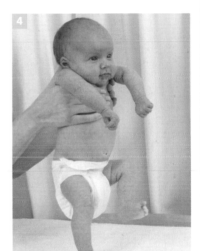

An easy-going baby will adapt to new people and places easily and have few sleeping and eating problems. However, if your baby's like this, it's possible for her to become overstimulated, because she's so easy to have around. If your baby averts her gaze rather than showing interest or if she suddenly falls asleep, it may be time to give her a break.

How your baby communicates

Initially, crying is your baby's only means of communicating her needs to you. Learning to understand her cries can be difficult at first, but with observation, patience and the experience of trying different things to comfort her, you can learn a lot about what your baby is trying tell you.

All babies have different crying patterns. Some babies cry some of the time, and others cry very little, while others cry a great deal. Some babies are easy to calm, while others are harder to soothe. Sometimes a baby cries for no apparent reason and nothing seems to console her. The way that babies cry can differ too – some may cry intensely, others may only whimper. The one common factor is that babies cry because they need something and they are asking for a response to this need (see page 346).

Your baby's growth

A newborn develops at an astounding rate over the first three months. Although most babies lose a small amount of weight after birth, they quickly regain this (see page 295). Once their original birth weight is achieved they gain, on average, 15 to 30 g (½ to 1 oz) each day for the first six months.

Although it may be hard for you to appreciate the daily change, friends who just saw your baby at birth may now marvel at her growth. Visits to the doctor will confirm this change, and allow you to see how much she has grown.

In addition to gaining weight, your baby will be developing her muscle strength. At birth, she will barely have been able to lift her head. By four weeks of age, she'll be able to lift her head up and turn it from side to side, although she'll still need you to support her head when you hold her upright. Just one month later, at eight weeks of age, your baby

will be able to lift her head and chest up when she's lying down on her front. Then, before you know it, at about 12 weeks, she'll be able to bring her chest up with her arms out straight.

DID YOU KNOW...

NEWBORN BABIES DON'T PRODUCE TEARS
Although they spend a lot of time crying, babies can't actually produce tears until they're about 3 to 12 weeks old. This is because the tear duct is very efficient at removing any excess fluid from the tear glands before they overflow.

By four or five months your baby will have developed some hand control and will be able to grasp objects. She will use her mouth to explore an item in her hand by gumming and sucking. By the age of around six months she will be rolling over and she will probably have learned to control her neck and head and will be beginning to try to sit upright.

Socially, your baby will become more and more interactive. When you first saw her at birth, she probably stared at you with a serious expression. Merely four to eight weeks later, there'll be an unforgettable moment when she looks at you and smiles – her first signal of sociability. At the same time, her schedule will be becoming more predictable and you may have an easier time interpreting her moods and needs.

She'll begin also to make cooing noises at about 8 weeks, the beginnings of her speech development. By 4 months your baby understands all the basic sounds that make up her language. Between four and six months she discovers how to make different sounds and starts to 'babble'. Babbling usually involves practising vowel sounds over and over again. But at this age she'll still communicate by crying.

14

CHAPTER

Taking care of your baby

Now there's a new baby – but also some new

parents. You have an awesome responsibility; this

tiny being is utterly dependent on you for

everything. Don't worry; every new parent wonders

whether he or she will do a good job, but you'll be

amazed at how soon you'll be comfortable with your

parenting skills. One of your first tasks, however,

will be to register your baby's birth. This has to be

done before he's six weeks old.

Feeding basics

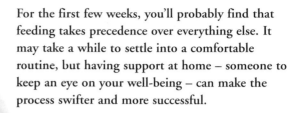

For the first few weeks, you'll probably find that feeding takes precedence over everything else. It may take a while to settle into a comfortable routine, but having support at home – someone to keep an eye on your well-being – can make the process swifter and more successful.

You'll probably have decided already whether you want to breastfeed or bottlefeed your baby (see page 190), but there are now other things to consider, such as how often and who should feed him. Initially, you may be concerned about whether you're doing the right thing and whether he's getting enough nourishment, but, as you see your baby grow and thrive, you'll gradually relax and learn to trust your own judgment.

How often should you feed?

Not so long ago, babies were fed on a rigid four-hourly schedule, regardless of whether they were screaming with hunger before the clock said it was time to feed them. Today, most health professionals recommend a more flexible schedule – that is, to feed your baby when he appears hungry. It's normal for a baby to want to feed frequently for the first few weeks, so if you accept that in the early days your breastfed baby may need nursing every two hours or your bottlefed baby every three hours, you can plan your day accordingly.

It may seem that you're doing nothing but feeding at first, but this period won't last forever – think of each feeding session as an opportunity for you to sit and rest. As your baby grows over the next few weeks, you'll probably find that the in-between periods get longer, and that your baby settles to a four-hourly routine of his own accord. Babies do vary in their ability to settle, however, so don't worry if your friend's baby seems to settle before yours.

Occasionally, smaller babies or babies who are sleepy – perhaps from drugs you were given during labour – don't always indicate when they need feeding. In this case, don't let your new baby go for longer than five to six hours without offering him your breast or the bottle.

Recognising that your baby wants to feed

Instead of waiting until your baby cries, which means he might have been hungry for some while, be alert to his signals. These usually involve your baby opening and closing his mouth, making sucking noises or sucking his fingers or hands, waving his hands and/or kicking his legs or turning his head or eyes to bring his mouth close to you.

How much does he need?

The needs of individual babies vary considerably and you'll probably find that your baby sometimes takes more milk and sometimes a little less. Let his appetite be your main guide, but as a general idea: if you're breastfeeding, your baby will take as much as he needs from your breast (see also page 299 to see how to ensure your baby breastfeeds well); if you're bottlefeeding, your baby will need 75 to 100 ml (2½ to 3½ oz) of formula for each 0.5 kg (1 lb) of body weight. Most bottlefed babies need six to eight feeds each day, so for a 3.5 kg (7 lb) baby, this would mean you need to give him 415 to 620 ml (14 to 21 oz) of formula in a 24-hour period.

Does my baby need water as well?

Breast milk contains enough water for your baby, so even in the hottest climate, if you're breastfeeding there's no need to give him supplementary drinks. Doing so could confuse him while he's trying to learn how to feed from your nipple. It also could overfill his tiny tummy, which may, in turn, interfere with his appetite.

If you're bottlefeeding your baby, you can give him a little extra water if it's very hot and humid and he's dehydrated or feverish. However, don't give him too much water or too often, as it may interfere

with his appetite. If you do give your baby water, make sure that it's boiled then cooled, until your baby is 6 months old.

Signs of a thriving baby

Whether you're breast- or bottlefeeding, you'll want to be reassured that your baby is thriving. One of the best ways to do this is to make sure that your baby is regularly seen by his healthcare providers. They will weigh your baby and plot his weight on a centile chart (a chart that compares your baby's weight gain to national averages). If you have any concerns about feeding, you will also be able to discuss them. However, you'll get an idea whether your baby is thriving if he:

- Is gaining weight steadily.
- Has a good skin colour.
- Is lively, with bright eyes and firm muscle tone.
- Is contented and seems satisfied after feeding.
- Has six or more wet nappies in 24 hours.
- Is passing soft stools.

Preventing wind

All babies take in some air when they feed, but some seem to suffer from wind more than others. If your bottlefed baby suffers from a lot of wind – you'll know because he'll seem upset and unsettled after his bottle – check that the holes of the teats are the right size. To test this, hold a bottle upside down and watch how the formula drips out – it should be at a steady flow of one drop per second. If the formula flow is slower than this, the hole is too small and your baby is having to suck hard to obtain the formula. This can mean that when your baby feeds he takes in too much air along with his formula. On the other hand, if your baby tends to gulp from the bottle, check that the holes of the teats aren't too large.

Make sure, too, that the bottle is always tilted enough when you feed your baby – the liquid should always completely cover the top of the bottle and fill the teat.

If you're breastfeeding, wind may be due to the fact that your baby isn't latching on properly (see page 301). It also may be due to irregular flow. If your milk tends to gush out before you put your baby to your breast, try expressing a little milk (see page 302) before you start to feed your baby.

Try also not to let your baby wait too long between feeding times. If he's hungry, he may cry too much and swallow a lot of air just before you feed him. He may also gulp down the milk too quickly, again causing wind.

Winding your baby

Some experts recommend you wind your baby after each meal to get rid of excess air; other experts maintain that it's not always necessary, particularly with breastfed babies. Babies have their own preferences about being winded and your baby may like to breastfeed or take the bottle without stopping and will scream indignantly if you try to wind him halfway through. Or he may need to stop in the middle to give a big burp. You'll soon get to know what your baby likes to do.

If your baby does have some discomfort from wind and is unable to bring it up by himself, sit him on your lap, leaning him forwards slightly and supporting his head by placing your hand under his chin. Alternatively, hold your baby upright against your shoulder (see picture, page 294). Have a clean towel at hand or draped over your clothing in case he brings up any milk. Also, it may be helpful to gently pat or rub your baby's back. If your baby can't bring up wind in these positions, try laying him face down across your lap and rubbing his back.

If your baby often has wind and finds it difficult to bring it up, you might like to learn some baby massage techniques from a health professional. One simple massage technique that can help with wind is called 'tiger in the tree' and is illustrated on page 346. Some mothers find that giving their babies colic drops can ease excess wind; other mothers find that these make no difference.

If your baby doesn't seem to suffer from wind, don't spend hours trying to get him to burp – some babies just don't. Or he may prefer to wait for an hour or so, before giving a big burp by himself.

Possetting

Most babies posset (bring up) small amounts of milk occasionally, usually when they're being winded or are lying down. This may simply be a result of physical immaturity: the muscles between the stomach and the oesophagus (the tube connecting the mouth to the stomach) lack coordination in some newborns. In other cases, babies may gulp a lot of air when they feed and then when they bring up wind afterwards, they simply regurgitate a little bit of their meal with it. As long as your baby is well, putting on weight and the vomiting isn't forceful, possetting is usually nothing to worry about. You can try to help to prevent it by winding your baby or by sitting him in a baby chair straight after a feed. You'll probably find that any possetting problems resolve once your baby is six months old, onto a more solid diet and drinking less milk.

If your baby is possetting frequently or forcefully or appears to be in pain, he may be suffering something more serious, such as a gastric infection or reflux disease. Contact your health visitor for further advice.

Starting to breastfeed

During pregnancy your body will have prepared for feeding your baby, and there's no doubt that nature's way gives your baby the best possible start.

Breastfeeding is a skill that has to be learned, just like riding a bike or driving a car, and it comes easier to some mothers and babies than others. But mothers who experience minor difficulties at first usually find that these can be overcome easily with patience and perseverance. If necessary, ask for help from your healthcare provider or contact a support group like the National Childbirth Trust to find out about breastfeeding counsellors in your area.

The first two days

Unless there have been any difficulties, such as an emergency Caesarean, you'll usually be encouraged to breastfeed your baby very soon after the birth. Many babies take to the breast immediately and begin to suck away happily without any problems. However, some aren't quite ready – for example, if the birth has been difficult or the baby is premature. If this is the case for you, you can still stroke your baby and get to know her until she's ready to feed.

Initially, it's also not unusual for babies to have a 6- to 8-hour gap between each feed. Don't worry that she's not getting enough food – babies don't need a lot in the first few days.

Producing breast milk

Understanding the milk production process can help you to breastfeed successfully. Each of your breasts is divided into 15 to 20 compartments called lobes. Within each lobe are several smaller compartments called lobules. These contain alveoli, which are grape-like clusters of cells that produce and store breast milk. Milk travels from the alveoli through the milk ducts. These ducts broaden out beneath the areola (the dark area around your nipple) to form milk sinuses, which release milk through the 15 to 20 openings in your nipple.

If practical, wear clothes that allow you to expose your breast easily, such as a loose top with a drawstring neck.

As your baby sucks, the nerve endings in your nipple and areola are stimulated and send signals to the brain telling it to release two hormones, oxytocin and prolactin. Oxytocin triggers your milk to flow, a process known as the let-down reflex (see below). Prolactin stimulates further production of milk in the alveoli, meaning your milk supply works on a supply-and-demand basis: the more your baby feeds, the more milk is produced.

The let-down reflex

When oxytocin flows into the blood vessels in your breasts, it causes the alveoli to contract, squeezing milk through the ducts, into the sinuses, and out through the nipple.

Some women experience this let-down reflex – also called the 'milk-ejection' reflex – as a sharp, needle-like sensation in the breasts, and their milk spurts out in jets. Other women simply feel a tingling or warm sensation and the milk drips out. The let-down reflex may also be triggered in response to the baby crying or during sex. Some women who breastfeed never feel the let-down reflex at all, but this doesn't mean that it isn't working.

THE STRUCTURE OF THE BREAST

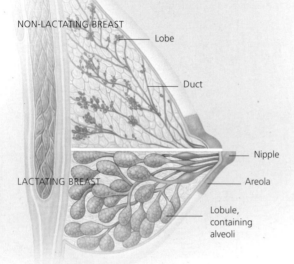

NON-LACTATING BREAST
— Lobe
— Duct
— Nipple
LACTATING BREAST
— Areola
Lobule, containing alveoli

If you find that your breasts leak milk when you're due to feed or when your baby starts crying, you may find it useful to wear breast pads inside your bra. If your milk starts leaking when you're not ready to feed, try pressing firmly on your nipples with the heels of your hands or your forearms to slow down the flow.

Changes to your breast milk

Unlike formula milk, the nutritional composition of breast milk changes – both during feeding and over the weeks that you feed. This ensures that your breast milk contains all the food and water your baby needs for at least the first 4 to 6 months of life.

Colostrum

The first food your baby receives from your breasts is colostrum. This is produced during late pregnancy in response to the hormones oestrogen and progesterone. It's a rich, golden-yellowish looking substance, which is produced for about two to three days. Although there's only a small amount of colostrum, it's a unique and valuable food for your baby. It contains a larger amount of protein than mature breast milk and all the minerals, fats and vitamins your baby needs in the first few days of life. Colostrum is rich in antibodies, which help to protect your baby from infections and build a strong immune system. Colostrum works as a laxative, too, clearing out the meconium (the first dark green stools) from your baby's bowels. Even if you don't intend to breastfeed for long, it's worth offering your baby the valuable colostrum for the first few days.

Transitional and mature breast milk

After two to three days, colostrum gradually becomes transitional milk. You might notice this change as a feeling of fullness in your breasts. You may experience this 'milk coming in' whether or not you breastfeed your baby. Transitional milk, which is thinner and whiter than colostrum, is a mixture of colostrum and mature milk.

After about two to three weeks, mature breast milk starts to come through. It has a watery, almost blue appearance when the milk starts to flow and changes to white as the fat content rises.

The changing appearance of mature breast milk has given rise to the idea that there are two types of milk: foremilk and hindmilk. In reality, however, there is only one form but because its creamier components are 'stickier', the milk that comes out when you begin to nurse your baby looks thin and watery. It's low in calories and fat and quenches your baby's thirst before she starts to feed.

As your baby continues to suck, the letdown reflex releases the milk, which is richer in fat, energy, and nutrients. Although there is less of it, this milk satisfies your baby's hunger and gives her the energy to grow. You can make sure that your baby has enough of this energy-rich milk by ensuring that she latches on properly and that she empties the first breast before you offer the other (this will also ensure a good supply overall). In time, the volume of milk produced will tend to decrease while the fat content will increase.

Maintaining a good milk supply

The production of breast milk is stimulated by the hormone prolactin, which responds to the touch of your baby's mouth on your nipple. So, if you feed your baby whenever she appears to be hungry or when your breasts feel full, you'll naturally produce all the milk your baby needs.

Some women are concerned that their supplies of milk are inadequate and try to 'build up' their reserves by restricting the amount of times that they breastfeed their babies. However, this can actually be counterproductive, as it reduces milk supply. If you worry that your baby seems hungry again shortly after feeding her, the solution may be as simple as feeding her more often and checking that she's latching on properly each time.

Ensuring baby feeds 'properly'

If you are worried whether your baby is getting enough milk (after all, you can't see it disappearing as with a bottle), ascertaining the following should help to reassure you:

◆ Your baby takes a large mouthful of breast; you should see more of the areola (the dark nipple skin) above your baby's top lip than below her bottom lip.
◆ That her chin touches your breast firmly and her cheeks stay rounded during sucking;
◆ She suckles rhythmically, taking long sucks and swallows with some pauses in between;
◆ She comes off the breast on her own when she finishes.

Occasionally, a baby is born with a tight piece of skin between the underside of her tongue and the floor of her mouth, which can make it hard for her to attach to the breast. Known as tongue-tie, it is easily treated so if you are worried that this is the case with your baby, mention it to your caregiver.

Sore nipples

Many women experience tenderness when they begin to breastfeed, and this may be accompanied by a pinching or burning sensation. In most cases, soreness can be cured simply by trying a different feeding position, perhaps changing it each time you breastfeed your baby. You also may have to make several attempts to get your baby to latch on correctly. If you want to change position, remember

---

ways to boost your milk supply

1 Feed more often. Try 'switch nursing', offering your different breast when your baby loses interest in the other, and 'breast compression' squeezing out a further mouthful when he's near finishing.

2 Expressing milk between breastfeeds, if necessary, will stimulate your breasts to produce more.

3 Take frequent sips of water. However, don't force yourself to drink large quantities (see page 332) or indulge in caffeinated and alcoholic drinks. What you eat and drink will pass through to your baby in your milk.

4 Watch your baby's reactions. If a food you normally eat seems to upset your baby, she simply may not enjoy it. Try replacing this food for another of similar nutritional value for a week.

5 If you can, refrain from offering a dummy for about a month or until breastfeeding is established; using dummies has been shown to reduce the amount of milk produced.

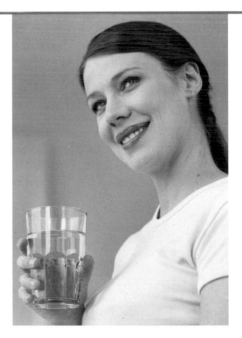

Before starting to breastfeed your baby, whether you're at home or in the hospital, try to make the atmosphere as calm as possible so that you can be as relaxed as you can. If necessary, take the phone off the hook or put a notice on the door asking not to be disturbed. Have a drink nearby to keep up your fluid intake.

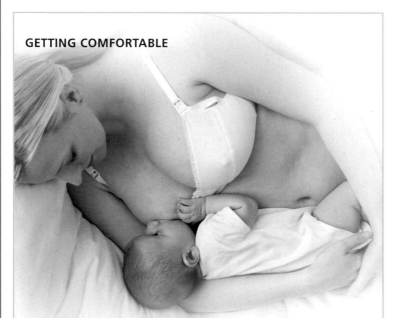

GETTING COMFORTABLE

A comfortable position can be the key to successful breastfeeding, so try out a few to see which work best. Generally, most women feed sitting upright on a chair, often with their feet raised and a pillow on their lap, but other positions can be adopted in certain circumstances. Whichever position you choose, your baby should be held close to you with her whole body facing your breast, her chest next to your chest. You should be able to bring her to your breast easily.

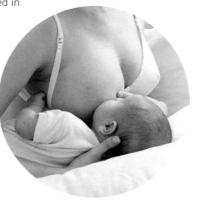

Your baby's mouth needs to form a tight seal over most of your areola. If this 'latching on' isn't achieved, your baby will chew or suck on your nipple, which can lead to problems such as nipple soreness (see page 299) or cracked nipples (see page 358). Some women find it difficult to get their babies to latch on at first. It often needs practice and patience in the early days.

POSITION YOUR BABY Before you begin feeding, make sure that you and your baby are both comfortable. If you're sitting upright you can either support her head and shoulders on your forearm or hold her head and shoulders with your free hand. Her head should be at the same level as your nipple and she should be able to reach your breast without any effort. For alternative feeding positions see box, left.

You may find it helpful to cup your breast with your hand or to support your breast by placing your fingers against your ribs just underneath it. Try not to place two fingers in a 'scissors grip' around your nipple, as it can prevent your baby feeding properly. Nor do you need to press your breast away from her nose so she can breathe – her flared nostrils allow her to breathe and feed simultaneously.

Your baby may instinctively start to suck as soon as she feels your breast against her cheek, or you can brush your baby's lips against your nipple to trigger her rooting reflex **1**. Once she opens her mouth wide, draw her quickly to your breast.

CHECK THAT SHE HAS LATCHED ON Your baby needs as much of your breast in her mouth as possible. If she's properly positioned, she'll have a mouthful of breast **2**, including your nipple and much of the underside of the areola, and her bottom lip should be curled back. Her jaw muscles will work rhythmically, as far back as her ears. If your baby's cheeks cave in when she's sucking, she isn't latched on properly. In this case, you'll need to reposition your baby and try again.

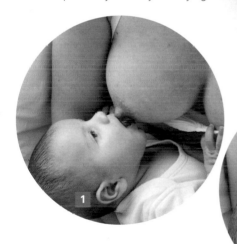

You can break the suction by inserting your little finger in the corner of her mouth **3**.

CHANGE BREASTS IF NECESSARY Your baby's sucking pattern will alter while she feeds, from short sucks to longer bursts, with pauses in-between. She'll let you know when your breast is empty by playing with it, falling asleep, or letting your nipple slide out of her mouth. You can then offer her the other breast. When you need to remove her from your breast, break the suction with your finger (as above). Don't worry if she refuses the second breast, but start with it the next time. It's important that your baby empties one breast before you offer her the other, because the last milk she'll get from your breast is the richer, calorie-packed milk.

to break the suction with your finger before removing your baby from the breast – pulling your baby away from your nipple will aggravate soreness.

Consider your nipple care, too. Very moist or very dry skin can cause soreness, so leave your bra off for a few minutes after breastfeeding to allow air to your skin, and make sure you wear bras made from natural fibres, such as cotton, which let your nipples 'breathe', and that aren't overly tight. Rubbing a little breast milk into your nipple after a feed or placing cool wet teabags on your nipples also can relieve tenderness.

If at any stage your nipples become red and shiny or you experience shooting pains in your breasts, consult your healthcare provider. You may have an infection such as thrush (see page 358). Other, less common, problems are discussed on page 357.

Engorgement

A few days after the birth, when the milk comes in, many women's breasts become engorged, feeling swollen, hard and painful with the accumulation of blood and milk. If this occurs, breastfeeding can become difficult, sometimes painful. Breastfeeding frequently – perhaps eight times or more in 24

hours – can help you to avoid engorgement. But if your breasts do feel full, try expressing a little milk before you a feed. Placing a cloth dipped in warm water on the areola before you begin to feed, and using a cold compress after you finish can help, too. Some women find that chilled cabbage leaves can offer relief: wash the outer leaves of a cabbage and place them on each breast for 10 to 20 minutes. Breast massage is another solution (see page 323).

Combining breast with bottle

If you want to give your baby breast milk from a bottle or intersperse breast milk with formula, do so after breastfeeding is established. To feed from a bottle your baby will need to learn a new sucking action, which can interfere with breastfeeding. If she is reluctant to feed from the bottle at first, it's often easier for someone else to feed her when you're out of the room. Alternatively, try a dropper or spoon.

If you want to stop breastfeeding altogether, do so gradually, interspersing breastfeeding with bottlefeeding. Not only will your baby need time to get used to feeding from a bottle, but your body also needs time to readjust. If you stop suddenly, there's a chance that you may become engorged (see above).

• •

HOW TO express your breast milk

• • •

At times, you may want spare breast milk, if, for example, your partner is taking a turn at feeding, or you're going out for a while. You can express milk using your hands or a pump.

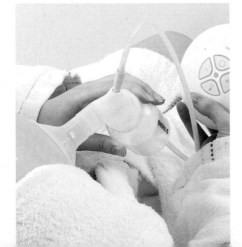

Your milk should be expressed straight into a sterile bottle, sterile plastic container, or breast milk freezer bag. You can store expressed milk in the coolest part of a fridge (not in the door) set at 4°C or lower for up to five days, in the freeze compartment for two weeks or in a domestic freezer set at 18°C or below for up to six months.

To express milk by hand, stimulate your milk flow by gently stroking downwards from the top of your breast toward the areola. Then place both your thumbs above the areola and your fingers below and begin

rhythmically squeezing the lower part of your breast while pressing toward your breastbone.

Many women, however, find using a hand, battery-operated or electric pump is quicker, more effective and easier. To use a syringe-style hand pump, simply place the funnel over your nipple, forming an airtight seal and then draw the cylinder in and out a few times. This sucks the milk out of your breast. You may need to try several pumps to find out what suits you, so see if you can borrow or rent a pump before buying.

Bottlefeeding your baby

Feeding your baby with infant formula milk from a bottle is a safe alternative to breastfeeding, as long as you maintain good hygiene and follow the manufacturer's instructions carefully.

Once you've made the decision to bottlefeed your baby, you'll quickly establish your own routine of cleaning and sterilising the equipment, preparing the formula and giving the bottle. It may seem like a lot of work, but all these processes have become much quicker and easier than they were in the past. If you haven't already bought all of your feeding, cleaning and sterilising equipment, see page 198 for some advice. There also are many different formulas on the market to suit individual parents' and babies' needs. Whichever you use, always keep in mind that bottlefed babies may be more prone to infections than breastfed babies, so you'll need to pay particular attention to hygiene.

Types of formula

The Department of Health advises that babies who aren't breastfed should be given formula milk until they're one year old. All baby formulas are carefully produced under government guidelines to ensure that they replicate human milk as closely as possible and contain the correct amounts of fat, protein and vitamins that your baby needs.

Babies under the age of one year shouldn't be given ordinary cow's milk, because it contains high levels of protein and minerals, which can put a strain on a baby's immature kidneys and cause dehydration. Cow's milk also doesn't contain sufficient iron for young babies. Goat's milk and condensed milk are also unsuitable for young babies.

If you're unsure as to which formula is best for your baby, your health visitor will be able to give you guidance. You can buy formula in powder, liquid concentrate and ready-to-feed forms at most supermarkets and pharmacies. Powdered formulas are usually the cheapest of these, while ready-to-feed

Keep your baby in a semi-upright position as he feeds. It will help him to swallow the formula more easily

forms are the most expensive but can be useful in the first few weeks, while you're getting used to feeding or if you're short of time.

There are two basic types of formula: those based on modified cow's milk and specialised formulas, usually based on soya milk.

Modified cow's milk

Most bottlefed babies are fed with a formula based on modified cow's milk; initially this will be one that is 'whey dominant' – proteins babies find easier to digest. (Casein-dominant formula or stage two or 'follow-on' milk contains proteins that are harder to digest and marketed as being able to keep babies satisfied longer). If your baby has fed on one while in the hospital without any problems, there's no reason to change when you get home. But if you're

In contrast to breast milk, which is always clean, it's possible for bacteria to get into baby formula and give a baby an upset stomach. To avoid this, thoroughly clean and sterilise all equipment before you make up a bottle. Feeding equipment can be washed and sterilised in a dishwasher or using chemicals, steam or a microwave.

It's best to feed your baby using freshly made formula milk; storing milk increases the likelihood of it becoming contaminated. If you need to feed your baby while away from home, use ready-to-drink infant formula.

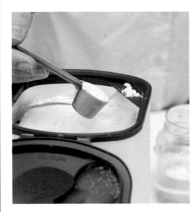

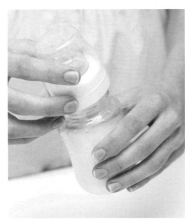

WASHING AND STERILISING

Fill the sink with hot, soapy water. Then clean the bottles, using a bottle brush around the thread at the top, and the teats, rings, discs and caps individually, removing stubborn milk deposits. Turn the teats inside out, scrub them with a teat brush and squirt water through the holes to check for blockages. Finally, rinse everything thoroughly in cold, clean, running water.

If using a chemical steriliser, empty the chemicals into the unit according to the manufacturer's instructions. Then immerse everything fully in the solution for the recommended length of time. If you're not using the items right away, you can keep them in the steriliser for up to 24 hours. Rinse with cooled, boiled water before use. Alternatively, you can use a microwave or stove-top steam steriliser or boil most of the items in a covered pan for 10 minutes – teats need only 3 minutes.

MAKE UP A FORMULA

Clean and disinfect your work surface then assemble your equipment and wash your hands. Stand the bottle on the surface and the teat and cap on the upturned steriliser lid.

Bring some fresh or filtered water to the boil and simmer for 1 to 2 minutes. Let cool to about 70°C (but no longer than 30 minutes). Don't use softened, bottled or repeatedly boiled water, as they may contain high levels of

mineral salts. If your tap water contains high levels of lead, consider buying a water filter.

Add the correct amount of cooled, boiled water to the bottle, then the correct number of scoops of formula, levelling each with a knife. Always use the scoop provided and add only the specified number of scoops per millilitres (fl oz) of water. Holding the teat by its edge, place it on the bottle and secure with the retaining ring. Cover with a cap. Shake vigorously until the powder dissolves.

Throw away any milk that has not been used within two hours.

SAFETY FIRST
PLASTIC BOTTLES The National Childbirth Trust (NCT) recommends not pouring boiling water for formula milk directly into a plastic bottle and discarding scratched or damaged bottles.

MEASUREMENTS Never heap or pack a scoop of formula or add an extra one. Make certain the amount of water is correct. If formula is over concentrated it may make your baby dehydrated; if it's too weak, your baby won't get enough nutrients. To make extra formula, add more water and powder in the correct proportions.

concerned that your baby isn't putting on enough weight or still seems hungry after you've given him his bottle, consider changing to another brand or type. However, always ask your health visitor's advice before you do this – the problem may not lie with the formula, but may be due to feeding techniques or an intolerance to a particular brand; or it may be caused by a medical condition that requires further investigation.

Specialised formula milk

Full-term, bottlefed babies who are diagnosed as intolerant to lactose or protein in cow's milk, or who have other feeding or medical problems, will be prescribed a hypoallergenic formula or soya milk, which has been formulated to provide babies with all the nutrients they need.

Feeding your baby

In the first few weeks, it can be a useful practice to prepare batches of formula in advance. Store prepared formula in the fridge for up to 24 hours, but keep bottles in the main body of the fridge, as it is slightly cooler than the door. You then can feed your baby as soon as he's hungry and he won't get upset while he's waiting and then refuse to feed. Also, avoid too many different people feeding him at first – let him get used to you and your partner. Feeding times should soon become relaxing and enjoyable occasions and you can help this by holding your baby close to you and maintaining eye contact with him (see page 345). By the time your baby is three months old, you'll see him starting to get excited when he knows his bottle is on its way.

Temperature of the milk

Although it's traditional to warm a baby's bottle to body temperature, most babies don't mind taking formula that's slightly colder, as long as it's at least at room temperature. To warm, use an electric bottle warmer, or place the bottle in a jug of hot, but not boiling, water for a few minutes. Don't use a microwave: the bottle may feel cool, but the formula continues heating after removal and may scald your baby's mouth. Always test the temperature before

giving a bottle by letting a couple of drops fall on the inside of your wrist – they should be just warm.

Once you've heated the bottle, feed your baby right away. Never keep formula warm for longer than an hour and always throw away unfinished formula. Bacteria can breed rapidly in warm formula and could result in your baby getting a stomach infection. If you're going out with your baby, take

---

SAFETY FIRST

CHOKING Even when your baby gets older, don't leave him on his own to feed from a propped-up bottle – there's always the risk that he could choke. You should inspect bottle teats each time you wash them to ensure that they're not clogged, worn or damaged. If fragments break off in your baby's mouth it can be dangerous.

---

bottles of prepared formula in a cool box and warm them for your baby when he's hungry.

Giving the bottle

Make yourself and your baby comfortable before you start and give him all your attention. Hold him securely in your lap with his head in the crook of your elbow and his back supported along your forearm (see page 303). Encourage the rooting reflex by touching your baby's lips with the teat of the bottle. When he's ready, insert the teat into his mouth. Keep checking that it doesn't slip out, as this may prevent him from sucking properly. While he feeds, keep the bottle tilted at an angle of about 45 degrees, so the top is full of formula and not air. If the teat becomes flattened, gently remove it from your baby's mouth to allow the air back in.

To help your baby relax, cuddle him close and talk or sing to him. Watch him all the time and respond to his demands. Some babies like to pause for air or to bring up some wind; others prefer to keep on feeding until all the formula has gone.

Meeting your baby's needs

Keeping an infant healthy and happy is a simple matter of meeting all of her daily needs. Besides feeding, she requires love, comfort, security, warmth and protection against infection.

As you get to know your baby, you'll start to recognize what's needed or wanted. Changing your baby's nappies or giving your baby a bath can be a little daunting at first, but using the following guidelines will make you an expert in no time at all.

Providing comfort

All babies cry at times, as it's their only means of telling their parents what they want. If your baby cries, it may be an indication that she's hungry, has a wet nappy, is overtired, or is too hot or cold. Attend to these things first, but if your baby is still crying, try the following to soothe her distress:

- *Holding* Pick up your baby and hold her close against you or carry her in a sling and talk, sing, sway, or gently dance.
- *Movement* Take your baby for a car ride or a walk in her buggy, put her in a baby bouncing chair, or sit in a rocking chair and gently rock her on your knee. But don't overdo it – too much jiggling can make a crying baby feel worse.
- *Noise* Music or sounds from machines, such as the vacuum cleaner or washing machine, can calm some babies, as can a musical toy.
- *Bathing* If your baby enjoys it, give her a warm bath. Once she's 2 months old, you can try adding one or two drops of essential lavender oil – it may have a calming and soothing effect.
- *Swaddling* Fold down the top-right corner of a light cotton blanket about 15 cm (6 inches). Lay your baby on her back with her head on the fold.

Pull the left-hand corner across your baby's body and tuck it under her back. Bring the bottom corner up under her chin. Finally, bring the right-hand corner across her body and tuck it under her back. The blanket should be secure but not tight and you can leave your baby's arms free if she prefers. Feel the back of your baby's neck regularly to check that she doesn't get too hot.

- *Massage* Lay your baby on her front across your knees and stroke her gently down her back and legs. Alternatively, hold her in the 'tiger in the tree' position (see page 346). To learn more techniques try attending a class in your area.
- *Dummy* If your baby likes to suck, a dummy can work wonders. Check with your health visitor what type to use and clean it between each use.

If your baby doesn't stop crying, no matter what you do, consult your doctor; persistent crying may be due to a number of causes. But if your doctor

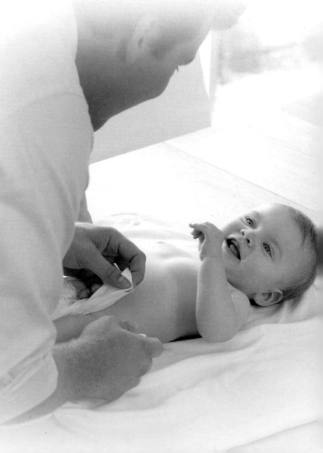

Involving your partner in the day-to-day care will give him an opportunity to get to know his baby.

pronounces your baby fit and well, don't blame yourself for the crying. Some babies will cry whatever you do and may just need to 'cry it out.'

Changing a Nappy

Newborn babies have very small bladders, so they can urinate up to 20 times a day in the first few weeks. Some babies also pass stools after every meal, so nappy changing is going to take up a big part of your early days as a parent (see page 316 for step by step advice).

Washing cloth nappies

While it's important that nappies are disinfected and washed thoroughly to prevent a baby from getting an infection, today, most parents choose to do so by simply washing them in sufficiently hot water (60°C) in a home washing machine. While it's important to remove any excrement on the nappies into the toilet and rinse them, it's possible to otherwise store them 'dry' in a lidded nappy pail. Some parents, however, add nappy soak or some tea tree oil. If you use a mesh laundry bag to hold used nappies, wraps and liners, you can simply put the bag and its contents into your machine although remember to turn them inside out. Another choice is to use a nappy-laundry service in your area, which may be more environmentally friendly than individual washing.

Keeping your baby clean

Your newborn has very sensitive skin and a limited potential for getting dirty, which means that on a daily basis you'll need to wash only her face, neck, hands, bottom and feet. This can be done by topping and tailing your baby (see page 312). After a week or two, you can start to bath your baby. However, at this stage you'll need to bath her only once or twice a week at most.

Until your baby is around three months old, it's best not to use any soaps or bath products for bathing. Plain water is sufficient. Some products may dry your baby's skin or cause nappy rash.

MORE **ABOUT**   your baby's excretions

One strange thing about becoming a mother is that you become obsessed with the contents of your baby's nappy. In fact, this is perfectly sensible, as they can tell you about your baby's health. In the first couple of days your baby will pass meconium. This sticky, greeny-black substance is left over from the amniotic fluid your baby swallowed in the uterus. Your baby's stools will then change, depending on how she's fed: if she's breastfed, they will be yellowy-orange and loose and won't smell very strong; if she's bottlefed, her stools will be pale brown, firmer and smell noticeably.

Immediately after the birth, your baby's nappy may also be stained dark pink or red. This is normal and a result of urates in her urine. If you're concerned about any change in the frequency, colour or consistency of her stools or urination patterns, tell your health visitor. Stools streaked with blood or frequent, pale, watery stools will need to be investigated.

However, baby oil or moisturiser may be useful for dry, flaky skin. Avoid baby powder; evidence suggests that it can choke a baby if inhaled.

When cleaning your baby, you'll need to take particular care when cleaning around the cord stump and, if your baby boy has been circumcised, you'll need to take care around his genitals (see page 313).

Care of the cord

Your baby's cord stump will turn black, shrivel up and fall off – normally within about 5 to 10 days. In the meantime, keep it clean and dry, using cooled, boiled water, surgical wipes, or antiseptic powder, depending on what your healthcare provider advises (see page 312). Leaving the stump exposed to the air as much as possible will help it to heal quickly .

Dressing your baby

The best clothes for your baby will be easy to put on, machine washable and made of natural fibres, such as cotton or wool, which are warm, but allow your baby's skin to breathe. For further information on the clothes your baby will need see page 200.

When dressing your baby, the objective is to keep her warm, not hot. For the first week or so after birth, she won't be able to regulate her body temperature, so it's important not to overdress or underdress her. Unless your home is very cold, she generally won't need to be dressed in more than a nappy and nightgown at night and a vest, nappy and all-in-one during the day (or a vest and nappy in warm weather). Outdoors, you may need to add a sweater and socks and in very cold weather, a pram

HOW TO treat skin irritations

Babies' skins are very sensitive and most experience minor irritations, such as nappy rash or cradle cap at some stage. You can successfully prevent and treat both these conditions at home with the following advice.

The first signs of nappy rash may be a mild red patch or small bumps on the buttocks. The skin may be angry-looking and moist, with open spots or blisters around your baby's buttocks or between the legs.

As nappy rash is mainly caused by prolonged contact with urine and faeces, the best way to prevent it is to change your baby's nappy as soon as it's wet or soiled. If your baby does have a rash, clean the area gently but thoroughly and apply a light nappy rash cream. Exposing your baby's bottom to the air for a while – perhaps after you've removed a soiled nappy – will help the rash to heal. If the rash doesn't clear up with ordinary

creams and the skin is bright red with white or red pimples in the folds, it may be infected with thrush (see page 364). In this case, consult your healthcare provider.

Cradle cap is a common and harmless condition that appears as greasy white or yellowish scales on a baby's scalp **1**. Cradle cap clears up of its own accord with time, but it can be unsightly. If you want to get rid of

the scales, try massaging aqueous cream or warmed baby oil into your baby's scalp. Leave the cream or oil on overnight, then brush **2** or wash it out. Never try to pick off the scales because you could cause an infection.

In severe or persistent cases of cradle cap, see your healthcare provider, as the cause of the skin problem may be a condition such as eczema (see page 364).

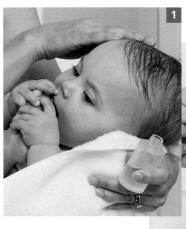

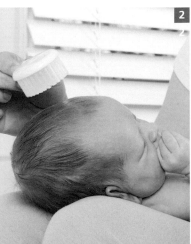

suit, mittens and hat. As a guide, dress your baby in the same number of layers that you dress yourself.

Unless it's less than 20°C (68°F) indoors, your baby does not need to wear a hat but she should wear one outdoors whenever your head feels a little cold. In summer, it's essential she wear a sun hat when outdoors.

Take care that your baby doesn't overheat if you're out shopping; in a car or a shop, remove her hat, mittens and outdoor clothing. Bear in mind, too, that if using a carrier or sling, this counts as an extra layer of clothing and a folded blanket or shawl is also two layers.

To help to protect your baby's delicate skin, wash her clothes using non-biological washing products designed for sensitive skins. Avoid fabric conditioner and bleach, as these have a potential to cause skin irritation. If your baby develops any rash or redness that may be related to the washing products, try running her washed clothes through an extra rinse cycle to remove any traces of soap or detergent. If the problem continues, talk to your caregiver.

Providing a safe place to sleep

For the first few weeks of her life your baby will sleep and wake at random. In these early days, you can choose to take your baby out with you in the evening or keep her up until you go to bed. Or, you may prefer to establish a regular bedtime routine from the beginning (see page 348).

Preventing SIDS

Whatever routine you decide, the way that you put your baby down to sleep is important. Most parents worry about sudden death infant syndrome – also called cot death (see page 383) – which happens when a baby dies suddenly, without any apparent explanation. Fortunately, cot deaths are rare and research has found that you can minimise the risks significantly by ensuring that your baby sleeps in the correct position and condition. Make sure you follow all the advice given below:

- *Let your baby sleep in the same room as you* Having your baby close is best for the first six months, or you can use a baby monitor.

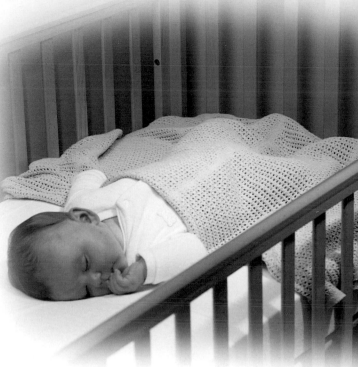

The feet-to-foot sleeping position, in which your baby's feet are at the bottom of the foot of the cot, allows her to move without getting tangled in the blankets.

- *Always put her to sleep on her back* This is the safest sleeping position unless the doctor has advised you otherwise. While your baby's awake, however, she should have time on her tummy to develop her neck, shoulder and arm muscles.
- *Tuck in any blankets and sheets* If there are covers in your baby's cot tuck them in around the mattress so that her face can't become covered. Also, place her in the 'feet-to-foot' position (see above) so that her feet reach the end of the cot, with lightweight blankets tucked under the mattress and reaching up only as far as her chest. Alternatively, dress your baby in a weight-appropriate sleeping bag and don't use any covers.
- *Check that the cot conforms to safety standards* and ensure your baby always sleeps in her own bed.
- *Make sure your baby's mattress is new and kept clean* Don't use a second-hand mattress and make sure the mattress is dry, firm and well aired.
- *Avoid placing soft items in your baby's cot* This

includes quilts, pillows, comforters, bumpers, sheepskins and soft toys.

- *Don't share your bed* and don't let her sleep on soft items such as a sofa, armchair, waterbed, beanbag or cushion. She can get buried under loose covers. It is especially dangerous to bed share if you smoke, have drunk alcohol or taken illegal drugs or medication that makes you sleepy.
- *Don't fall asleep breastfeeding your baby* Or while holding her on a sofa or armchair.
- *Don't overheat the room* and don't let your baby get too hot. The room should feel comfortable for a lightly clothed adult – between 16 to 20°C. Your baby should never sleep with a hot water bottle or electric blanket nor next to a radiator, heater, fire or in direct sunlight.
- *Don't smoke* and always keep your baby in a smoke-free environment.
- *Encourage your baby to use a dummy for sleeping* This has been related to a reduced risk of cot death. One possible theory is that the bulky handle of the dummy may help air to get to the baby's airways, even when bedclothes are over her face. Do not worry if your baby's dummy falls out while she is sleeping or if your baby does not want to use one. If you are breastfeeding, wait until this is established before offering a dummy. Not all babies take to dummies; never force your child to use one if she rejects it.
- *If your baby is unwell, seek advice promptly* For signs that your baby needs to be taken to the doctor, see box, right.

Safeguarding your baby's health

Young babies are susceptible to bacterial infections, which can have severe consequences for their well-being, and are also at risk from colds and flu. Therefore, while your baby is young, make sure you limit the number of people who handle her and ensure they wash their hands thoroughly before doing so. Anyone with a cold or cough should not be permitted near your baby.

After your baby's birth, you'll be invited to take her for regular checks at a baby clinic, usually held in your GP's surgery. At each visit, your baby's weight, height and head circumference will be measured to make sure she's growing properly. Routine physical and developmental checks will also take place when she's six to eight weeks old and then at around eight to nine months, at one year and at 18 to 24 months. The purpose of all these checks is to detect as early as possible any problems that may affect your child's health and development. They also provide an opportunity to discuss any concerns you have about your baby's health and well-being.

At the age of eight weeks, most babies start their routine immunisation schedules (see page 370). These are vital in protecting your baby's health and that of the people around her. Your doctor or health visitor will discuss any possible side effects of immunisations before they are given.

HEALTH FIRST

SYMPTOMS Babies often have minor illnesses and it can be hard to tell whether medical help is needed. Below are guidelines for when to call the doctor – these are slightly different for newborns (see page 360) – but if you're ever in doubt, err on the side of caution. Seek help if your baby:

- Has convulsions (fits) or is floppy.
- Has difficulty breathing, turns blue, or has stopped breathing.
- Cannot be wakened or is unusually drowsy or unresponsive.
- Has severe vomiting or diarrhoea, appears to be in severe pain, or passes blood in her stools.
- Refuses to feed twice in a row.
- Develops a purple-red rash, similar to bruises, anywhere on the body.
- Has a high fever – a body temperature above 100.4ºF (38ºC).
- Has a high pitched or unusual cry, or screams or cries inconsolably.

PICKING UP YOUR BABY

It's natural to feel a little nervous when you first pick up your baby, but he's tougher than you think. You do, however, need to support his head.

SUPPORT YOUR BABY Slide one hand under his head **1** and the other beneath his back and bottom.

BRING HIM TO YOUR CHEST As you stand upright, bring your baby close **2**. Keep his head slightly raised.

REST HIM IN YOUR ARMS Slide the hand under his bottom up to his head. Bend your other arm so that his head rests in your elbow **3**. Use your free hand for support.

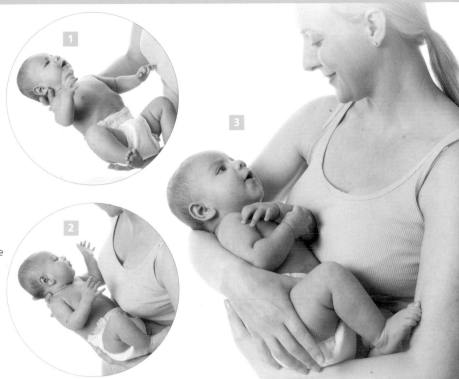

HOLDING YOUR BABY

Your young baby can appear fragile, but you shouldn't be afraid to hold him firmly. Babies like to feel secure when they are held and yours will enjoy the closeness and warmth of your body. As well as being cradled in your arms, he may enjoy these holds:

FACE DOWN Position your baby's head just over the crook of your elbow with your forearm supporting the length of his body **1**. Place your other hand between his legs so that you can support his tummy.

AGAINST YOUR SHOULDER Holding your baby upright allows him to feel and hear your heartbeat. Use

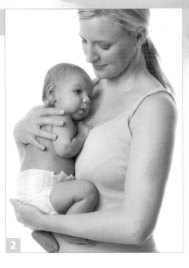

one hand to take your baby's weight under his bottom **2**, and the other to support his head and neck.

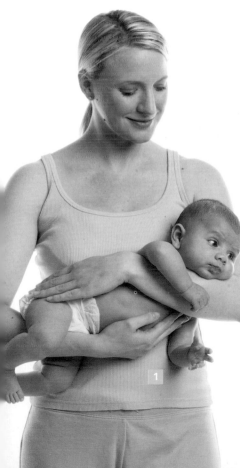

Until the cord stump falls off you only need to wash your newborn's face, neck, hands, feet, genitals and bottom each day.

To top and tail her, have on hand a bowl of cooled, boiled water, some cotton wool and a soft towel. To avoid the spread of infection, always use a fresh piece of cotton wool for each part of your baby's body. If she gets cold, keep her nappy on while you clean her top half, then put a vest on her while you clean her bottom half.

CARE OF THE CORD

Until the cord stump falls off, wash it each day to prevent infection. Incorporate this into your topping and tailing routine. To clean the cord, dip some cotton wool into the cooled, boiled water, then wipe the stump and the area around it gently. Dry thoroughly with a fresh piece.

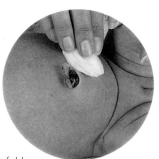

When putting on your baby's nappy, fold it back below the stump to keep it dry from urine. If the area around the stump is red or there is any discharge, consult your healthcare provider.

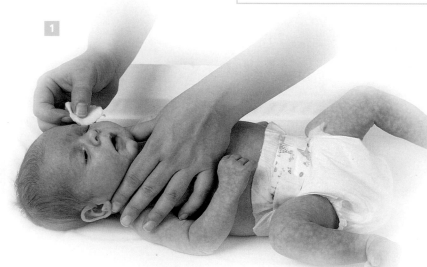

CLEAN YOUR BABY'S FACE Dip a piece of cotton wool in the water and wipe one of your baby's eyes, moving from the inner to the outer corner **1**. Using a fresh piece, repeat on the other eye. Using more moistened cotton wool, wipe the rest of her face, including her nose and ears – but avoid wiping inside these sensitive areas. Clean in her neck creases, then gently pat her skin dry.

CLEAN HER HANDS AND ARMS Gently un-clench each of your baby's hands and wipe clean **2**, particularly between her fingers. Lift her arms and using fresh cotton wool, wipe the armpit areas. Gently pat these areas dry with a towel.

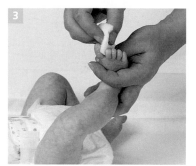

CLEAN HER FEET Use more moistened cotton wool to wipe the top and bottom of your baby's feet and between her toes **3**. Dry each foot carefully.

REMOVE YOUR BABY'S NAPPY If your baby has had a bowel movement, take her nappy off slowly, using the front to remove as much of the mess as possible **4**. Fold the nappy over, place in a plastic bag and put it aside for later disposal.

CLEAN HER TUMMY AND LEGS

Holding your baby firmly but gently, wipe her tummy area with some wet cotton wool. Using fresh cotton wool, clean along the folds of your baby's legs **5**. Wipe downwards and away from her body to avoid transmitting any infections to her genital area.

CARING FOR A CIRCUMCISED BOY

If your baby boy has been circumcised, avoid giving him a bath until the wound has healed. If he has a dressing, you may need to apply a new one when you change his nappy for the first day or two. Use a light dressing such as gauze and put petroleum jelly on the gauze so that it won't stick to his skin.

It will probably take around seven to ten days for the wound to heal. During this time the tip of the penis may be red and raw and there may also be a yellow secretion. It may even become ulcerated if it comes in contact with wet nappies. If there's persistent bleeding, fever, pus-filled blisters or swelling, consult your baby's doctor.

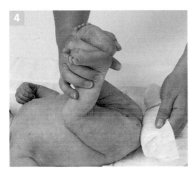
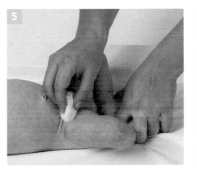
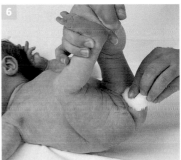

CLEAN HER GENITALS AND BOTTOM When cleaning a girl, hold her ankles gently with one hand, put your finger between her ankles, and lift her bottom slightly. Using fresh cotton wool, clean the outer lips of her vulva – but don't clean inside **6**. Always wipe downward when cleaning her genitals so that you don't transfer bacteria from her anus to her vagina. Then, keeping her bottom raised, clean her buttocks using fresh cotton wool. Clean the backs of her thighs and up her back if necessary. Dry the whole area thoroughly.

CLEANING A BABY BOY

Your baby boy may urinate when you remove his nappy, so do so slowly.

Using fresh cotton wool, wipe his penis using a downward motion – don't pull the foreskin back. Clean around his testicles as well. Holding your baby's ankles, lift his bottom gently and clean his anal area and the backs of his thighs. Pat the whole area thoroughly dry.

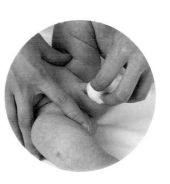

Most babies love bath-times but, as your baby won't be getting very dirty, she won't need a bath more than about once a week. As some babies do feel the cold, it's best to warm the room and have everything ready before you start. You'll need two soft towels, a bowl of cooled, boiled water for washing her face, cotton wool, mild baby shampoo, a plastic baby bathtub or basin and a clean nappy and clothes.

FILL THE BATH AND TEST

Place the bath on a secure surface, and make sure that it won't slip. Try to keep the bath away from draughts.

To avoid scalding, always put cold water in the tub first then add the hot water. Mix thoroughly and check the water with your elbow or the inside of your wrist to make sure that it's comfortably warm – it should be about body temperature.

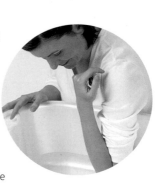

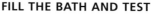

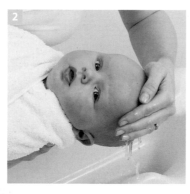

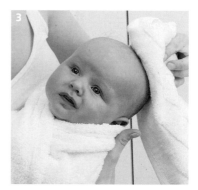

WASH YOUR BABY'S FACE To avoid any risk of infection, it's best to wash your baby's face with a separate bowl of warm, previously boiled water. Moisten some cotton wool and gently wipe your baby's eye from the nose outward **1**. Using another fresh piece of cotton wool do the same with the other eye. Use fresh cotton wool to wipe around his mouth, nose, ears, and neck – but don't wipe inside his ears and nose.

WASH HIS HAIR Wrap your baby a little tighter in the towel, making sure his arms are covered. Hold his legs between your arm and side so you can grip them under your armpit. Support his body along the length of your forearm and hisr head with your hand. Hold him over the bath or basin. Use your free hand to take some of the water over his hair. Gently apply some baby shampoo. Rinse it off with handfuls of water **2**.

DRY HIS HAIR Pat – rather than rub – your baby's hair dry using the edge of a soft towel **3**. Don't press the soft fontanelles too hard and avoid covering his face, as he might panic and cry.

SAFETY FIRST
STAY WITH YOUR BABY

Bath your baby in a baby bath or basin until he can sit up on his own. Never leave him alone, even for a minute – babies can drown in just a couple of inches of water. If you have to leave the room, wrap your baby up and take him with you.

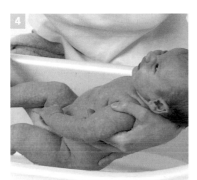

PLACE YOUR BABY IN THE BATH
Unwrap your baby. Place one arm behind his back and grip the arm farthest from you. Support his legs and bottom with your other hand and gently lower him into the bath **4**.

WASH YOUR BABY'S BODY
Supporting your baby's head and shoulders with one hand, wash his body with the other **5**. Pay particular attention to the areas under his arms and at the tops of his legs. However, at this young age, he won't need much washing. As he gets older, you'll need to move him around a bit more to clean him more thoroughly.

LIFT YOUR BABY OUT To remove your baby from the bath, keep one arm around his shoulder and slide the other hand under his bottom. Lift him out of the water in the same position as you put him in.

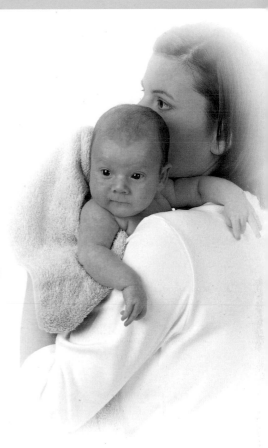

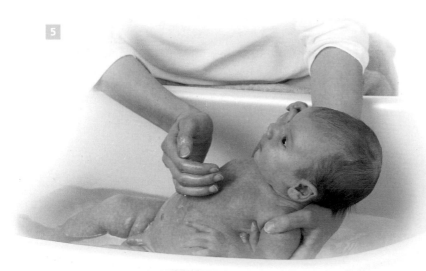

DRY YOUR BABY As soon as you've lifted your baby out of the bath, place him on a large, soft towel. Fold over one side and then the other, but avoid covering his face. Gently pat him dry **6**, paying particular attention to his neck, under his arms, and around his legs, genitals and bottom.

DRESS YOUR BABY Once your baby is dry, put on a clean nappy. Then dress him, while keeping exposed parts of his body covered with the towel.

To avoid nappy rash and to keep your baby comfortable, try to change her nappy as soon as it's wet or soiled. You can change your baby on the floor or a changing table. If you use a table, always keep one hand on your baby, and never leave her alone.

When removing a soiled disposable nappy, use the front of to clean up as much mess as possible; you should use a liner with a cloth nappy. Once the nappy's off, clean your baby thoroughly as you would when topping and tailing (see page 312).

POSITION AN OPENED NAPPY

With your baby on her back and an opened out the nappy beside her, lift your baby's ankles with one hand and slide the nappy under her bottom with the other **1**.

BRING UP THE FRONT Let go of her ankles and place the front of the nappy across her tummy **2**. If you are changing a boy, place his penis pointing down so he doesn't urinate on you.

FASTEN THE SIDES Smoothe the nappy down on her tummy then unpeel the protective backing and attach the tabs to the nappy **3**. Tuck in the waistband neatly.

TO REMOVE Unfasten the tabs, take the nappy down between her legs then roll up and place in a sack.

WASHING NAPPIES

To ensure used nappies are sanitised, machine wash them (plus any wrappers or cloth liners) at 60°C. Store them in a mesh bag in a dry nappy bucket until ready to wash then put the bag and its contents in the washer on their own. Remove as much excrement as possible into the toilet beforehand. Use half to two-thirds the recommended amount of non-biological detergent. Hang to dry on a rack or place in a tumble dryer.

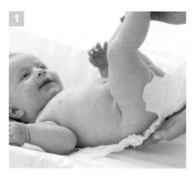
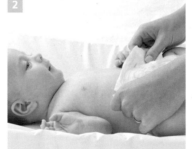
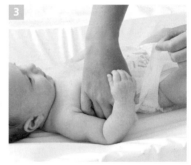

USING A REUSABLE NAPPY

Cloth nappies come in many different styles although one-piece pre-shaped ones are most like disposables and can be put on similarly. They have self-stick or popper closings with elasticated legs.

Pocket nappies have a separate waterproof outer layer (known as a wrap) and a fleecy inner layer and require an absorbent insert or liner to soak up wetness or excrement.

Flat nappies must be folded before use and then covered with plastic pants.

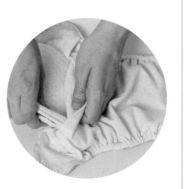

PUTTING ON A VEST

Your baby will probably enjoy the contact she has with you while you dress her. If she's less enthusiastic, make dressing fun, with smiles and cuddles. Save time by gathering her clothes together before you start.

OPEN THE NECK Stretch the neck opening wide, and place the back of it at the crown of your baby's head. Gather up the fabric, keeping it clear of her face **1**.

PULL IT OVER YOUR BABY'S HEAD AND FIT THE SLEEVES Gently pull the vest over her face without 'catching' her ears. Adjust the fabric. Reach in to gently hold your baby's wrist then guide it through a sleeve. Pull the sleeve down with your other hand Repeat with the other side **2**.

NEATEN AND FASTEN Gently pull down the vest. Fasten the poppers, if appropriate **3**.

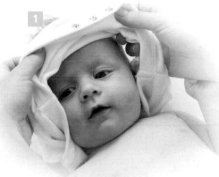

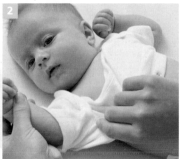

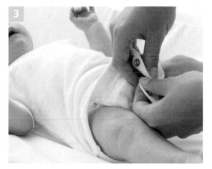

PUTTING ON AN ALL-IN-ONE

Open all the poppers of the suit before you start, then lay your baby on top.

INSERT YOUR BABY'S LEGS Gather the leg material and slide it over her foot **1**. Pull the material up her leg. Repeat with the other leg.

INSERT YOUR BABY'S ARMS Gather up one sleeve, and slide it over her wrist **2**. Repeat on the other side.

FASTEN THE POPPERS Straighten the sides **3**, then do up the poppers, starting at the bottom.

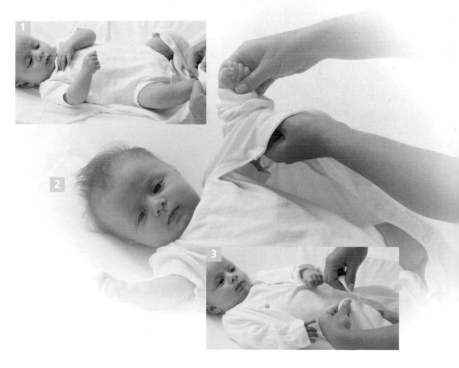

IN THE CAR

Your baby must travel in the appropriate infant car seat, which must be correctly fitted. If you're fitting it yourself, follow the manufacturer's instructions carefully, and make sure that the seat is suitable for your make of car – some require a special anchorage system.

FIT THE CAR SEAT Infant car seats are best placed in the middle of the rear seat, but some are suitable for the front passenger side, provided there is no air bag fitted. Current recommendations are that your baby should face the rear until she's four years old.

If not using an Isofix system (which fixes to the chassis), strap the seat in place with your car's seat belt, checking that the straps aren't twisted. The seat belt buckle must not rest on the frame. Check that the belts are tight enough to prevent excessive movement.

STRAP YOUR BABY IN THE SEAT
Place your baby in the seat and fasten the straps securely. Check them each time as fit will be affected by the different clothes your baby wears. As you drive, keep checking on your baby. Consider fitting a second mirror so that

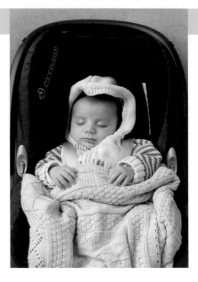

you can keep an eye on her without turning your head.

The inside of cars can get very hot. Check your baby regularly for overheating and use a sun diffusion screen on the window, if necessary. Never leave your baby alone in a car.

USING A CARRIER

Until the age of 4 months, place your baby in a carrier facing your chest so that her head is supported and she can feel your heartbeat. An older baby will enjoy facing forward, looking out at new surroundings.

If using a sling, make sure your baby is held upwards as in your arms and that her face is uncovered and she can breathe freely.

No matter how much support the carrier provides, always protect your baby's head with your hands when bending forward or to the side. Never leave your baby unattended in the carrier or use it as a cot.

PUT ON THE CARRIER Strap yourself into the carrier, following the manufacturer's instructions **1**. Fasten one side.

EASE YOUR BABY INSIDE
Supporting your baby's head, lift her into the carrier. Support her weight on the open side with one hand while you ease her legs into the holes with your free hand. Fasten the straps and buckles, then adjust them so that your baby's weight is evenly supported **2**. When you've finished using the carrier, always take your baby out of it and put her down somewhere safe before you take off the carrier.

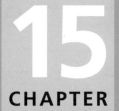

CHAPTER

Looking after yourself

Your baby's here at last and you're euphoric – if not a little exhausted. You may be feeling unexpectedly uncomfortable, perhaps even a little bit down. But relaxation, a nutritious diet and gentle exercise will help your body to readjust to its non-pregnant state and give you the energy to focus on being a mum.

about making haemorrhoids worse (see page 69). Your abdominal muscles, which you use to eliminate waste, may be temporarily ineffective because they have been stretched.

The more pressure you feel to have a bowel movement the less likely you are to perform. So the best thing you can do is not worry. Although your first few bowel movements are likely to cause discomfort, your stitches won't be affected, and you should be back to normal within a few days. Eating plenty of fibre – whole grains and fresh fruit and vegetables – and drinking fluids will help to get your bowels moving again. Gentle exercise and pelvic-floor exercises will help to ease any discomfort. However, if you are constipated your healthcare provider may suggest stool softeners or a laxative.

Breast discomfort

Even if you choose not to breastfeed, the hormonal changes that prime the breasts for breastfeeding will still take place. The pituitary gland begins the process of lactation (milk production) by producing and releasing the hormone prolactin. Once this process has begun, your baby encourages milk production by her frequent sucking. Two to four days after the birth, your breasts will become larger and firmer and may be painful as they prepare to provide milk. This is referred to as engorgement.

While your breasts are engorged, wearing a well-fitting, supportive bra will make you much more

---

HEALTH FIRST

PERSISTENT SWELLING If swelling persists after the birth or you experience bad headaches or pains in your legs, call your healthcare provider, as these are signs of high blood pressure (see page 253). If you experience swelling in one leg accompanied by severe pain, this could signal deep vein thrombosis (see page 252); seek urgent medical attention.

---

comfortable. Some experts recommend wearing a bra 24 hours a day during the engorgement period. Before breastfeeding, it may help to stand under a very warm shower or put warm compresses on your breasts. The moist heat will dilate the milk ducts and, when your baby sucks, the milk will flow more freely, and your breasts will be relieved of pressure.

If you're not going to breastfeed, try putting a cool compress on your breasts and take an analgesic such as paracetamol or ibuprofen. Don't stimulate your breasts or try to express milk to relieve pressure, as this will only cause your body to produce more milk. Engorgement lasts around two to five days – lack of stimulation by a sucking baby will gradually slow and then stop the production of milk. There's no need for special care for healthy breasts. Washing your breasts with mild soap and rinsing well is all that is necessary. If your breasts are inflamed, extremely uncomfortable or if you have cracked nipples, see page 358 for care instructions.

Body shape

On average, giving birth results in a 5-kg weight loss, which sounds great, until you check your shape in the mirror to see huge breasts, a distended stomach and sagging skin. However, this is exactly how a postnatal body should look. Your breasts are preparing to feed your baby; your stomach sticks out because of fluid retention and because your uterus hasn't yet contracted, the sagging is caused by overstretched skin and loss of muscle tone. Over time, your body will get closer to its pre-pregnancy shape. Your waist may be slightly bigger, but a healthy, nutritious diet and the right exercise regime will do wonders. However, now is definitely not the time to put yourself on a diet (see page 333).

Skin changes and hair loss

Altered hormone levels after the birth can be hard on your skin, making it spottier, drier and more sensitive. Skin pigmentation such as the linea nigra and chloasma (see page 66) should fade gradually, but some may never completely disappear. To prevent dark areas from getting darker, avoid excessive sun exposure or use a good sunscreen.

MASSAGING ENGORGED BREASTS

If you're breastfeeding, your baby's frequent sucking will help to diminish engorgement, but in some countries, like Japan, women are encouraged to massage their breasts to relieve discomfort. Cup your breasts, supporting them from below and thrust your chest forwards while pushing your breasts together with your hands. The flow of milk from the base of your breasts will be much freer. Hold your left breast and gently move your hands on the breast, in a circular action around your nipple. Repeat on your right breast. Repeating this massage daily while engorged should help to alleviate discomfort.

Stretchmarks will fade in time. Retin-A cream or gel and laser treatment may slightly reduce their appearance, but before you embark on any treatment, make sure it's safe, if you're breastfeeding.

You can expect to sweat a lot after the birth as your body gets rid of the extra fluids accumulated during pregnancy. This can continue for up to six weeks. You'll perspire more if you're breastfeeding, as it speeds up your metabolic rate. Make sure you drink plenty of fluids to help to accelerate the process. Wearing natural fibres, such as cotton and wool, will allow your skin to breathe. If you are concerned about your sweating, take your temperature. If it's over 37°C, talk to your healthcare provider, as you may have an infection.

Some women are alarmed to find their hair falling out in handfuls after the birth. This is perfectly normal and nothing to worry about. During pregnancy, hormones arrest the normal cycle of growth and loss. When hormone levels plummet after the birth, the resting phase goes into overdrive, resulting in what can seem like a massive loss of hair. However, this amount of hair is simply what you would have normally lost over nine months.

Within six months your hair should have resumed its normal pattern of growth and loss. Until it does, handle your hair gently. Only wash it when necessary, using a mild shampoo and a nourishing conditioner. Don't use heated rollers, hair dryers or straightening irons, as these may cause damage. Avoid chemical-based hair treatments, such as perms or hair-relaxers, until your hair is back to normal.

Back pain

This is very common after the birth and can last for months. During pregnancy your back had to support the weight of your growing baby, as well as compensate for weaker abdominal muscles. Relaxin made ligaments and joints looser, and you more prone to backache. Pregnancy also shifted your centre of gravity, so you had a tendency to lean back and push your tummy forwards. Giving birth can exacerbate back problems, especially if labour was long and exhausting. If you had an epidural, you may experience pain where the anaesthetic was injected. Once your baby's born, bending to pick him up or put him down, or sitting for long hours breastfeeding can make matters worse.

How long back pain lasts depends on your individual circumstances, but gentle exercise that builds up muscle tone in your abdomen (see page 336) and back can help alleviate a lot of problems. However, consult your caregiver before starting to exercise. He or she may want to check that any pain doesn't stem from a more serious underlying condition such as a bruised, or even broken, coccyx.

To check your posture when standing, imagine that a wire is pulling your head towards the ceiling. Relax your shoulders so that your chest isn't too tight. Gently pull your tummy in and lengthen your spine. If you're sitting down for long periods, make sure that your lower back is always supported. Slowly roll your neck to the front and the side to relieve tension in your shoulders.

Getting your periods back

If you aren't breastfeeding, your periods will probably start within about four to six weeks. If you're breastfeeding, you may resume menstruation

RECOVERING FROM A CAESAREAN

A Caesarean is major abdominal surgery so it's inevitable that you'll experience some pain after delivery from the incision as well as from after-birth contractions. You will also produce lochia and may have a sore perineum if the Caesarean occurred late in labour.

Care following a Caesarean differs slightly from that given for a vaginal birth. For example, you will be offered injections, support stockings and early mobilisation to reduce the risk of blood clots (DVT).

When you can be moved, you'll be brought to the maternity unit. You may be encouraged to get up later that day, with assistance. Moving around will help you to feel better and recover sooner.

PAIN RELIEF Medication will be offered to you after the surgery and for the next few days. Depending on the pain-relief protocol in your

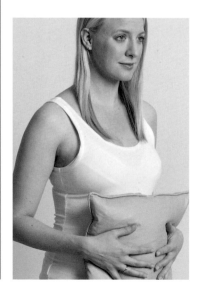

hospital, you may get continuous pain relief by a special intravenous (IV) line that you control, called patient controlled analgesia (PCA). Don't be afraid to give yourself adequate medication. Short-term postnatal medications won't significantly affect your baby and the analgesia will help you to move about more and sooner, speeding up your recovery. Also, inadequate analgesia – and continued pain – can interfere with breastfeeding.

If you had an epidural or spinal, morphine analgesia can sometimes be given through the epidural catheter to help you through the first 24 hours. You also could receive injections of a narcotic. After the first day, you may be given medication by mouth or some hospitals use suppositories, which last for 12 to 18 hours.

EATING AND DRINKING For the first 24 hours you'll have an intravenous line through which fluids are given. You may have a liquid diet on your day of surgery and progress to solids depending on your medical condition and healthcare provider.

GOING TO THE TOILET Your urinary catheter will usually be removed within 24 hours. On the second or third day after surgery, you may find that you experience gas pains. This is because it usually takes a few days for your bowels to start functioning normally. Rocking gently backwards and forwards

while sitting in a chair, taking short walks as often as you can and changing your position frequently can all help your bowels work more quickly.

CARE OF THE INCISION Using a pillow or abdominal binder can ease incisional discomfort. While walking, stand as straight as possible and have someone with you in case you feel dizzy. Supporting your stomach by holding it with your hands can provide support and comfort.

The dressing should be removed about 24 hours post op and your sutures or clips will be removed before you go home or at your GP's surgery, within four to seven days. While you're in hospital, the staff will gently clean and dry the wound and the incision should heal within about a week. At home, you or your partner should look at it daily to make sure it's healing properly. If you have inflammation or any pus-like drainage from the incision, consult your healthcare provider.

After the bandage is off, you can wash the area with mild soap, rinse well and pat dry. For a few months after the wound has healed, you may experience a decrease in sensation on or near the scar. Most sensation will return and the scar will get less noticeable as your abdominal strength increases. It's also not unusual to experience a tingling sensation as the nerves in the skin begin to regenerate. It's generally believed that the internal uterine incision heals in six weeks although the scar itself can take up to a year to heal completely and that you keep it out of the sun for at least 6 months.

MANAGING BREASTFEEDING You should start as soon as possible, although finding a comfortable position will be key. Either in bed or a comfortable chair with a pillow supporting your back and another over your incision, lay your baby on your lap in the 'football' hold, lying alongside your body, and support her head with your hand. Alternatively, you can lay her across the pillow on her side so that her mouth is level with your breast. If you find it difficult to sit, lay your baby facing you with her mouth in line with your breast and your arm supporting her head. Make sure that you have plenty of pillows to support you. A specially designed breastfeeding pillow will make feeding easier.

SITTING UP Begin very slowly and gradually ease yourself into each position. Roll gently onto your side and bring up both knees. Use your hands to push yourself up into a seated position; it will be painful so keep pushing with your arms until you are stabilised. Then wiggle your hips backwards underneath you and bring your arms forward, suppoting yourself on your hands.

GETTING OUT OF BED Once you are sitting, swing your legs slowly to the side of the bed, and place your feet on the floor. Use your hands to push yourself forwards and take your weight on your feet. You'll crouch over at first. Press a cushion against your incision to support the scar. Try to straighten up. Once you feel comfortable on your feet, take a few small steps. Keep your head up and try and breathe in and out through your mouth.

RETURNING HOME Most women stay in hospital for two to four days after a Caesarean, depending on what help they have at home. Once you're home, avoid heavy lifting or returning to work until you've had your check-up, usually in four to six weeks. You also should avoid driving until you can move without pain and are able to make an emergency stop. You should plan to have help with other children, housework and cooking.

REGAINING STRENGTH Once home, you should concentrate on resting whenever you can and doing some gentle exercises to strengthen your abdominals. These can be done in bed. Good ones to try and do several times a day are pelvic tilts. This is where you contract your abdominals and press your lower back into the bed. Do about 4–8, holding each one for 2 seconds.

Leg slides, which consist of you lying on your back with your knees bent then pressing your ankle down and sliding the foot down the bed are also effective abdominal strengtheners. Do 4 pushes with each heel and rest between sets if you need to.

Slowly lifting your hips off the bed and then doing the reverse – adopting an all-fours position and then slowly lowering and raising your abdomen up to 5 times a session, are other gentle ways that prepare you for being more active and able to care for your baby. For more about exercising after a Caesarean, see page 335.

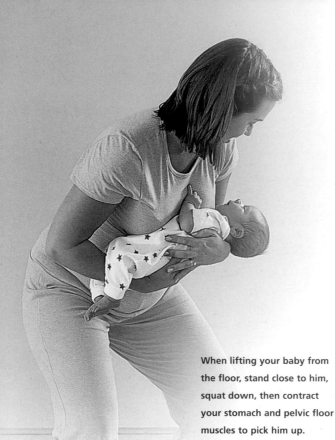

When lifting your baby from the floor, stand close to him, squat down, then contract your stomach and pelvic floor muscles to pick him up.

If you're not breastfeeding, you can start taking birth control pills about two to three weeks after the birth. If you are breastfeeding, oestrogen-based pills can affect milk production. In which you case, you may be able to take a progesterone-only pill. Avoid using barrier contraception if you have had stitches or until your cervix is completely healed. Your healthcare provider will be able to advise you in detail about your choices.

Postnatal check-up

To make sure that you're recovering well, you will need to see your healthcare provider about six weeks after the birth; however, you may want to see him or her earlier if you have any medical worries, are suffering from depression or have had a Caesarean and need to have sutures or clips removed.

At this visit, your weight and blood pressure will be checked, and a pelvic examination will be done to see if your uterus has reduced sufficiently.

If you have not had a cervical smear in the last three years, you will be advised to have one at three months after the delivery. Any incisions – Caesarean or episiotomy – will be checked to see if they are healing properly. You will be asked about your bowel and bladder function, breast changes, any pains you might have and how your baby is feeding.

Keep a list of questions to ask at your visit. This is also the time to talk about how you're getting on emotionally, especially if you're feeling unusually tired or sad, if you've experienced a significant change in your appetite, or if you're just not feeling the way you expected. You also can discuss suitable contraception. Make the most of these visits, that's why they're there.

at around this time, or you may have irregular periods or no periods until you have stopped breastfeeding – everyone is different. Like many women, you may find that your menstrual cramps are less severe than those you experienced before you were pregnant. It's unclear why this is but it's definitely a change for the better.

The amount of menstrual flow for the first few cycles can range from light to quite heavy, but should soon settle down. You may find it helpful to mark on a calendar when the flowing occurs and the type – heavy, light or spotting – to show to your healthcare provider. You also should describe any cramping or discomfort that occurs.

Choosing birth control

You will begin to ovulate before you have your first period following childbirth, so having unprotected sex could result in another pregnancy. To prevent this, you'll need to use some form of contraception as soon as you start having sex again.

Enjoying motherhood

Being a mother is one of the most important roles you will have in life and is fulfilling in a way you probably couldn't even imagine before your baby was born. Although your new baby will take up a lot of your time and energy, you still need to make time for you.

A new baby is a 24-hour-a-day responsibility, which can be a bit of a shock at first. Many new mothers start to feel that they're losing their identity in the early weeks and just see themselves as an extension of this tiny, but extremely demanding new baby. But making time for you and your partner is important, too. So enjoy all the happiness that comes with motherhood, but don't allow being a mother to completely take over your life – remember you are still a person in your own right.

Your new baby will take up a lot of your time, but don't forget to find time to enjoy yourself. Friends will keep you connected to the outside world.

You may want to spend a few days after the birth alone with your new family before your mum and dad or other family members come for a visit. You and your partner are the best judges of your family dynamics, so talk about whether or not to have visitors, who they should be, how long they should stay and how they can help. If you tell your family and friends what your feelings are before the birth and are very clear about what you want and need, the likelihood of rising tensions is reduced.

Your relatives and friends will all be keen to lend a hand as soon as the baby arrives and you may find their enthusiasm a little overwhelming. Let them help you with some of the babycare, but don't be obliged to 'play hostess' – you should be resting as much as possible. You could arrange for your mum or a friend to come in for an hour or two during the first few days to help with other housework such as washing, cleaning and cooking. Or you could employ a postnatal doula (see page 184).

Don't try to force your baby to fit into your schedule – you'll find it far less frustrating to stick to hers, at least for the first few weeks. Try to sleep when she does so that you don't get overtired.

Learn to relax

As you try to determine what will help you to relax, don't forget what worked for you during your pregnancy – massage, meditation or deep breathing, for example (see page 124). You can modify such techniques to work for you now – choose a different mantra to fit in with the way you're feeling, such as 'silence' or 'energy'.

Exercising on a regular basis will help you to relax more easily. But don't do anything too energetic just before you go to bed – you may find it difficult to get to sleep. You'll still need to hold on to your strength for your baby, so don't choose an exercise routine that takes too much of your energy. Use this time to focus away from your daily chores and concentrate on you and the way you are feeling.

Build up relationships

Another way to relax is to nurture relationships. Your time and energy will be limited, so this may not be the best time to develop new friendships, but you could re-establish contact with old friends. Don't try to do too much – concentrate on the relationship, not activities. This may mean calling more often, e-mailing or inviting old friends over for a snack and a chat. Enjoying loving relationships will help you to get through times of stress.

You may prefer not to leave your new baby with baby-sitters for long periods, but as she grows stronger and breastfeeding becomes less frequent, it can be good for you and your partner to get out of the house for a short time. Find ways to fit fun days out between feeding times, like a trip to a café or a lazy walk through the park – you can always keep in contact with your baby-sitter at home via a mobile phone so that you don't worry.

Depression after the birth

Postnatal blues, also called 'baby blues', and postnatal depression (PND) aren't the same. The former is common and short-lived, the latter may be emotionally debilitating and can have lasting effects on both mother and child. Being able to distinguish between them is vital.

Up to 85 per cent of mothers suffer from the baby blues and it's considered by many to be normal. The symptoms can include mood changes, irritability, anxiety, confusion, crying spells and appetite disturbances that occur a day or two after birth and last for about 10 to 14 days. Although it's not known what causes the baby blues, rapid hormone shifts and sleep deprivation are commonly suspected – all the more reason why you should nap whenever you can and try some relaxation techniques. As your baby gets a little older and establishes a feeding routine, she'll drink more and sleep a little longer at a time.

Recognising postnatal depression

After 10 to 20 per cent of all births, baby blues evolves into postnatal depression. In more than half of these cases it begins in the first six weeks and peaks at ten weeks after the birth. Common symptoms of PND include loss of interest in usual activities, difficulty concentrating or making decisions, fatigue, feelings of worthlessness or guilt, recurrent thoughts of death or suicide, significant weight gain or loss, changes in appetite or sleep and excessive anxiety about your baby's health.

PND is often identified by health visitors and general practitioners when you visit them about the baby rather than about yourself. But don't hesitate to talk to your family doctor if you think you are depressed, because not only are you at risk of recurrent depression later in life, but your condition may have long-term effects on your child's development and behaviour. In the short term, a baby can become withdrawn and stop expecting or demanding attention from his mother. Some try harder and harder to get attention, crying incessantly and displaying anger at being neglected.

More serious long-term effects include a difficult and insecure relationship between mother and child and the child having behavioural problems later in life. There is also thought to be a link between PND and lower IQ, particularly affecting boys.

CHECK IF YOU HAVE POSTNATAL DEPRESSION

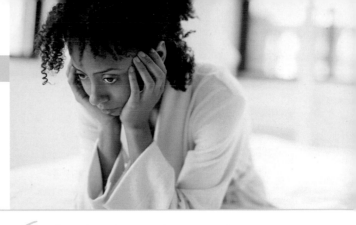

You may feel uncertain about whether you're depressed or not. Answer the following questions from the Edinburgh postnatal depression scale, a questionnaire especially devised to detect PND. It's best to do this at about six to eight weeks after the birth of your child. In the past week:

1 **I have been able to laugh and see the funny side of things...**
As much as I always could.
Not quite so much now.
Definitely not so much now.
Not at all.

2 **I have looked forward with enjoyment to things...**
As much as I ever did.
Rather less than I used to.
Definitely less than I used to.
Hardly at all.

3 **I have blamed myself unnecessarily when things went wrong.**
No, never.
Not very often.
Yes, some of the time.
Yes, most of the time.

4 **I have been anxious or worried for no good reason.**
No, not at all.
Hardly ever.
Yes, sometimes.
Yes, very often.

5 **I have felt scared or panicky for no very good reason.**
No, not at all.
No, not much.
Yes, sometimes.
Yes, quite a lot.

6 **Things have been getting on top of me.**
No, I have been coping as well as ever.
No, most of the time I have coped quite well.
Sometimes I haven't been coping as well as usual.
Yes, most of the time I haven't been coping at all.

7 **I have been so unhappy that I have had difficulty sleeping.**
No, not at all.
Not very often.
Yes, sometimes.
Yes, most of the time.

8 **I have felt sad or miserable.**
No, not at all.
Not very often.
Yes, quite often.
Yes, most of the time.

9 **I have been so unhappy that I have been crying.**
No, never.
Only occasionally.
Yes, quite often.
Yes, most of the time.

10 **The thought of harming myself has occurred to me.**
Never.
Hardly ever.
Sometimes.
Yes, quite often.

The four possible answer choices are scored 0, 1, 2 and 3 according to increased severity of the symptom. If you choose the first answer, give yourself 0 points; the last scores 3 points. Add the scores together for each of the ten questions – if your score is 12 or over, there's a strong possibility that you're suffering from depression, and you should talk to your healthcare provider as soon as possible.

What causes PND?

The most common theory is that it results from a fluctuation in hormone levels after pregnancy. As yet, no-one has identified a biological basis, but women can experience thyroid changes during pregnancy that, if treated, will help their depression. Your healthcare provider may suggest a thyroid test if he or she suspects PND. You're at higher risk of PND if you have twins or triplets, suffer from bi-polar disorder, have a family history of depression or if you had PND after a previous birth and stress from external sources, such as financial problems or lack of family support. This is important information to give to your healthcare provider – identifying the symptoms allows for early treatment, which can help to shorten the course of this illness.

What treatments are available?

You may find it difficult to talk about your feelings with your healthcare provider or even with a family member, particularly because there is a general assumption that new mothers should be happy. But don't be embarrassed, PND is an illness – so let your healthcare provider know. He or she may suggest counselling (available from mother-and-baby units attached to psychiatry clinics or sometimes at home) and medication. There are several self-measures that you can take, such as gentle exercise (see page 334 and below). Make sure that you let your healthcare provider know if you're breastfeeding, to ensure that safe medications are prescribed. Sometimes counselling or medication can be used alone, but most frequently a combination is recommended.

9 ways to help yourself to overcome PND

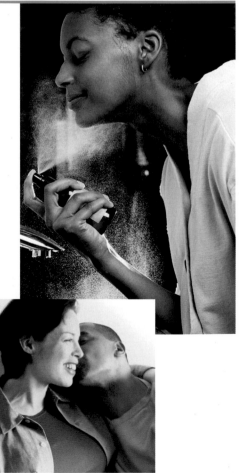

1   Try not to feel guilty or inadequate. There is no such thing as a perfect parent – or a perfect child. Like all mothers, you will learn as you go along and even once you learn, don't expect perfection.

2   Eat heathily and avoid sugar, chocolate and alcohol, as these can all have a depressant effect.

3   Make time for things that make you laugh, such as watching your favourite comedies. Laughter is a great way to relieve depression.

4   Try meditation or other relaxation techniques (see page 124).

5   Pay attention to your appearance. If you look good, you'll feel better.

6   Get out and about. Take the baby for a walk, or get your partner to look after the baby while you go out with a friend.

7   Join a new mothers' support group or a postnatal exercise class. Sharing experiences may help to lift your spirits.

8   Don't force yourself to do things that you do not really want to do or which upset you. Treat yourself with a little kindness, and be occupied doing things which do not cause you anxiety.

9   Don't shut your partner out. Communication is very important for you both during the immediate postnatal period. If he understands how you feel, he will be able to support you.

A healthy postnatal diet

You should continue to eat well and healthily after pregnancy in order to restore your nutritional status and boost your general well-being.

The demands of pregnancy and birth can leave you short on nutrients, particularly if you had a long labour or lost a lot of blood. Although you don't have to eat anything special, a balanced diet will maintain your health and give you the energy you need to care for your new baby. Similar to when pregnant, you should aim to eat

- *5 portions of fruit and vegetables a day* Make sure you eat a variety including fresh, frozen, tinned, dried and juiced;
- *starchy foods,* such as wholemeal bread, pasta, rice and potatoes, as the bulk of your diet. Contrary to popular opinion, complex carbohydrates are not themselves fattening, it's the butter, oil and cream with which they are normally served that adds the calories;
- *plenty of fibre.* Found in fruits and vegetables, wholegrain bread and breakfast cereals, pasta, rice and pulses, this can help prevent constipation and/or other bowel problems;
- *protein* in the form of lean meat and poultry, fish, eggs and pulses;
- *2 portions minimum of fish each week,* one of which should be oily;
- *dairy foods,* such as milk, cheese and yogurt.

However, looking after a new baby may mean that you have little time to cook or to eat as healthily as you did during pregnancy. If this is the case, keep some healthy snacks on hand so that you can grab them when you get the chance (see box, page 332). Freshly made juices, smoothies and soups also can supply needed nutrients quickly and easily.

When you do get the chance to cook, make enough for several nights and freeze the surplus, so that you can just defrost meals when you need to. It may be worth considering topping up with a broad based, well balanced multivitamin and mineral supplement. Consult your caregiver if you have any concerns about your diet.

Vegetarian and vegan mothers may need to take vitamin B_{12} supplements.

Breastfeeding mums

Although breastfeeding is demanding activity, it may be reassuring to know that your baby will be supplied with nutritious milk no matter what you eat (or even how much). Research has proved that babies gain weight and thrive even when their mothers are on poor or restricted diets. The 2011 report by the UK's Advisory Committee on Nutrition suggests an increase of around 330 calories per day (for normal weight breastfeedng mums), but NHS guidelines centre around what a mother eats rather than how much. That being said, you're more likely to feel hungrier than usual when breastfeeding, so you should let your appetite during the first few weeks after birth be your best guide to how much you should be eating. If you feel like a snack or second helping, don't deny yourself.

Your diet needs to provide your baby with the nutrients she needs and with tastes she likes. If you find that your baby becomes fussy about feeding after you've eating something identifiable, cut out that food and see whether that solves the problem.

Peanuts

Many breastfeeding mums worry about eating peanuts as they are one of the most common causes of food allergy. Unless you, any family members or your baby's father have a food allergy or other allergic condition such as hayfever, asthma and eczema, peanuts are safe to eat unless your caregiver advises otherwise.

Key vitamins and minerals

The concentration of vitamins in your breast milk is largely influenced by what you consume and you should get all that you need from a healthy diet. The exception is vitamin D. Breastfed babies need extra vitamin D because, like all babies, they are no longer exposed to sufficient sunlight to generate it themselves (the main source of vitamin D is from the action of sunlight on the skin) because they are protected against skin cancer by being kept them out of the sun. (Formula-fed babies are protected in that Vitamin D is routinely added to formula.) A lack of vitamin D can cause rickets, a crippling bone disease, so you will be prescribed a daily 10 mcg supplement. You may even be eligible for free vitamins; ask your health visitor or GP.

If your intake of some minerals – in particular iron and calcium – is low, your natural body stores will be used to maintain your breast milk levels and these may already be depleted following pregnancy, so it's sensible to try to have sufficient to keep you and your baby healthy. Your increased needs can be provided by a well-balanced diet. Iron can be found in lean red meat, fish, wholegrain cereals, spinach, fortified breakfast cereals and pulses. Calcium-rich foods include dairy products, tofu and green leafy vegetables. If you're lactose intolerant, however, you should consider taking calcium supplements to help to prevent losing calcium from your bones.

Fluid intake

Make sure that you drink plenty of liquids; aim for at least 1.2 litres or six to eight 250-ml glasses a day. It's especially important to drink when you're breastfeeding, as you're supplying your baby with 0.5 to 0.6 litres (1 to 1⅓ pints) of fluid each day. Always have a glass of water, milk or unsweetened juice beside you when you're breastfeeding and take frequent sips. However, don't force yourself to drink too much water – drinking more than 12 glasses of water a day will actually slow milk production.

Any alcohol you drink will pass into your breast milk. It will alter its smell and may affect your baby's ability to feed and sleep. Excessive alcohol consumption may cause drowsiness, irritability and slow growth in your child. For these reasons, it's best to avoid alcohol while you're breastfeeding. If you drink any at all, limit your intake to one or two

6 nutrient-packed snacks

1 Ready-to-eat and dried figs, apricots and currants, are a source of iron and a good source of energy. Bananas are rich in potassium, which controls water balance within the body.

2 Smoothies made with fresh or frozen fruit not only contribute 2 of your 5 portions of fruit but also fibre.

3 Yogurt and fromage frais – reduced fat if you prefer – will help you to get your calcium levels back up to prime.

4 Fortified breakfast cereals are a good source of many B vitamins and sometimes iron.

5 Sunflower seeds contain zinc, a nutrient that will help you to heal.

6 Strips of pepper, florets of broccoli and cherry tomatoes will boost your levels of vitamin C to help your body to fight off any infections.

units (a unit is 25ml of spirits, half a pint of beer, half a 175ml-glass wine) – once or twice a week and do so after the last feed of the day or when you won't be feeding for at least two hours.

When you drink caffeine-containing coffee, tea, cocoa, cola or an energy drink, your baby is less well able to eliminate caffeine than you are, so it may accumulate in her system. This can result in poor sleeping patterns and irritability, so try to drink no more than one cup of coffee or tea a day, and always at least two hours before you breastfeed.

Cutting back on calories

You're no doubt anxious to get your figure back and be rid of those extra pounds, but don't be too hasty. Diving into a restricted or crash diet is not only unhealthy, particularly if you're breastfeeding, but is also likely to prove counter-productive. If your diet

doesn't contain sufficient vitamins and minerals, you run the risk of not being healthy and fit enough to care for your new baby. Watch your intake of fats, oils and sugars. Fill up on fresh fruits and vegetables and unrefined carbohydrates, such as brown rice and wholegrain bread, cereals and pasta. Don't have more than two portions of oily fish a week.

Breastfeeding is claimed to help you lose weight, but this may not be the case for every woman.

If you aren't breastfeeding, you can return to your pre-pregnancy requirement of 1950 to 2100 calories a day but do it gradually, over a period of some weeks, and don't be too strict with yourself too soon.

Once breastfeeding is well established, you can start losing weight moderately but take things slowly and sensibly; wait until six to eight weeks after the birth before cutting back to no fewer than 1800 calories a day.

MENU PLANNER FOR BREASTFEEDING MUMS

Here are a few meal ideas for keeping up your essential breastfeeding vitamins and minerals, healthily and deliciously.

BREAKFAST
- Muesli topped with apricots and low-fat milk.
- Boiled egg with wholemeal toast.
- Strawberry and banana smoothie.
- Bagel with soft cheese and smoked salmon.

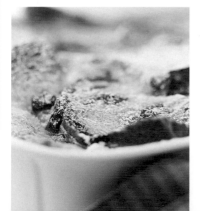

LUNCH
- Pepper and olive-topped pizza.
- Tuna and baby spinach sandwich with low-fat mayonnaise.
- Avocado, red pepper and feta cheese wrap.
- Falafel with tahini dip.
- Pea and spinach soup with tomato-topped bruschetta.

DINNER
- Grilled lamb or beef steak with baby carrots and green beans tossed in olive oil.
- Pasta primavera with a tomato-and-mozzarella salad.
- Thai-spiced salmon with new potatoes and broccoli.
- Chicken and Chinese vegetable stir-fry.
- Grilled turkey cutlets topped with barbecue sauce.

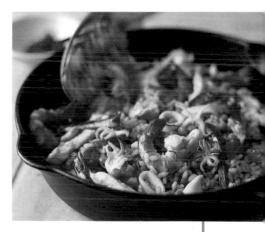

DESSERTS
- Seasonal fruit with natural yogurt.
- Passionfruit or mango sorbet.
- Meringue nests filled with apricots or strawberries and low-fat creme fraiche.
- Rice pudding or creme caramel.
- Slice of date and walnut bread.

Getting back into shape

The key to regaining your pre-pregnancy figure is to combine healthy eating with a strengthening and toning exercise regime. But take it easy – your body has been through a tremendous upheaval and needs time to recover.

Some weight gain during pregnancy is unavoidable as are overstretched abdominal muscles. However, excessive weight gain or prolonged retention of the extra weight after delivery can be harmful both to your health and your self image.

Begin gently

If lochia is still present, don't start even a moderate exercise programme until the bleeding subsides and you get the go-ahead from your healthcare provider, at your postnatal check-up. Until then, if you feel up to it and had no complications during your delivery, you can take your baby for walks. Then you can begin some simple exercises to target particularly weakened areas – those that need the most work to get back to the way they were. But listen to your body; when you feel tired, rest.

Check you're ok to exercise

Before embarking on any exercise programme, check the integrity of your abdominal muscles. A common condition, called *rectus diastasis*, occurs when the vertical muscles of your abdominal wall separate down the middle during pregnancy to give your uterus room to expand. After your baby is born, the muscles are still quite stretched.

Lie on your back with your knees bent. Place three fingers horizontally on your stomach below your belly button. Take special care if you've had a Caesarean. If you can move your fingers more than two fingers' width laterally, then you have separation. Recheck every three to five days until the separation has healed. If it doesn't heal within 12 weeks after the birth, contact your healthcare provider for a referral to a specialist. Meanwhile use the 'hug technique' to strengthen your abdominal muscles. Lie on your back with your knees bent and cross your arms at your waist as you raise your head and shoulders off the floor.

Modified sit-ups

It's important to exercise to regain abdominal muscle tone and a little toning now can save a lot of problems later. Sit-ups done as early as the day after birth will improve your posture and decrease the risk of lower back pain without straining your muscles.

Lie on your back on a firm surface and slowly raise and then lower just your head, looking at the ceiling and keeping your shoulders on the floor. You also can contract and then releasing your abdominal muscles.

Pelvic-floor exercises

Your pelvic-floor muscles will probably be quite sore immediately after delivery, but as soon as you feel up to it you can start a few gentle exercises. The sooner

Check regularly for separation of your abdominal muscles (rectus diastasis) by pressing in your middle three fingers just below your navel and raising your head. If you feel a gap, notify your caregiver.

EXERCISING AFTER A CAESAREAN

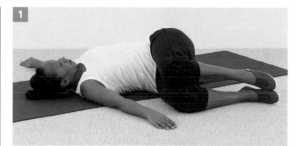

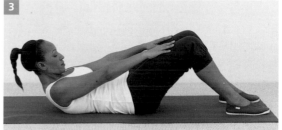

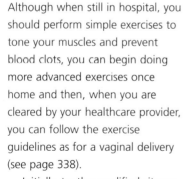

Although when still in hospital, you should perform simple exercises to tone your muscles and prevent blood clots, you can begin doing more advanced exercises once home and then, when you are cleared by your healthcare provider, you can follow the exercise guidelines as for a vaginal delivery (see page 338).

Initially, try the modified sit-ups and pelvic floor exercises described on the opposite page, then, when you feel able, include some simple leg exercises – bringing your knees up and over to each side and then bringing them up to your chest and hugging them before returning your legs to the floor **1**. Follow this with gentle leg circles **2**.

By weeks 7–12, you should try working your abdominals more. Intensify your moderate sit-ups by curling your head and shoulders off the floor, sliding your hands up your thighs as you do so **3** before releasing back down. As your muscles strengthen, try a knee curl, raising your head and shoulders off the floor and bringing one knee into your chest. Repeat on the other side **4**.

Your growing baby can help with your recovery by acting as an ever increasing weight when you perform certain exercises – and he will enjoy being part of your routine.

YOUR EXERCISE PROGRAMME

You need to ensure that the different components are catered for in your regime. The exercises illustrated will help you to tone those areas that will need the most work.

MUSCLE CONDITIONING

After having a baby, you will need to get slack abdominal muscles back in shape and build up those in your arms and legs in order to care for your baby more effectively.

If you have a baby-sitter and access to a fitness club, you may want to start a muscle-conditioning programme at the gym. Some gyms offer childcare while you exercise and others have special postnatal exercise programmes. But it's also to do this type of exercise at home. Whether you use free weights or gym equipment, safety and proper technique are important. Speak to a qualified instructor to find out exercises that will be safe for you to do. Keep to low weights – you should be able to lift them for two sets of 12 to 15 repetitions comfortably. In a pinch, you can use cans or filled water bottles.

FLEXIBILITY

It's important to include some stretching at the end of a session to lengthen your muscles and return them to their pre-exercise state. You can extend flexibility by increasing the amount of time you spend in each stretch.

CARDIOVASCULAR FITNESS

As during pregnancy, you should use the FITT principle (see page 121) when considering your aerobic exercise programme, whether it be a workout class or an activity in which your body weight is supported, such as cycling, swimming or aquafit classes. Begin your first session with 15 minutes of activity at your target heart rate then increase your time by 5 minutes every week. Most people use 40 minutes to one hour as a maximum target time for working out. However, if you get tired or only have time for 20 minutes of activity at your target heart rate, work yourself up to that level and then maintain it.

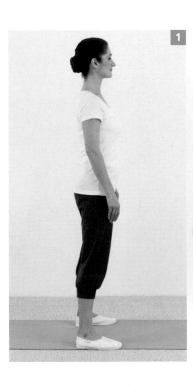

1

2

BOTTOM Stand tall with your shoulders pulled back and down, your ribcage lifted off your waist and your tailbone pulling down towards the floor **1**. Then bend your knees and lower yourself down, pushing your bottom out behind you. Extend your arms to balance yourself **2**. Then, with back straight, straighten your knees and press your hips forward. Lower your arms.

THIGHS Start on all fours then extend your right leg out behind you. Lift his leg off the floor as high as you can. Touch the foot back down to the floor then lift to repeat. After 10 repetitions, bring your right leg in and extend your left leg. Lift and lower this 10 times. Take care not to swing your leg but to lift it using your buttocks muscles.

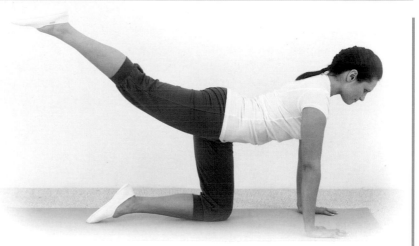

ARMS Start on all fours, with your legs bent and crossed and your arms out to the sides. Have your weight mainly on your arms. Slowly bend your arms, lowering your entire body until your nose and hips and just off the floor. Straighten your arms to lift up and repeat 10 times. Make sure your bottom doesn't stick up and your hips and shoulders are in a straight line.

ABDOMINALS You can do this with your baby. Lie on your back with your knees bent and hold your baby carefully on your abdomen. Slowly raise your head and shoulders. Try to keep your neck straight and don't bring your chin into your chest. Lower your head to the floor and repeat ten times, rest, and do two more sets of ten. When you feel stronger, you can curve your lower spine off the floor and lift, taking baby with you. If you like, you can do a few pulses in the raised head position before carefully lowering your hips to the floor.

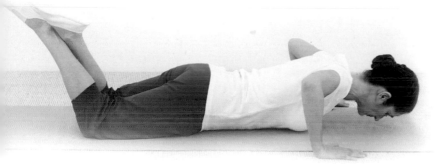

you start, the sooner your vaginal muscles will be strengthened. Clench your pelvic-floor muscles ten times in succession. You'll find the exercise easier each time you do it. If you're experiencing perineal pain, clenching your pelvic floor and maintaining the clench as you sit down will make it more comfortable to sit. The sore perineal muscles will be drawn upwards and inwards, and the pressure of the chair or bed will be directed onto your bottom. Most of the swelling will go down within a few days and the soreness will subside in about a week.

Pelvic-floor exercises should become a part of your regular exercise programme for the rest of your life – they will help to decrease your risk of developing urinary incontinence now and in the future and will help to maintain your vaginal tone after menopause.

Resuming an exercise routine

After a straightforward, uncomplicated birth, you can usually start an aerobic exercise programme in about six to ten weeks. If you had a Caesarean section, you may need at least ten weeks to heal and not feel sore from the incision. When your healthcare provider thinks that you're ready, you can start your exercise programme.

Remember to start slowly. If you're breastfeeding, you should wear a good support bra – not a sports bra, as this binds the breasts and may hinder lactation – or wear two bras so that your heavy, and possibly tender, breasts are supported during the activity. If you're breastfeeding, you may want to

SAFETY FIRST
SIGNS YOU SHOULD STOP As with any exercise, you may experience some soreness until your conditioning returns. You shouldn't, however, experience any pain. If you do, or if you feel dizzy or faint, you should stop. If pain or dizziness persists, call your healthcare provider.

exercise after you feed your baby or after you express milk so that your breasts aren't full. Try not to do anything too strenuous until you've stopped breastfeeding completely because lactic acid – a by-product of exercise – can build up in your milk.

Choose loose-fitting, inexpensive lightweight garments in which to exercise and layer them as necessary. Avoid body-hugging lycra until you're in better shape.

Exercise options

As well as a personal trainer or classes specialising in post pregnancy fitness, books and dvds are available that can be easily followed at home. There are also many neighbourhood mum-and-baby groups that have a fitness component; working out using a buggy is a popular choice as well as mum and baby yoga and pilates classes.

Just 30 minutes three to five times a week can make a difference, although you will see quicker results if you're able to exercise more often. If it's more manageable, you can even split your session into 10- or 15-minute segments. When time is short, try and exercise several big muscle groups at once – say, concentrating on the abdominals, buttocks and legs.

Whichever form of exercise you choose, it should have at least three components – building muscle strength and endurance, improving flexibility and building heart and lung fitness.

Warming up and cooling down

Don't forget that every aerobic activity must have a good 5- to 10-minute warm-up and cool-down, so you may have to adjust your total activity time accordingly. You can incorporate stretching and relaxation exercises as a warm-up and cool-down to muscular conditioning activities or to your aerobic conditioning work out.

Remember, too, to stay hydrated throughout. Keep some water handy and stop to take sips throughout and a further half glass at the end. It's a good idea to eat a couple of hours before exercising as this reduces the risk of indigestion and ensures you have sufficient energy.

Enjoying parenthood

Becoming a parent affects you in ways you can't

imagine, and the learning curve in the first few

weeks is particularly steep, as you adjust to the

realities of having a new baby at home. Everyone has

to learn to be a parent, but if you stay as calm, cool

and collected as possible, you'll soon find you'll

adopt the role with ease.

Early days as a parent

Adjusting to a new arrival might not always go according to plan – family life with a new baby takes a lot of getting used to, and there are no universal signposts for success.

On top of the physical after-effects of the birth, you're bound to experience a whole range of emotions – some of which may not be quite what you expected. Some parents, buoyed up by joyful emotions and an 'easy' baby, launch into parenthood with great enthusiasm and ease, while others are more cautious now that the reality of being a parent is upon them. Everybody is different.

What might the early days bring?

In addition to coping with physical discomforts, such as episiotomy stitches or a Caesarean scar (see page 324), your regular routine will be affected immediately by the following:

- *A sense of responsibility* It suddenly dawns on you that you are now in charge of a helpless being who is totally dependent on you to feed her, change her, bath her, care for her, diagnose any problems and love her.
- *A lack of routine* Your day was reasonably predictable before the birth, but now it's topsy-turvy, as you lurch from one feed or one nappy change to the next. You'll soon establish a new routine around your baby's needs but, in the meantime, accept that your life will be chaotic.
- *New demands* Looking after your new baby is extremely draining, both physically and mentally. Lack of your usual amount of sleep, the effort of learning new skills and the new worries of parenthood, can put you and your partner under considerable physical and mental stress.
- *Visitors* Everyone wants to see the new arrival and you'll probably get terrific pleasure from showing her off to friends and relatives.

However, this may mean that you have little free time to rest and to recharge your batteries.

- *A change of lifestyle* Perhaps you held down a full-time job before the birth, and maybe you and your partner often went out without planning ahead. You're now in a new phase, one in which you both have to sacrifice personal freedoms because there is an extra person to consider.
- *A period of adjustment* Like any parent you want to do a good job, to get things right for your baby. Be patient with yourself, however, and don't let the occasional minor upset rock your confidence in your abilities. You'll soon adapt to these changes in your life, and within a few weeks you'll wonder what you did with all that free time you used to have. The 'downs' of parenthood will quickly be submerged by the 'ups'.

Highs and lows

One minute you may feel excited because your baby gulped down her milk without complaint, while the next you may be tearful because she is crying and you don't know what could be troubling her. At times, you might feel uncertain, vulnerable, even overwhelmed, but don't worry – minor mood swings like these are commonplace.

Small wonder, then, that almost four out of five women – and some men – have mild feelings of depression and anxiety in the first few weeks following their baby's birth. Known as the 'baby blues' (see page 328), these emotions are so widespread that they are regarded as entirely normal. Depressed feelings may be connected to the huge drop in pregnancy hormones in your body following the birth, but they also are a predictable reaction to the huge responsibility of caring for a new baby, as well as the other changes to your body and lifestyle. Whatever the cause, the baby blues should soon pass as your confidence in yourself as a parent grows.

To help you to cope with your fast-changing emotions, don't keep them bottled up, share your feelings with your partner or a close friend. Also, try to spend some time doing things that you enjoy, such as watching a funny movie, reading a good book, having a friend to visit or lazing in the bath and pampering yourself.

Reactions to the birth

Many women react to the birth itself in ways that they didn't expect. Some find that the experience didn't quite meet their expectations, and this response is often more marked when the birth didn't go exactly according to plan – for example, because forceps had to be used. Any interruption to a smooth delivery can be traumatic – even when the

HEALTH FIRST

POSTNATAL DEPRESSION (PND) If you continue feeling depressed for more than a couple of weeks, it's important to talk to your healthcare provider, as it's possible that you may be suffering from PND (see page 329). Other symptoms, which you might experience, include lethargy, difficulty sleeping or feelings of panic, detachment, inability to cope, indifference towards your baby or even a fear that you may harm your baby.

baby arrives safe and well – and this can leave you feeling unsettled. Some women experience feelings of failure if, for example, there was a need to use pain relief when they'd planned a 'natural' delivery. These reactions to childbirth are normal and will soon pass. It may help to talk to your partner or other mothers about what you are feeling. If you find that you can't stop thinking about the birth, then talk to your healthcare provider.

What being a parent is all about

Having a baby unleashes all kinds of new experiences, which is partly why it's so exciting to be a new parent. But, alongside this exhilaration is the reality that the responsibility of caring for your new baby can be very daunting – restrictions on your time mean that you can't please yourself so easily. There are many daily decisions to be made about every aspect of your baby's life, ranging from the choice of babygrows to the frequency of her feeds. Of course, there will be times when you're not sure what's the best thing to do, but the chances are that you'll get it right most of the time.

Parenthood is also about commitment. In these early months, your baby needs you to be there for her. Whether she's hungry, tired, bored or sick, the fact that you're busy or exhausted makes no difference to her. Finding that extra strength to be able to care for her when she depends on you will encourage a strong emotional attachment between you and your child.

Amid the stresses and strains of new parenthood lie many moments of fun and fulfilment. Holding your clean, warm, satisfied-looking baby close to you, as she stares earnestly into your face, makes it all worthwhile. So will all the exciting new skills that she acquires over time. It's a lovely feeling to know that she's content.

You may be surprised to find that being a parent also involves discovering characteristics in yourself that you never knew you had. Many parents discover that they can do a lot more in a day than they previously thought, and that they possess a hidden strength and determination that had never surfaced before. They're often also surprised by the depth of love and protectiveness they feel for their new son or daughter.

Trusting in your partner

If you have another person in your life, then resist the temptation to keep everything to yourself. Initially, you may want to spend all of your time

5 ways for dad to get involved

1 Help with feeding time. If your baby is breastfed, make sure you attend to her at night, bringing her to your partner or ask your partner to express some breast milk so that you can give your baby the occasional bottle.

2 Sing your baby a lullaby when you put her down for her afternoon nap or evening sleep.

3 Give her a bath. If you're anxious about holding her at first, bath her with your partner until you build up your confidence.

4 Take an interest in her playtime – sit down and have fun with her. The delighted expression on her face will be a lovely reward.

5 Dress her and change her nappies whenever you're around.

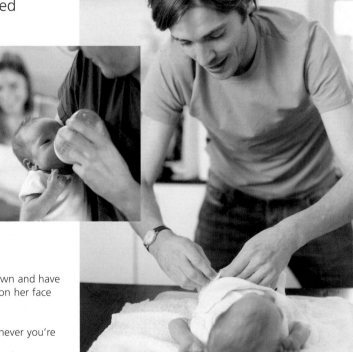

with your baby or you may feel that you are better at caring for her than your partner is, but you'll soon gain enough confidence to share the care of your baby without worrying about loss of control. Insisting that you do everything yourself can make your baby too dependent on your particular way. Bear in mind, too, that your baby learns different things from each of you. Whether your baby is breastfed or bottlefed, both partners can take a turn. Breast milk can be expressed, and both parents are equally capable of giving a bottle. The same applies to the routine caring tasks such as bathing, changing and dressing. Your baby will enjoy love and attention from both of her parents – it doesn't have to be the same one each time.

Keeping in control

The reality of parenthood doesn't always match up to expectations, and you may find it more demanding than you'd anticipated. It can be hard always being on call to respond to your baby's needs – whether that's feeding, nappy changing or cuddling. But you can be a responsive parent without losing control, without letting your baby take the upper hand.

To be in control, you should always have confidence in yourself and your ideas. This doesn't mean that you never have any doubts or that you'll never make any mistakes when looking after your baby. Of course you will – everybody has moments of uncertainty and at times wishes that he or she had done something differently. Don't let these occasional moments affect your self-confidence. You might think that every other parent is more capable than you, but you can reassure yourself that other parents have the same thoughts, too.

Always make a point of sharing your ideas and feelings with your partner or with a close friend. Explaining your ideas to someone else helps you clarify your thoughts, even if the listener doesn't offer any advice. And if advice is given, listen to what the person has to say and discuss the matter together. You may not change your mind at the end but you should feel more confident about the decisions you've made.

Making use of others' advice

Problems can arise, however, if you are showered with too many opinions – possibly conflicting – from well-intentioned relatives and friends, who are all convinced that their perspectives are best. They only want to help you, but too much advice can have the opposite effect and can totally confuse you. If you're struggling to make sense of all sorts of different babycare advice, it might be helpful to consider the following:

- *There's more than one 'right' way to bring up your baby* While there are some principles of child-rearing that apply to every family – for instance, every baby should be loved – many issues come down to personal opinion. Feeding is one of these. Some parents stick to a rigid schedule, while others prefer a less structured approach on this and many other matters.

- *What suits your friend's baby might not suit yours* Although your friend's baby falls asleep when driven about in a car for half an hour, the same strategy might not work with yours. Listen to suggestions from other parents, but don't automatically assume that their tips will have the same impact on your baby.

- *There are fashions in parenting* Years ago, parents believed that 'children should be seen and not heard', whereas nowadays most encourage their children to express their views clearly and confidently. Views on parenting often change, and this could lead to conflict between you and your parents or in-laws. You might feel that your parents are criticizing you or worry that they will think you don't want their advice, so make sure you thank them for their help, but explain why that method doesn't suit you.

- *There's no point attempting to follow advice that you dislike* Suppose, for example, someone suggests that you should feed your baby every time she cries in order to get peace and quiet. This won't be right for you if you're the sort of person who likes to follow a more structured routine. You may follow it at first, but you won't stick with it for long. Only try techniques with which you feel comfortable.

The best strategy for coping with advice from friends and relatives – whether solicited or not – is to listen to the advice attentively, evaluate the suggestions very carefully, talk over the problem with your partner or a close friend and then decide what you want to do.

Give something time to work

Once you've decided on a plan of action for looking after your baby, such as helping her to sleep by singing her a lullaby, make sure that you follow your plan. If your strategy doesn't work immediately, you may be tempted to give up and try something else. Stick with your initial idea for at least a few weeks before considering a change of tactic.

Accept that you're only human and that you won't always get it right the first time. This doesn't mean that you're a poor parent or that you won't ever get it right. What matters is that you learn from your experience. Make sure to applaud yourself when your efforts do succeed.

Make time for yourself

Your new life can have plenty of free moments, if you know how to make them. The more you can plan the better, so try to establish a basic routine for your days together, such as taking your baby out for a walk in the afternoons and giving her a bath or wash in the evenings.

Whenever you get a free moment take advantage of it. Relax and put your feet up – there's no law that says that you have to be on the go all the time. Make a point of having a 10 to 15 minute break a few times each day while your baby is asleep or while your partner cares for her. Use this time to do something you really enjoy. Or if your baby is settled after her feed and you feel like grabbing forty winks while she sleeps next to you, go ahead – you'll feel much better for it. If you get a chance to practise some relaxation techniques (see page 124) in your free time, you'll feel even better.

Divide the housework

Following childbirth and with a newborn to care for, you'll probably find yourself less able to carry out household tasks that you previously tackled with vigour. Try not to take this as a sign that you can't cope. You and your partner may simply want to rethink the housework and how you divide it up. Look at each of the following together and decide who will do them:

◆ Cooking.
◆ Shopping.
◆ Cleaning.
◆ Washing.
◆ Ironing.
◆ Feeding your baby.
◆ Changing dirty nappies.
◆ Bathing your baby.
◆ Dressing your baby.
◆ Attending to your baby at night.
◆ Caring for older siblings.
◆ Gardening.
◆ Caring for pets.

If you find that you and your partner can't cope and you're feeling tired and stressed, consider enlisting some help. Don't be afraid to accept offers of help from friends or relatives – ask them to go shopping for you or iron a pile of clothes. Also consider hiring a nanny or a cleaner, even if only for a couple of hours a week. You could talk to other parents and find out how they sorted out the workload that comes with a new baby. And don't worry if you have to cut corners on the less essential housework – no-one will notice if you let the dust settle for a while – it's far more important for you and your partner to have time to relax into parenting.

Overcoming problems

An infant will constantly challenge new-found parenting skills. Three areas however – feeding, crying and sleeping – are of prime importance in your baby's life – and in yours – and most actual problems arise in these areas.

In the months leading up to the birth, you'll have been given a lot of information about different babycare methods, and some tried-and-tested techniques are provided in Chapter 14. However, you need to make sure that the methods you choose are not only right for your baby but right for you, too. If it feels wrong, then it will become a source of anxiety for you, and, in turn, a source of anxiety for your baby. So go with your natural instincts. If you decide, for example, that you'd rather bottlefeed than breastfeed (see page 190), don't then become concerned that bottlefeeding will have a detrimental effect on the emotional bond that you have with your baby – what matters with feeding is the sensation of relaxation and comfort that you create. Try to remember that feeding isn't just about physical nourishment, it's about emotional nourishment, too.

Relax into feeding

Many feeding problems that parents experience in the first few months start off as very minor difficulties – perhaps the baby has trouble latching on or possets some milk during a feed – but these can soon grow into major problems if they are fuelled by parental anxiety and tension.

Your baby is highly sensitive and will know if you are anxious – tension can cause your muscles to tighten, and if you're tense, your milk may flow less than when you're totally relaxed. This, in turn, can

HOW TO enjoy feeding time

If feeding times aren't going as well as you'd like, your first priority is to trust yourself. Have confidence in your abilities, and tell yourself that minor difficulties aren't the end of the world – you'll soon be able to establish a good feeding pattern.

Allow plenty of time for feeding so that you don't have to rush; don't schedule another task too soon after. Until you and your baby both get used to feeding, it may help to feed him in a quiet room where you won't be disturbed. Prepare yourself calmly and without hurrying, pick up your baby gently and softly. Then get comfortable in a position that suits you and your baby (see page 300).

Make sure that you connect with your baby during feeding times by looking into his eyes, talking to him in a soothing voice, and holding him close against your body.

If your baby is taking his time to feed or won't latch on, take a break, and try again after 5 or 10 minutes – if you're getting stressed, it will give you both a chance to calm down. No matter how successful or fraught you find the feeding process, ask your partner to take a turn occasionally so that you can have a rest.

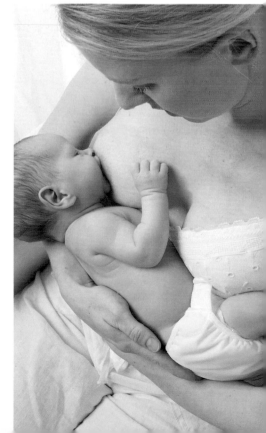

agitate your baby if he can't get enough milk and at the rate that he wants. This can set up a vicious circle, in which your and your baby's anxiety upset each other more and more, until you dread the prospect of feeding.

Assuming that your baby is in good health and that you've tried different practical strategies such as changing the feeding position or, if you're bottlefeeding, changing the formula – with your healthcare provider's advice – what can you do if feeding times continue to be troublesome? Practical solutions won't work unless your whole approach to feeding is relaxed. If feeding times have evolved into a psychological struggle – because, for example, your baby feeds too slowly or feeds hurriedly then sleeps before finishing – then step back and have an objective look at the whole process.

Ask yourself the following questions: do I look forward to feeding times? Do I enjoy holding my baby while I feed him? Does he look very settled and comfortable in my arms and when taking the breast or bottle? Does he seem satisfied when he's finished? If the answer to any of these questions is 'no', it's time to consider the emotional dimension of feeding. The box on page 345 gives some ideas for creating a relaxed atmosphere and is useful for both breast- and bottlefeeding.

Coping with crying

A big challenge facing you in these early months is getting used to your baby's cries. You were so delighted to hear him cry moments after delivery – because that was the signal that he had arrived safely – but now that he's home, his repeated cries can

EASING COLIC

Colic is the term often used to describe piercing crying that often occurs at around the same time each evening, reaching its peak around 12 weeks old. Nobody knows for sure why a baby gets colic – explanations include poor feeding, milk allergies, weak digestion, wind and parental stress.

If your baby howls the place down and seems inconsolable, by all means call your doctor. But if you're told 'he's just got colic', caring physical contact is still the best way to ease his distress.

A great way to help to relieve your baby's anxiety is the 'tiger in the tree' massage. Pick up your baby with his back to you and your left arm along his front **1**. Bring your right hand between his knees and place your palm flat on his tummy **2**. Tuck his foot under your arm and turn him over onto your hand **3**. With your right hand, gently knead his tummy.

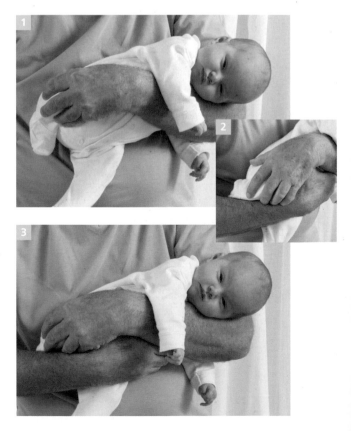

wear you down. Try to bear in mind that crying is your baby's main way of communicating; it's his primary form of language and is a sign of healthy development. In fact, you'd probably be more worried if he didn't cry at all.

Your baby's crying is natural and doesn't mean that you're doing something wrong. Many parents experience guilt feelings when their babies cry, especially in the beginning, as though it's their fault their newborn is so tearful. Try to avoid such negative thoughts.

Learn to communicate

If your baby seems to be crying all the time, you can easily become overwrought and distressed yourself. In most instances, the main reason you become upset is that you don't know what your baby's crying means. You feel frustrated and worried watching his discomfort without knowing immediately what to do to help him to settle. But, once you tune into his cries, you'll get to know what he's trying to tell you. Always look for an explanation – babies rarely cry just for the sake of it.

When your baby's screams pierce the air, think about what he might be trying to tell you and how you can respond:

- I'm hungry – feed him.
- I'm hot/cold – adjust his blanket or the room temperature.
- I'm uncomfortable – change his nappy.
- I'm bored – play with him.
- I'm lonely – give him some loving attention.
- I'm tired – rock him gently to help him to sleep.
- I'm ill – take him to the doctor.

The common theme in all these suggested solutions is that he needs you. Of course, your being there won't stop him crying if, for example, he's hungry. But your loving, gentle touch should ease his discomfort until food arrives.

Be patient

Everyone has a favourite 'recipe' for success on ways to soothe a crying baby, and some are given on page 306. It's far better to try out a new idea for soothing your sobbing baby than to sit helplessly with him.

DID YOU KNOW...

THERE ARE PATTERNS OF CRYING
The peak period for crying is in the first three months of life, and babies cry most frequently when they are 6 or 7 weeks old. The typical baby cries heavily in the early evening, although he will also cry at other times of the day. Studies have found, too, that almost a quarter of all babies have periods of constant crying when there's no obvious reason for their tears. Finally, there are no gender differences when it comes to crying – boys and girls cry the same amount.

But whatever strategy you use, stick with it for a couple of weeks. Unless you're particularly lucky, a new method is unlikely to have an immediate effect. Only change tactics when you have seen no positive response after two or three weeks.

Your self-confidence as a parent plays its part, too. If you're tense and anxious when you pick up your crying baby – which you probably will be at first – he'll sense this and become even more tense himself. He'll cry more strongly, which will, in turn, increase your tension, and the spiral of parent–baby anxiety will escalate rapidly. That's why it's important that you try to take a relaxed approach when soothing your tearful baby. Remind yourself that his sobbing is just his way of telling you that he wants loving comfort from you. If you're becoming too tense, take a short break. Share the burden with your partner or a friend, where possible – a few minutes' respite may be all that's needed to put you in a more positive frame of mind.

If the crying occurs predictably at the same time each night, your baby may be suffering from colic (see box, opposite). However, if you're really worried about your baby's incessant distress, see your doctor.

GETTING A GOOD NIGHT'S SLEEP

Between birth and the age of 3 months, your baby's sleeping habits will change constantly. You'll probably long for those earlier pre-baby times when you could fall asleep at night with total confidence that you wouldn't wake until the alarm sounded the following morning. Those days are over, at least for the time being. For the first three months, your baby's sleep and your own sleep are less than predictable.

According to research, your new baby will result in you losing 400 to 750 hours of sleep in his first year. Up until his 5th month, you'll lose about two hours a night, gradually falling to about one hour a night until he's two years old.

Be philosophical and accept that lack of sleep is part of parenthood at this stage in your baby's life. You will quickly learn to catnap when ever you can; this can be a great way to recharge your batteries. If you have a partner, consider taking turns so that you comfort your baby one night and your partner goes to

him the next – that way each of you gets some quality sleep at least every other night.

Your emotional and physical adjustment to this new state of affairs will be quicker if you understand that a great deal of your baby's changing sleep pattern is part of his natural development. When he's a couple of weeks old, he may only spend one or two hours awake each day; around the age of 3 months, he spends roughly 14 to 16 hours of his time asleep within 24 hours, but this is spread evenly throughout the day and

night – it's not until later that he'll start to sleep more during the night and less during the day. Not only that, research also reveals that he'll sleep for a maximum of only four hours at any one time.

This means that lots of his naps, and lots of waking periods, are scattered evenly throughout the day and night. The fact that you want him to sleep longer at night makes no difference to him.

Although they may not work immediately, you can take some positive steps to encourage your baby to sleep more soundly during the night. The following suggestions will help you to create the best atmosphere for him to gently drift off to sleep:

MAKE HIM COMFORTABLE He's more likely to sleep when he's clean and dry with a fresh nappy, when his blankets are tucked securely

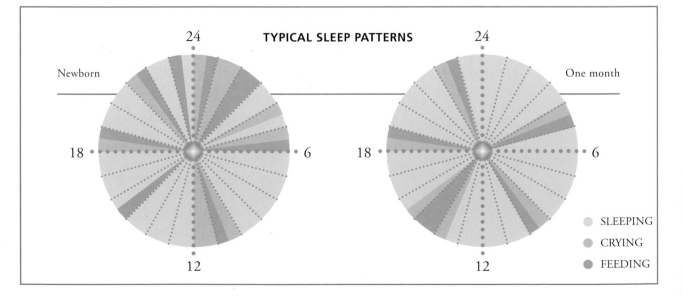

TYPICAL SLEEP PATTERNS

Newborn

One month

24

24

18 · 6

18 · 6

12

12

● SLEEPING

● CRYING

● FEEDING

RESPONDING TO YOUR BABY'S CRIES

There's considerable debate among psychologists about the best way to respond to a young baby who won't sleep. Some claim that a sleepless baby should be picked up and cuddled until he's relaxed enough to close his eyes. Others argue that picking him up each time will encourage him to stay awake the next time, as he'll quickly learn that this is the best way to get his parents' attention.

The challenge facing you is to make him feel relaxed and secure with you so that he's ready for sleep, but not so comfortable that he would rather stay awake in your company. If you pick him up every time he cries and refuses to sleep, he'll cry a lot more. Certainly, you need to soothe him when he wants to remain awake, but consider doing this without actually picking him up. The solution may be as simple as feeling his tummy to see if he's too hot and adjusting his blankets accordingly **1**, or comforting him by providing him with a dummy, playing with his mobile or singing softly to him **2**.

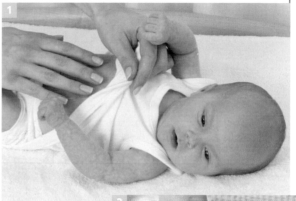

around him, and when the bedroom is warm but not too hot – 16 to 20°C (61 to 68°F) is ideal.

PROVIDE A SERENE ENVIRONMENT

He's much less inclined to fall asleep if there are loud, sporadic noises in your house. Although you don't need to tiptoe from room to room, aim for relative peace and quiet. A pleasant, peaceful bedroom atmosphere induces sleep.

STICK TO A ROUTINE

He may only be a few months old but he can respond to routine. Try to follow the same procedure each night before putting him in his cot. For example, you could feed him, bath him, cuddle him and then read him a story or sing him a lullaby.

TRY TO BE RELAXED AND CALM

This greatly increases the chances of achieving your goal. As you encourage him to nod off, your baby responds to your emotional state, either positively or negatively.

CONSIDER FEEDING TIMES

Your baby will want to sleep soon after he has been fed at night. So think about feeding him after you've bathed him, changed him and got him ready for bed.

ENCOURAGE COMFORT HABITS

From very early on many babies begin to associate certain items or patterns with sleeping times. A musical mobile, a dummy or a night-light can become a signal that the baby is expected to sleep, and also provide comfort while your baby is alone.

Settling into family life

Caring for your baby can be all-consuming, but it's important not to lose sight of yourself as an individual. It's also important, too, that other family relationships – between you and your partner and between your baby and the grandparents – are maintained.

Within a relatively short time, you may be keen to re-establish your own lifestyle, return to work or pursue other interests. Don't feel guilty for thinking about yourself. Your partner or a trusted relative can look after your baby for a couple of hours so that you can spend time on your own, relaxing or going out with friends.

To work or not to work?

Probably the biggest decision to make over the next few months is whether or not you'll return to work. Take your time thinking about this and move forwards in a way that suits you and your partner.

Opting to stay at home

If you decide to care for your baby full time, this may well provide you with all the satisfaction you used to get from your job. Some women, however, worry that by staying home they will somehow lose their individuality. If you start to feel like this, focus on the fact that the job you have now – that of bringing up your baby – is equally, if not more, important than your previous one.

If you have the opportunity to stay at home, you may discover a whole new you. Many women point out how enjoyable it was discovering things with their babies and watching all the incredible changes they go through. And you can share all these with other new mothers who may become new friends.

Opting to go back

The first thing you'll have to consider if you decide to return to work is when. This will depend on how you're feeling and the arrangements you made for

any maternity leave. Then, you must make your final decisions on childcare – whether a nanny, childminder or nursery is necessary (see page 193).

When the time comes to return to work, it's the rare woman who doesn't feel a bit sad or guilty, thinking about the precious times she could be spending with her baby or wondering what will happen if the baby has an accident. Try not to let feelings such as these get you down. Concentrate on the notion that you'll feel more independent and fulfilled while working, and you'll pass on these qualities to her. Working will benefit your baby also by providing her with a stable financial background. And try to calm any worries that nobody can care for her as well as you can. If you've found a good caregiver, your baby will be fine.

Your baby should develop a close bond with her caregiver, but this won't affect the relationship she has with you. Of course, you need to find time to spend alone with her and build this into your routine. After you get home you can feed her, play with her and then put her to bed – times that will be comforting for both of you.

Don't be surprised if you find returning to work very difficult at first. Many women today feel under pressure to be Supermum, but accept that you will be tired and that it'll take time to get used to your workload and responsibilities at home. Now's not a good time to take on extra work or do overtime; decide what housework you can delegate.

Remaining a couple

Amid the hubbub of this busier way of life, you need also to maintain your life together with your partner. After all, you're not just parents to your new baby – you both have your own emotional needs.

Living with a baby affects each partner in different ways. Maybe one of you now stays at home, whereas before you held down a full-time job, or maybe one partner resents the attention the other gives to your baby. Unexpressed, these concerns can create barriers between you. Honest communication is the best way to maintain a strong relationship, and for it to evolve as your family grows.

Re-establish your social life

Caring for your new baby normally leaves little energy for a social life, but make the effort anyway. When you feel ready, try leaving your baby with a reliable sitter. You don't need to go out for the entire evening at first; just taking in a movie or visiting some friends will provide a welcome break.

Be open with each other

Share your ideas about parenting with one another, as well as any concerns about your new role. Listen to your partner's hopes and fears, and make sure you voice your own. Bear in mind, too, that being a new mother is like falling in love all over again – except that the person you feel so passionate about is tiny and totally dependent on you. Even if your partner is also passionate about the baby, the apparent switch in your affections can make him feel hurt and left out – as if he no longer figures in this new relationship. The only way through this is to talk about it. Both of you should be honest – the worst thing you can do is pretend everything's fine.

Put sex back on the menu

Sex can become an issue in the early weeks. Exhausted, battered and bruised from giving birth, it can be the last thing on your mind. Your partner, however, may feel quite differently and be very keen

. . . .

HOW TO enjoy sex after the birth

. . .

If you've had stitches or are sore, the idea of penetrative sex can be disturbing. But there are plenty of other ways to express love. Kissing and cuddling sound obvious, but it's surprising how you can overlook each other's need for closeness when you're so focused on your newborn. Massage, mutual masturbation and oral sex can be satisfying until you feel ready for penetration.

After the birth, when your oestrogen and progesterone levels plummet, you may temporarily experience a loss of vaginal lubrication, as well as hot flushes and sweats. These may continue for some time. So, when you're ready for intercourse or want to try masturbation, use a water-based,

vaginal lubricant. Don't use petroleum jelly, because this is oil-based and can lead to an infection.

Make love in a position in which you can control the depth of penetration of your partner – with you on top or lying side to side – so that if the pressure becomes uncomfortable, you can ease away. Avoid the missionary position until you feel completely comfortable and pain-free.

If you have any worries or concerns about sex, don't be embarrassed to seek advice from experienced professionals – they'll be able to help you to decide when you're ready to restart your sex life.

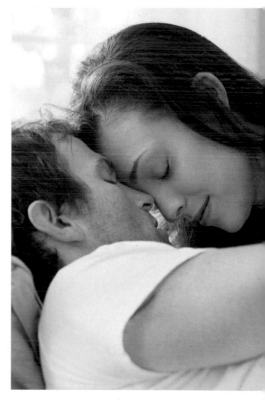

to get your sex life back to normal. Or you may feel keen to resume relations but your partner may be somewhat traumatized by what you went through to have your baby.

Although many healthcare providers advise waiting six weeks before having sex, it really depends on your individual circumstances and when you feel ready. If you had a relatively easy birth and don't have any discomfort, there's no reason to wait; if you had a difficult birth and had to have stitches, six weeks will seem far too soon. If you're unsure, your healthcare provider can help you to decide.

When you do feel ready, take it at your own pace. When you're in bed together, tactfully explain what feels good and what doesn't. You don't have to go into graphic detail – gently moving your partner's hand to a particular spot may be all that's needed. If you're tense at the prospect of intercourse, you may just want to start by snuggling together – that's fine. You'll have more later on when you're ready.

Guard against feeling guilty if you don't want to make love. It's very common for your sex drive to decrease after childbirth, and not surprising when your body's busy adapting to the physical aspects and while you're experiencing exhaustion, lack of sleep and the massive adjustment that a new baby demands. You may simply need to accept that with a baby needing constant room service, sex might not be as spontaneous as it was before.

Don't forget contraception

Ovulation can start even if you're breastfeeding and your periods haven't returned, so you need to use some form of contraception when you resume sex. Condoms are probably your best option at first. If you want to use other forms of contraception, you'll need to speak to your healthcare provider. You shouldn't take an oestrogen-based pill if you're breastfeeding, as it can block your milk production (see page 326). However, it is usually safe for you to take the 'mini-Pill', which contains progesterone only. If you want to have an IUD fitted, you'll need to wait until your cervix has recovered, which may take around six weeks. If you previously used a diaphragm, you'll need to get a new one fitted.

Considering existing children

If this is your second baby, the early weeks will be different from those with your firstborn. For one thing, you didn't already have another child to look after, and for another, you and probably your partner will already have experience of caring for a newborn. This will give you confidence, but bear in mind that you will probably feel more tired caring for two or more children.

Happy families?

With a second baby, the issue of sibling rivalry arises (see box, left). Jealousy between children in the same family is very common but it can be disruptive and cause havoc in family life. Fortunately, there are steps you can do to tackle the problem.

The first meeting of your existing child and the new arrival needs careful handling. Let your older child buy the baby a present and, when he visits you in the hospital, make a big fuss of him and try to make him feel important. Tell him how much the new baby loves him.

DID YOU KNOW...

THE AGE GAP INFLUENCES SIBLING RIVALRY
Studies have found that if the gap is less than 18 months, your first child is unlikely to be jealous, because he won't fully understand what is happening. If the gap is around two years, sibling rivalry is often extreme. Your first child is old enough to know that a new baby affects him, and he may feel insecure. However, this age gap is healthier from a mother's point of view. With a gap of three or more years, feelings of jealousy are less likely. Your first child's life won't be significantly affected by the presence of a baby brother or sister and he'll probably be proud of the new family member.

6 ways to encourage grandparents

1 Some grandparents stay away from their grandchild, fearing that they'll be considered too dominant. A positive welcome will help to put them at ease.

2 Involve them in your baby's care. If they are concerned that they're 'out of practice', give them a simple task to start with, such as reading your baby a story. It will help them to build their confidence.

3 Ask for their advice. Even though you may not agree with your parents' views about everything, they'll be flattered when you ask for their opinion.

4 Make them feel wanted. Tell them how fond of them their grandchild is and how you all look forward to their visits

5 Don't make assumptions. It's easy to take it for granted that your parents will baby-sit for you at a moment's notice; they may need plenty of warning and they deserve thanks also when helping you out.

6 Conflicts frequently arise about discipline, with some grandparents being too lenient. So talk about discipline and make your expectations clear.

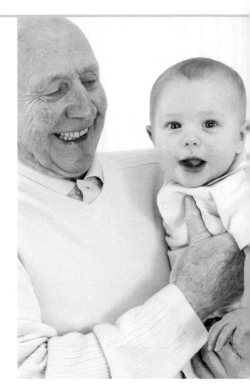

One strategy to encourage harmony when you're home is to get your older child involved in caring for the baby – this helps also to form a connection between them. How much your older child can do depends on his age, but you could ask him to fetch nappies, pick out clothes for the baby or share toys. In addition, spend at least half an hour every day alone with your first child, perhaps when the baby is asleep. This special time boosts his self-esteem. Keep your older child's normal routine where possible – the less disruption, the better. And remember to continue days out together as a family.

Including the grandparents

Grandparents can be very important to a baby during her formative years. Although they are traditionally considered to spoil their grandchildren or to interfere with their upbringing, they can be ideal buffers between you and your children.

Today's grandparents are more likely to be active in later life and so can be more involved when their grandchild comes along. How much involvement your parents and in-laws have will be up to you – and it'll probably take some time before you're able to strike the right balance between accepting their help and discouraging any interference. Your baby's grandparents are probably aware of this, too, so try to discuss their level of help calmly and openly.

Grandparents as caregivers

If your parents or in-laws are willing and live nearby, they may be able to help with childcare arrangements, which can be especially useful when considering a return to work. This option can save you a lot of money but does give them a huge responsibility, which can create family disharmony. You and your partner should sit down with your parents and discuss this fully as a family, sorting out as many potential problems as you can – such as how you prefer to feed your baby or put her to bed before starting the arrangement.

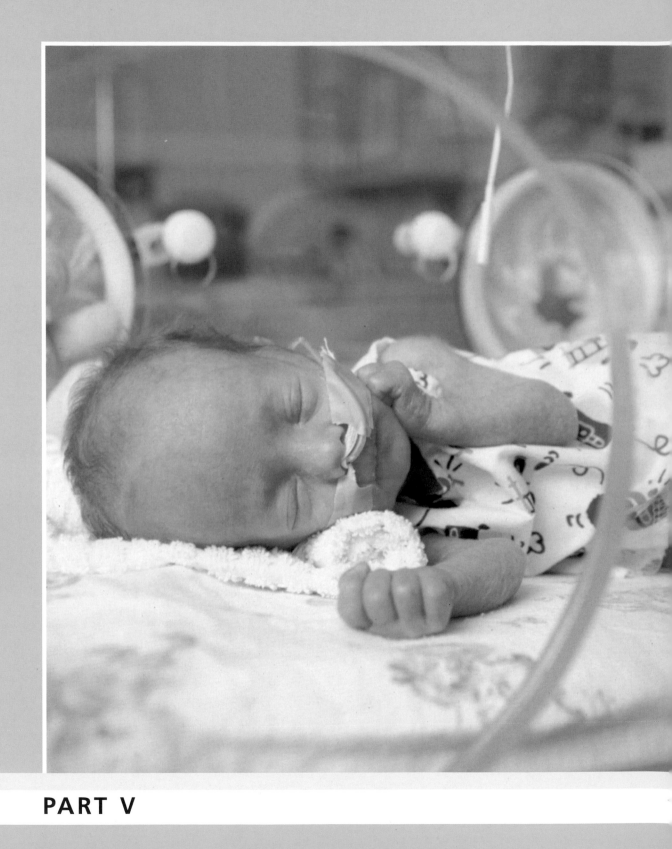

PART V

Postnatal Directory

Maternal complaints and treatments

After birth, many mothers experience some discomfort from stitches – if they've had an episiotomy or tear – and until breastfeeding is successfully established, breasts may be achy and tender. But major problems are normally rare. Always seek advice from your healthcare provider if you have any concerns.

Complications after the birth

Postnatal infections

It's estimated that 1 to 8 per cent of all births will be followed by an infection. Factors that increase the risk include: premature rupture of the membranes and prolonged labour, frequent internal examinations, internal fetal monitoring, an infection already present during pregnancy, diabetes and being overweight. The most common infection, endometritis, affects the endometrium (the lining of the uterus) but infections also can occur in the cervix, vagina, vulva and perineum.

What to look out for

- Fever
- Abdominal pain
- Offensive vaginal discharge
- Inflammation, redness, and swelling

Treatment

Most infections that occur after a birth require medical treatment, usually with antibiotics. Endometritis may require hospital treatment, in which intravenous antibiotics will be given for two to seven days. Once treated it usually resolves within one to three days. Other infections may vary in their response to treatment, but most will clear up within seven to ten days. Breastfeeding can be continued during most treatments.

Postpartum haemorrhage

It's normal to have some vaginal bleeding, whether you had a vaginal birth or a Caesarean, for several weeks after the birth. Postpartum haemorrhage refers to excessive bleeding after delivery. There are many different causes of abnormal bleeding. The most common is that the uterus doesn't contract well. Other causes include retained placenta (where fragments of placental tissue have not been expelled) or unrecognized tears that occur in the cervix or vagina.

While postpartum haemorrhage usually occurs in the days following the birth, it also can develop several weeks later, if fragments of placenta remain attached or if an infection develops internally.

What to look out for

- Heavy, bright-red blood loss for 4 days or more
- Passing large numbers of clots
- Foul-smelling vaginal discharge
- Feeling faint, breathless, and light-headed

Treatment

Some women are given medication for a day or two to help the uterus to contract. Occasionally, a minor operation – called an evacuation of retained products of conception – is needed to remove any tissue left behind in the uterus. Anaemia caused through loss of blood may be treated with iron supplements and a diet that includes iron-rich foods (see page 108).

Prolapse

During pregnancy and birth, the pelvic-floor muscles that support the pelvic organs can be weakened, leading to incontinence (see page 359) and, in extreme cases, prolapse, where organs in the lower abdomen drop downward. The most common form of prolapse is where the uterus descends into the vagina.

What to look out for

- Dragging sensation and feeling of heaviness in the lower abdomen
- Leaking urine when coughing or sneezing
- Pain in the lower abdomen or back
- Uncomfortable or painful sex
- Constipation

Treatment

Strong pelvic floor muscles can help prevent prolapse so re-starting your pelvic-floor exercises (see page 122) as soon as possible is a good idea. Eating plenty of fibre will guard against constipation and therefore straining, which puts pressure on the pelvic floor. Moderate uterine prolapse can be helped with ring pessaries – similar to the diaphragm contraceptive. Surgery such as a repair operation may be needed once your family is complete.

Stitch complications

It is possible for episiotomy stitches to become infected, causing a great deal of discomfort. Bacteria can invade the site of a wound despite the best precautions and hygiene.

What to look out for

- Red, painful, swollen perineum
- Unpleasant odour from the area

Treatment

Infected stitches usually resolve with careful hygiene and frequent baths, but an infection of the perineum may require treatment with antibiotics, so you should seek advice from your healthcare provider. Occasionally, stitches come apart prematurely. Further stitches may be required, but simple hygiene procedures are often sufficient for healing to occur.

Breast problems
Blocked milk ducts

Anything that restricts milk flow in the breast – such as a too tight bra – can cause blocked ducts. Commonly experienced by women who, for some reason, have a build-up of milk, the cause may be the production of excess milk or a baby not latching on properly, not emptying the breast, or sleeping through and missing out being fed.

What to look out for

- Tenderness
- Redness, with or without heat
- Lumpiness, which reduces with massage or after feeding

Treatment

Apply heat, such as a face cloth dipped in warm water and squeezed dry, to the affected area, along with massage before each breastfeeding session to

Pelvic-floor muscles, weakened by a rapid delivery, a long labour, or a large baby, can fail to support the uterus in its normal position so it drops down into the vagina. Other organs – the bladder, urethra, rectum, and abdominal lining – also can drop, put pressure on the vagina, and cause vaginal prolapse or vaginal wall descent. Different prolapses can occur in combination.

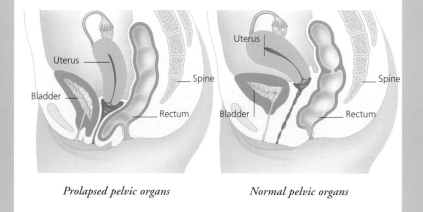

Prolapsed pelvic organs   *Normal pelvic organs*

help to relieve the problem. Feed frequently and use a breast pump at the end of a session if your breasts have not been completely emptied. Try different positions at each feed and make sure your baby is latched on correctly (see page 301).

Mastitis

If bacteria find their way into a blocked milk duct – often through a cracked nipple (see below) – the milk within may become infected, resulting in inflammation of the duct. This is called mastitis. The most usual site is the upper, outer segment of the breast. Women may be predisposed to mastitis by engorgement, stress and a change in feeding patterns – for example, if your baby starts to feed at longer intervals or is having occasional bottles.

What to look out for
◆ Inflamed, painful lump
◆ Shiny, red skin over affected area
◆ Feverish, flu-like muscle aches
◆ Nausea

Treatment
Mastitis requires treatment with antibiotics, analgesics and the self-help measures given for blocked milk ducts. The medicines prescribed will be safe to use while breastfeeding, because an important part of the treatment is continued breastfeeding. If there is no improvement after 24 hours of taking antibiotics, ask your healthcare provider for advice, as there is a risk of an abscess.

Cracked nipples

While sensitive and sore nipples are very common during the first few days of breastfeeding, vigorous sucking, incorrect positioning and milk left on the nipple can cause the nipple to crack. Cracked nipples are very painful and may become infected.

What to look out for
◆ Small cracks on the nipple, which may bleed
◆ Sharp, piercing pain during feeding

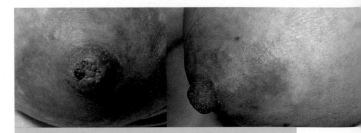

A cracked nipple (left) and mastitis (right) may make breastfeeding uncomfortable but neither condition precludes continuing to breastfeed. Cracked nipples are more common in fair-skinned women, although the reason for this is not known.

Treatment
Continue breastfeeding, making sure that your baby is latched on correctly (see page 301). Use a breast pump to empty your breasts if they still feel full when your baby has finished feeding. Expose your nipples to the air for a short while after each breastfeeding session. Always wash your nipples with plain warm water – never use soaps or disinfectants, which are drying – and gently pat dry. If using breast pads, avoid plastic-backed ones and change them after each feed. It can help to put a thin smear of white soft paraffin or purified lanolin ointment on the crack. Breast shields may also help.

Thrush

Cracked nipples often become infected with the yeast *candida albicans* resulting in thrush. Women who are prone to vaginal thrush yet have no problems with breastfeeding also can develop thrush on their breasts. Thrush also can be encouraged by antibiotics.

What to look out for
◆ Itchy, irritable, pink or red nipples
◆ Tiny white spots on nipples
◆ Stabbing pain deep in the affected breast

Treatment

Thrush can be passed between mother and baby, so both of you may need to be treated, usually with an antifungal medication. Although it is likely to be painful, breastfeeding should continue during any treatment.

Let-down failure

If you are unable to produce adequate milk or if your milk does not flow freely, this is failure of the let-down reflex, usually a result of unrelieved breast engorgement in the first week after birth. Sometimes let-down failure occurs if a baby has problems immediately after birth and stays in the nursery, or is very small or premature and cannot or will not suck vigorously. Depression and emotional upset also can reduce milk production.

What to look out for

- Your breasts don't leak between feeds
- No let-down sensation (mild uterine contractions immediately after birth, then pins and needles in breast after two weeks)
- Baby seems unhappy and appears hungry
- Baby does not gain adequate weight
- Baby urinates infrequently

Treatment

Feed frequently in a quiet and relaxed place, sitting in a comfortable position with your baby correctly latched on (see page 301). Use a breast pump if your baby isn't providing adequate stimulation in terms of pressure or time at the breast. Discuss depression or emotional problems with your healthcare provider.

Urinary and bowel problems

Urinary incontinence

Physical changes that occur in the body during pregnancy – rather than weak pelvic-floor muscles, as was previously thought – are now believed to cause urinary incontinence.

A common problem after a vaginal delivery, urinary incontinence may last for a few weeks or months.

Stress incontinence (a type of urinary incontinence caused by laughing, coughing and straining), is very common and can last up to a year after delivery. It usually improves over time.

What to look out for

- Leaking small amounts of urine
- Feeling of fullness and an urgency to pass urine
- Inability to control urine flow

Treatment

Whatever the cause, regular pelvic-floor exercises (see page 122) are the best method of combating incontinence. It may take a few weeks before any improvement in bladder control is noticed, but you should persevere. Wear sanitary pads or protective underwear to forestall leaks.

Faecal incontinence

A forceps delivery, severe tearing or an episiotomy can damage nerves and muscles of the anal sphincter, the muscles responsible for opening and closing the bowel. This can lead to loss of control over bowel movements. The duration of faecal incontinence depends on how much damage has been done. Women who are affected can take from six weeks to four months and more to regain control of their bowels after childbirth.

What to look out for

- Involuntary bowel movements
- Passing excessive wind

Treatment

Pelvic-floor exercises (see page 122) can strengthen your pelvic-floor muscles and increase blood flow to the perineum, which may help recovery. If the incontinence doesn't improve with these exercises, it's important to discuss the problem at your postnatal check. There's no need to feel embarrassed about it. It is far better to get the problem treated as soon as possible.

Newborn medical problems

Most babies are born perfectly healthy, but problems occasionally arise and medical intervention is required. Although this can be upsetting, most problems can be treated successfully. Your healthcare providers will be able to explain any procedures that may be required.

Intestinal problems
Constipation
This is the production of hard, dry stools, which may be passed less frequently than normal. It's very unusual for babies to be constipated in the first few weeks. If your newborn is constipated, vomits or has abdominal distension, he may have a disorder of the digestive system.

What to look out for
- Hard, difficult-to-pass stools
- Less frequent stools
- Stools streaked with blood on the outside
- Abdominal pain or discomfort, leading to excessive crying and drawing up of knees

Treatment
A young baby with mild constipation should be offered plenty of extra fluids. Constipation that results from dietary changes, such as a different formula, usually resolves itself within a few days. More serious constipation, with hard and painful-to-pass stools, requires medical treatment. Babies should never be given laxatives, unless they are prescribed by the doctor. Sugared water should also be avoided, as it can cause your baby to develop a sweet tooth.

Diarrhoea
This is a sudden increase in the amount of stools, with looser, more watery stools than usual. The stools may be a greenish colour and foul-smelling. Sometimes diarrhoea is accompanied by vomiting.

The most common cause of diarrhoea is a viral infection, although there are also bacterial causes, which can cause blood to appear in the stools. Diarrhoea may also be associated with: a urinary infection; an upper respiratory tract infection, such as a cold or ear infection; or a more serious illness. In these cases it's often accompanied by a

WHEN TO SEE THE DOCTOR

Newborns can become unwell very quickly, so it is important to be aware of the symptoms that could indicate illness. If a baby develops any of the following, or appears unwell, urgent medical advice is required:
- Paleness or a bluish colour around the mouth and on the face
- Fever with a temperature of 100.4°F (38°C) or more
- Body becomes floppy or stiff
- Eyes are pink, bloodshot, have a sticky white discharge, or eyelashes that stick together
- White patches in the mouth
- Redness or tenderness around the navel area
- Nose blocked by mucus, making it difficult for the baby to breathe while feeding
- Diarrhoea – more than six to eight watery stools per day (see page 307).
- Projectile vomiting
- Vomiting that lasts for six hours or more, or is accompanied by fever and/or diarrhoea
- Refusing to be fed
- Crying for unusually long periods
- Blood-streaked stools

Relieving abdominal discomfort

Massage can comfort a fretful baby. If you suspect your baby has tummy ache, try the following procedure, making sure that the room where you massage your baby is warm and draught-free.

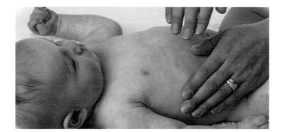

1 Massage hand-over-hand down the right side of the abdomen, from between the hip and the lower rib to below the navel. Repeat on the left side.

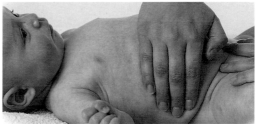

2 Cup your hand and gently knead your baby's tummy from side to side. Don't push downwards as he will tense up and keep it playful.

3 Using your cupped hand, massage your baby's tummy in a circular motion, clockwise from your left to your right. If your baby's tummy is hard, gently tickle it before you begin so that it relaxes.

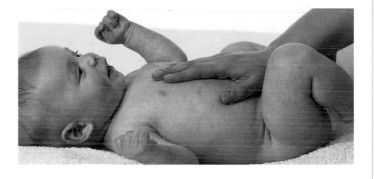

fever. Problems with feeding also can cause loose stools. Other causes of diarrhoea in early infancy include an intolerance of a particular type of formula milk and the use of antibiotics.

What to look out for

- Very soft, watery, foul-smelling stools
- Vomiting
- Abdominal pain
- Fever
- Refusing to be fed
- Floppiness

Treatment

Avoid dehydration by offering more milk. You can give your baby cooled, boiled water between feeds. If he becomes dehydrated, he may require hospital treatment so that fluids can be given to replace the salt, electrolytes and sugar that have been lost. If a bacterial infection is the cause, your baby may be put on antibiotics. If a milk allergy is suspected, a change of formula may be suggested.

Diarrhoea caused by an infection usually gets better over a period of a week or so. Finding the right formula may require more time to resolve.

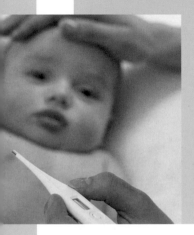

TAKING YOUR BABY'S TEMPERATURE

A young baby's temperature should be taken under his arm. If you're using a digital thermometer, wipe under your baby's arm to remove any sweat, then place the bulb into the fold of his armpit and hold his arm against his side to keep it in place. Leave for 3 to 4 minutes or until the thermometer beeps. Contact your healthcare provider if the temperature is raised to 38°C (100.4°F)) or more. Always mention that it is an axillary temperature (one taken under the arm), as this has a slightly lower reading.

Vomiting

Many babies bring up relatively small amounts of milk while or shortly after being fed, and if your baby is otherwise growing and doing well, this is probably related to reflux of milk from the stomach, which will resolve itself in time. When a baby vomits, however, he forcefully throws up large amounts of milk, and he may do so quite suddenly. Vomiting can be the result of milk allergy. Anatomical abnormalities of the intestine, such as pyloric stenosis (see page 379) or a narrowed digestive tract, prevent babies from keeping milk down. As with diarrhoea, bacteria and viruses also can cause vomiting. If it is caused by an infection, your baby may also have a fever.

What to look out for
- Large amounts of milk being expelled
- Fever and/or diarrhoea
- Persistent or forceful vomiting
- Blood in vomit

Treatment
You need to see your healthcare provider urgently if your baby has any of these symptoms so that the cause is identified quickly. If an infection is suspected, tests will be carried out and, if confirmed, antibiotics may be given. If the vomiting is related to a blockage in the intestine, an X-ray or ultrasound may be performed, and your baby may require surgery. Consult your healthcare provider immediately if your baby appears to be dehydrated, with a dry mouth and lips, lethargy, sunken fontanelle (see page 283), or a dry or dark yellow-coloured urine-stained nappy.

Infections and skin disorders

Fever

If your baby is under 3 months, most doctors would consider a temperature of more than 38°C (100.4°F) to be a fever. There are several reasons why a baby may develop a fever right after birth. The mother may have an infection that has been passed on to her baby. Even if the mother has a normal temperature, an infection can cause a fever in her baby. Less likely, a raised temperature can be related to the baby's environment: if the delivery room or nursery is too hot, a baby's temperature may increase.

What to look out for
- Skin that is warm to the touch
- Signs of a possible infection, such as a cold
- Lack of interest in feeding
- Lethargy

Treatment
No matter what the cause, an elevated temperature in a baby should never be ignored; it may be the first indication of a more serious problem. A raised temperature in a new baby usually indicates an infection of some kind. He may have caught a bacterial infection during birth or may have become infected with a cold virus from a visitor. Either way, a healthcare provider should always see a young baby with a suspected fever, as treatment may be required.

Colds

These are infections of the upper respiratory tract and are almost always caused by viruses. Colds are very common in babies. Some colds are mild and only last for a day or two; others are more severe, lasting for several weeks. Sometimes complications develop, such as an ear infection or a sore throat.

What to look out for

- Runny or blocked nose
- Clear, yellow, or green nasal discharge
- Sneezing
- Red, watery eyes
- Cough
- Fever
- Lack of appetite

Treatment

There is no cure for a cold. Antibiotics are ineffective against viral infections, although they may be used to treat any complications. A blocked nose makes sucking difficult, so encourage frequent breast- or bottlefeeding. Additional fluids should be given, as these will help to loosen any congestion. Using a vaporizer or humidifier in the nursery may make your baby more comfortable. If he's having trouble breathing, his cold may have developed into a more serious problem, so contact your healthcare provider immediately.

Group B streptococcus (GBS)

Also known as Strep B, this can cause a very severe bacterial infection in newborn babies. The bacteria is found in the vaginas of approximately 10 per cent of all women, and a small percentage of babies are infected with it during vaginal delivery. Many healthcare providers now check for the infection during pregnancy. In early-onset infection a baby becomes sick within hours after birth. In late-onset infection (a week or more after the birth), meningitis (see right) frequently ensues.

What to look out for

- Grunting noises
- Poor feeding

- Lethargy or irritability
- Abnormally high or low temperature
- Rapid heart rate
- Rapid breathing

Treatment

GBS is potentially fatal, so an infected baby will require urgent medical attention. If you tested positive during pregnancy, antibiotics will probably have been given during your delivery to decrease the risk to your baby. Late-onset Group B strep requires immediate hospital treatment. With both types of infection, early intensive treatment could prevent potentially serious consequences.

Meningitis

This is an inflammation of the membranes that line the brain and spinal cord. It's usually caused by a viral or bacterial infection. Viral meningitis may be caused by a number of different viruses, and is commonly mild, with no long-term side effects. Very occasionally it can be severe and cause serious problems.

With a newborn, bacterial meningitis is usually caused by Group B streptococcus. In babies over 3 months the three most common forms of meningitis are: haemophilus influenzae Type B (Hib); meningococcus Groups A, B and C. Group B is the most common, but Group C is the most severe and requires immediate hospital treatment, as it can be fatal if not treated early.

What to look out for

- High-pitched crying
- Drowsiness or lethargy
- Bulging fontanelle (soft spot) on the top of a baby's head
- Vomiting
- Refusal to feed
- Pale skin and cold limbs
- Sensitivity to light
- Fever and a blank, staring expression
- Stiffness of the neck
- Difficulty breathing
- A convulsion with stiffened body and shaking

One possible symptom of meningitis is a rash (left), which may start as pin-prick red spots and develop into large purple marks. If you press a glass tumbler against the rash (top) and it does not fade or turn white take your child to the doctor or a hospital immediately.

- Reddish-purple spots that don't go away if pressed with a glass and that develop into bruises under the skin

Treatment
If you suspect meningitis, call a doctor without delay or take your baby to the hospital for urgent evaluation. Meningitis may be hard to diagnose, so your healthcare provider my perform a lumbar puncture to confirm any diagnosis. Antibiotics will be given if bacterial meningitis is suspected. A hearing test may be carried out after 4 weeks, as deafness is the most common side effect of bacterial meningitis. If the infection is viral, your baby should recover within a few days.

Oral thrush
Thrush is caused by a yeast (fungus) called *candida albicans*. This fungus also causes nappy rash. A baby may come into contact with the infection when he passes through the birth canal if his mother has a vaginal yeast infection.

What to look out for
- White patches on the tongue and on the insides of the mouth
- Feeding is uncomfortable
- Severe nappy rash

Treatment
There are a number of oral medications that can treat thrush. If you are breastfeeding, you need to use anti-fungal cream on your nipples. All teats, dummies and bottles should be thoroughly sterilized each time they are used.

Infantile eczema
Also known as atopic dermatitis, this is the most common form of eczema in babies under 12 months. Eczema is an allergic condition related to asthma and hayfever. It can be inherited but also can exist in isolation. It commonly appears on the face and scalp or behind the ears. Your baby may only have a few patches of dry skin; but if the eczema is severe, your baby's skin may become sore, inflamed and weepy. This is unbearably itchy, so your baby will scratch continuously, leaving his skin open to infection.

What to look out for
- Severe itching
- Oozing, crusty patches of inflamed skin
- Patches of red, dry skin
- Flaking skin and occasional blisters

Treatment
Though it can only be managed, not cured, most children do grow out of atopic eczema. It is important to maintain a strict skin-care regime under medical supervision. Emollients will prevent your baby's skin from getting too dry and itchy. Steroid creams can reduce inflammation, but are generally only used if your baby's eczema hasn't responded to emollients. Antibiotics may be prescribed to clear up infection in severe cases.

Wearing mitts will help to stop a baby scratching. Breastfeeding for the first six months may give some protection against allergens.

Eye problems
Blocked tear ducts

About 5 per cent of babies are born with a blockage in their tear ducts. Many newborns have a partial blockage that gradually clears so, by the time they are 18 months old, the tear ducts are normal. Blocked tear ducts predispose your baby to eye infections.

What to look out for

- Weepy, constantly running eye
- Nostril remains dry when baby cries

Treatment

Keep your baby's eyes clean by wiping with cooled, boiled water using a fresh piece of cotton wool for each eye. Massaging the area just under the eye right next to the nose where the duct is located will help. Antibiotics may be needed if there is an infection. Rarely, surgery is required to clean and dilate the ducts.

Conjunctivitis

An inflammation of the membrane covering the eyeball and the inside of eyelid, conjunctivitis – also known as sticky eye – is usually caused by a viral infection accompanying a cold. It also can be caused by a bacterial infection. Bacterial conjunctivitis occurs more commonly in babies with blocked tear ducts (see above). Rarely, conjunctivitis is a symptom of gonorrhoea or chlamydia infection, which has been passed from mother to baby.

What to look out for

- Mucus or 'matter' in corner of eye
- Discoloured – yellow or green – eye discharge
- Eyelids stuck together
- Dislike of bright lights
- Swollen, red eyelid

Treatment

Keep your baby's eyes clean by wiping away any sticky discharge with cooled, boiled water using a separate piece of cotton wool for each wipe. Seek

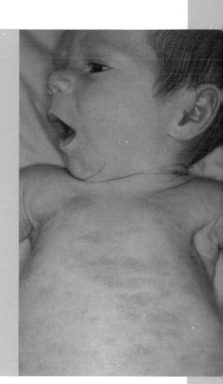

Eczema is diagnosed from your baby's inflamed, red scaly skin. The condition causes intense itching and constant scratching can lead to the skin being split, leaving it prone to infection. Common affected areas include the face, trunk, groin, knees, hands and underarms.

medical advice if the eyes remain red and swollen for longer than three days or the eyelids are stuck together. Antibiotics may be required.

Blood disorders
Neonatal jaundice

Fifty per cent of babies develop jaundice at birth. Usually this is because a baby's liver can't process bilirubin (a natural waste product of the baby's blood) fast enough, which results in a build up of yellow pigment in the skin. The yellow colour appears first on the head and passes down the body as the bilirubin level rises.

Babies who were bruised during birth can have jaundice, as extra blood is broken down in the bruise and more bilirubin is formed. Premature babies also are likely to become jaundiced, because their livers haven't matured. Other, less common, causes of jaundice include infections, liver problems and rhesus incompatability.

What to look out for

- Yellow tinge to skin
- Whites of eyes become yellow

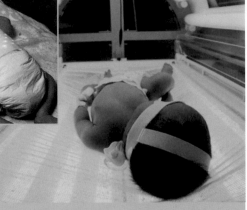

Jaundice may be treated with phototherapy while the baby is in an incubator (above). A new treatment is a bilirubin wrap (top left) where the baby can remain in a normal cot.

covering since the light doesn't shine directly from above. In most cases, jaundice goes away for good.

Jaundice in infants after the early newborn period can be serious and of a different nature than newborn jaundice.

Hypoglycaemia

This is a condition in which the amount of glucose (sugar) in the blood is lower than normal. Although reasonably common in newborn babies, there are certain babies who have a higher chance of having problems. Babies born to mothers who have diabetes during pregnancy may have problems controlling their blood sugar levels. Both particularly large babies and those who are small for their age also are more likely to have difficulties with blood sugar levels. Premature babies, babies who won't eat for long periods after birth and those who have bacterial infections may also experience problems.

What to look out for
- Sweating
- Pale skin
- Rapid breathing
- Increased heart rate
- Jitteriness and jerky movements

Treatment
Simply feeding your baby may be all that is required to improve his blood sugar levels. Occasionally, if your baby doesn't respond, sugared water may be given intravenously to achieve adequate levels.

- Excessive weight loss
- Baby appears very sleepy and may have poor sucking ability

Treatment
Your baby's bilirubin levels will be monitored to make sure they don't become dangerously high, which can damage his nervous system. Blood can be drawn from your baby's vein or heel. Newer ways of checking bilirubin levels without drawing blood include a special light sensor that can be placed on the baby's skin.

Neonatal jaundice usually clears up by itself over a few days or weeks, but if bilirubin levels are high, phototherapy may be given. This is a very safe treatment, during which a baby is exposed to controlled amounts of ultraviolet (UV) light – not the kind that burns. The UV light breaks down excess bilirubin so that it can be disposed of through your baby's liver. Your baby will be placed in an incubator under lights for a couple of days, wearing just his nappy and with his eyes covered by a protective mask.

Newer bilirubin wraps or blankets allow a baby to sleep in a normal cot, stay in the hospital room with his mother, and avoid wearing an eye

Monitoring your baby's health and development

Within a few days of your baby's birth, you will be given a personal child health record (PCHR). In it, both you and others will record important information about your child, so you should bring it with you whenever you see anyone about your child's health and development. In it, you can note special milestones, such as a first smile or tooth, along with important medical information such as immunisations that have been given and any illnesses suffered.

Your baby's growth

Your baby's head circumference, weight and height are a good indication of her general health and well-being during the first year. Although the range of 'normal' at any age is very wide, there is an 'average' range, into which most children fall (see page 368). Special allowances will be made if your baby is premature.

At each check-up your baby will be measured, and her healthcare provider will plot the numbers on a chart of national averages for children of the same age and sex. You will then be told what percentile your child is in. For example, if your 2-month-old is in the 75th percentile for weight, that means that 75 per cent of the 2-month-olds in the country are lighter and 25 per cent are heavier than her.

Parents sometimes worry needlessly about these percentiles. Keep in mind that your child is an individual and will develop at her own pace. These measurements are only a general guide to assess your baby's developmental progress. The most important thing to watch for is that your baby is growing steadily.

How the measurements are taken

- *Head circumference* Unlike other vital organs, which are fully formed at birth, your baby's brain – and, therefore, her head – continues to grow during her first year. Your baby's healthcare provider will measure her head by placing a measuring tape just above her eyebrows and ears, and around the back of her head where it slopes up from her neck.
- *Weight* After your baby is completely undressed she will be placed on a scale (either a traditional beam scale or an electronic model). Both types should be set to zero before the baby is laid down.
- *Length/height* Until your baby is old enough to stand still on her own, she'll be measured lying down. Sometimes a special device with a headboard and movable footboard is used to make sure the results are accurate.

Taking the measurements yourself

Your baby's healthcare provider may give you percentile charts to fill in at home. However, it is important to remember that your measurements may not be as accurate as when a he or she takes them. Once you have plotted the measurements on the growth percentile charts you will be able to see how your baby is growing and how she compares to her other babies of her age.

If you have concerns

Sometimes a baby has feeding problems, or you may be concerned that she is not getting enough milk at each feed. By weighing her regularly and plotting her weight gain on a percentile chart you will soon be able to see whether there is a problem. If you are concerned about any area of your baby's development you should discuss your worries with your child's healthcare provider.

Charting your baby's growth

The solid line in the middle of the grey band indicates the average growth rate in the first year. The grey band shows the range of normal measurements.

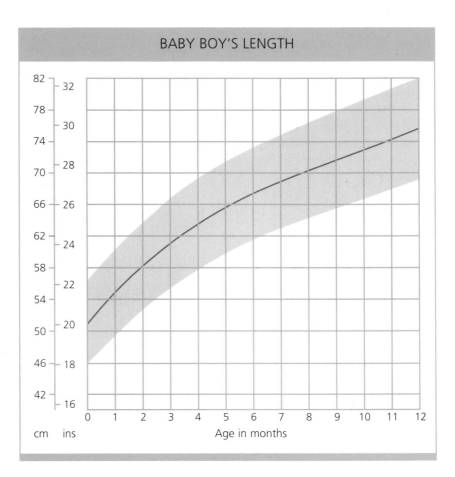

BABY BOY'S LENGTH

cm   ins

Age in months

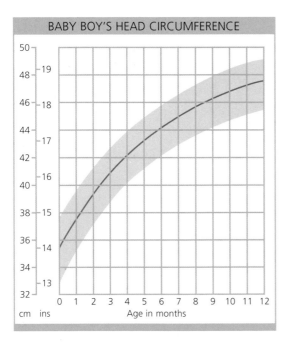

BABY BOY'S HEAD CIRCUMFERENCE

cm   ins

Age in months

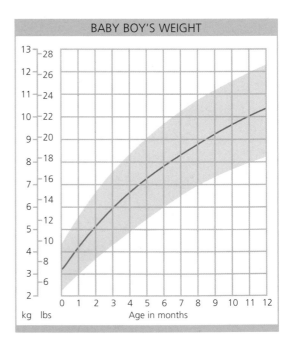

BABY BOY'S WEIGHT

kg   lbs

Age in months

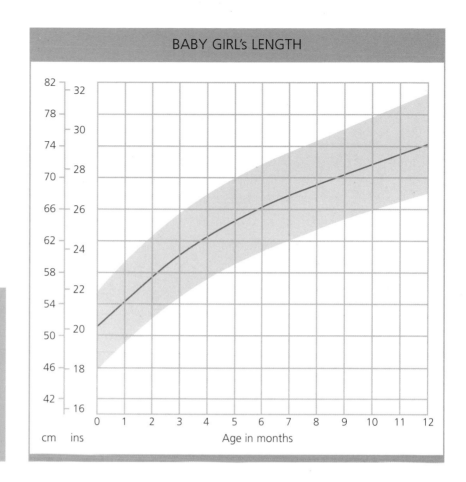

BABY GIRL's LENGTH

Your child's growth curves should fall somewhere within the grey band and should follow the shape of the curve of the solid line.

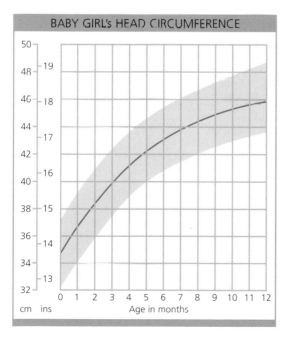

BABY GIRL's HEAD CIRCUMFERENCE

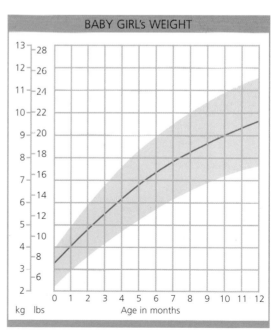

BABY GIRL's WEIGHT

Vaccination may be delayed if your child is sick with anything other than a mild cold or if her immune system is weakened by immune-suppressing medications.

AGE	VACCINE/HOW GIVEN
Newborn	BCG if at risk of TB - One jab
2 months	DTaP/IPV/Hib against diphtheria, tetanus and pertussis (whooping cough), polio and Haemophilus influenzae type B - One jab
	PCV against pneumococcal infection - One jab
	Rotarix against rotavirus - Drops
3 months	DTaP/IPV/Hib (2nd dose) - One jab
	MenC against meningitis C - One jab
	Rotarix against rotavirus - Drops
4 months	DTaP/IPV/Hib (3rd dose) - One jab
	MenC (2nd dose) - One jab
	PCV (2nd dose) - One jab
12 to 13 months*	MMR against measles, mumps and rubella (German measles) - One jab
	Hib/MenC (4th dose of Hib, 3rd dose MenC) - One jab
	PCV (3rd dose) - One jab

*Parents who don't want their child to have three vaccinations at the 12 to 13 month visit should be offered the Hib/MenC at a later visit.

Giving protection from disease

Immunisation is one of the most important steps you can take to ensure your baby's current and future health. Since immunisation was first invented, it has saved hundreds of thousands of children's lives. This simple procedure involves the use of vaccines, which protect children from serious, and sometimes fatal, infectious diseases by strengthening their immunity (the body's ability to fight off these diseases).

Natural immunity

Your baby is born with a degree of natural, inherited immunity, which she acquired before birth. That immunity is reinforced if you are breastfeeding, as breast milk is rich in antibodies, especially in the first few days after birth. But this type of passive, inherited immunity is only temporary – it wears off during your child's first year of life. This leaves her vulnerable to a host of serious diseases. Vaccinations give your child protective immunity against these diseases.

Generally, vaccines are safe and very effective. The benefits of immunisation far outweigh any risks. Typical side effects may include a mild fever or slight rash, depending on the vaccine. More serious side effects are rare, but if other symptoms develop or fever is high, consult your child's healthcare provider.

Keeping an immunisation record

It's a good idea to keep a record of the immunisations that your child receives. Record sheets are often provided by healthcare providers. They're valuable if you move or changes doctors, or if you need proof of your child's protection against certain infectious diseases, for example, when you travel abroad. The immunisation record should specify the types of vaccine, and be dated and signed by your child's healthcare provider each time an immunisation is given.

How to stop an infant from choking

Babies under 12 months old usually choke because they have breathed in a foreign object, which can lodge at the back of the throat and cause muscle spasm. This may block the airway and will need to be removed immediately. If you suspect your baby is choking but she can still cry and cough, allow her to continue coughing. watch carefully but do not pat her back or give her water.

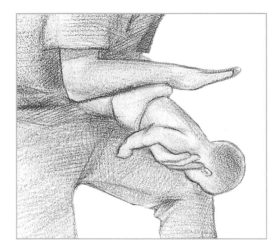

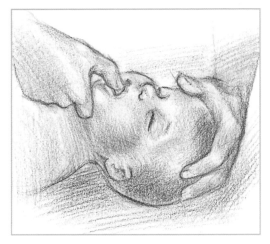

1 If your baby cannot cry, cough or breathe, or is making high-pitched noises, lay her along your forearm on her tummy; rest your forearm on your upper thigh with your baby's head extending past your bent knee. With the heel of your other hand, give your baby up to five back blows between her shoulder blades.

2 Check your baby's mouth quickly after each blow and remove any obvious obstruction: Place her on her back and tilt her forehead back slightly. Using a single finger, carefully feel and remove any obstruction from her mouth.

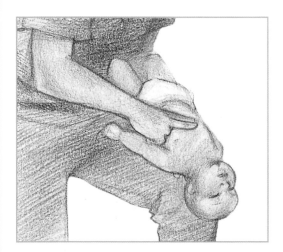

3 If your baby is still choking, carefully turn her over and using two or three fingers, push inwards and upwards in the middle of her chest up to five times. Check her mouth quickly after each thrust (see above). If the obstruction does not clear after three cycles of back blows and chest thrusts, dial 999 (or 112) for an ambulance. Continue cycles of back blows and chest thrusts until help arrives. If your baby is breathing but loses consciousness, place her in the recovery position: hold her on her side, head tilted as if you were giving her a cuddle with her head lower than her tummy. You must seek medical advice if you have given your child abdominal thrusts. If your baby is not breathing, perform CPR, see page 372.

How to give cardiopulmonary resuscitation (CPR) to babies under one year of age

Learning CPR and other life-saving techniques is best done from an expert e.g., a St. John's Ambulance course. The following steps should only be performed if your baby is not breathing. If you have someone with you, send him or her to dial 999 (112) for an ambulance immediately. If you are on your own, carry out CPR for 1 minute before carrying the baby to the phone to call for an ambulance.

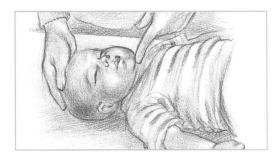

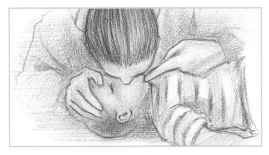

1 Lay your baby down on a firm flat surface such as the floor or a table, then gently tilt her head back with one hand, and lift her chin with the other to open her airway. It's important not to tilt her head back too far as this could kink her airway. Put your ear to her mouth and nose, and look, listen and feel for breathing.

2 If your baby is still not breathing, give her 5 Rescue Breaths: fill your cheecks with air and seal your lips around her mouth over her nose and lips. Give one small breath every three seconds looking along her chest as you breathe. As her chest rises, stop blowing and allow it to fall.

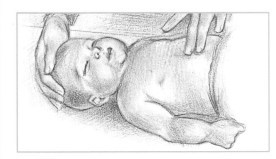

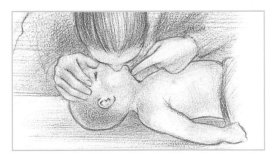

3 Then give chest compressions: place two fingers in the middle of her chest and press down one-third of the depth of her chest. Press 30 times at a rate of 100 per minute.

4 After 30 compressions, give 2 Rescue Breaths. Continue resuscitation (30 compressions to 2 rescue breaths) without stopping until help arrives.

Babies needing special care

Most babies who are too small at birth – weighing less than 2.5 kg (5½ lbs) at birth – or are born too early will need some form of special care to enable them to catch up. A premature baby will most probably be treated in a special care baby unit (SCBU).

Newborns are said to be premature if they're born before 37 weeks of age. Babies born after 24 to 25 weeks of gestation (pregnancy) may be mature enough to survive, but will be in intensive care for a while. Babies born at less than 23 weeks of gestation aren't usually mature enough to survive. Apart from age, other factors boost the outcome for a premature baby, including being female and African-American.

While premature babies face early difficulties, it is important to keep in mind that nearly two thirds of premature babies who survive will either grow up to be completely normal or will have only mild or moderate problems.

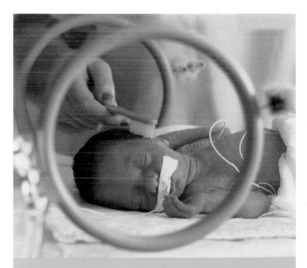

This premature baby, seen here in an incubator, is so tiny his hair is being brushed with a soft toothbrush. Electrodes have been attached to him to monitor his heartbeat and breathing.

The care your baby will receive

A premature baby may need to be on a ventilator, as his lungs will not have matured. As infections often cause premature birth, your baby will be given antibiotics and intravenous fluids, either through an IV or umbilical central line. A premature baby may be placed in a special bed with a radiant warmer to help to maintain his body temperature, plus a cellophane wrapping to minimize the loss of heat and fluids through his thin skin. He also will probably be on a cardiorespiratory monitor with a pulse oximeter to measure the oxygen in his blood, and he may have a feeding tube if he is mature enough to eat.

Unless the baby is over 32 to 34 weeks, he probably won't be able to breastfeed or drink from a bottle but will have a tube in his mouth or nose that goes down to his stomach. A mother of a premature baby can express milk and store it in the SCBU until her baby can take it.

Most premature babies are not ready to be discharged until some time around the date they were originally due. So for a baby born at 26 weeks, that can mean three months in the hospital. In general, a baby will need to be gaining weight, breathing well on his own – although he may need oxygen – and eating to be able to leave the SCBU. After that his progress will be checked regularly by a team of specialist doctors.

Birth abnormalities

Although the great majority of babies are normal, about 1 per cent will have some form of congenital defect. Babies can be affected by a large number of things during their development in the uterus, and many of the resulting defects can be treated before or after birth.

Congenital heart problems

The heart is a complex organ and much of its structural development occurs between 3 and 7 weeks after conception. Congenital heart defects are the most common group of abnormalities, affecting nearly 1 in every 100 babies born. The range of defects is very wide.

A mother with a congenital heart defect, or who has had an affected child, has a slightly increased risk of having a baby with a heart problem. Many heart problems are also associated with other genetic problems such as Down's syndrome (see page 249) and testing for such problems may be offered if a heart defect is found.

How heart defects are diagnosed

Most problems are detected on an ultrasound scan at 18 to 22 weeks. Many defects are not visible earlier than this. If there's a history of a heart problem, regular scanning may be carried out during pregnancy. However, some heart problems may not be seen at all on an ultrasound scan, even with experience; as many as 40 per cent of problems can be missed.

Treatment

Intrauterine surgical techniques are being developed so that in the future some defects can be treated before birth. After birth the management of a heart defect will depend on the severity of the diagnosis. For mild problems, a newborn baby can usually remain with her mother and will be assessed by a paediatrician in the hospital. More serious problems that can lead to a lack of oxygen will require specialist care. This means that the birth should take place where specialist care can be offered. Many heart

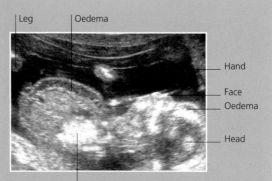

On an ultrasound scan for fetal hydrops, oedema appears on the entire body, due to an accumulation of fluid in the tissues. In this case the oedema is caused by a mass in the chest obstructing blood flow.

problems are amenable to surgery, although there are some that will not allow the baby to survive outside the uterus.

Fetal hydrops

This is heart failure in the baby, and on a scan the skin appears swollen, and there is evidence of fluid within the chest and abdomen. The causes are many, including blood group incompatibility, which can be diagnosed in pregnancy.

How fetal hydrops is diagnosed

Through ultrasound scans

Treatment

Treatment will depend on the severity and cause of the condition. Some causes, such as anaemia, can be treated, but others, such as those associated with severe heart defects, cannot. Babies with a blood group incompatibility may be treated with intrauterine blood transfusions. Whether a baby diagnosed with hydrops will survive depends on the diagnosis and how ill the baby is at the time of discovery. All babies who have reached this stage are very ill indeed, and many do not survive.

Septal defect

This is commonly known as a 'hole in the heart.' It may occur in the dividing tissue between the smaller or larger chambers of the heart. A small defect may not be detected and sometimes the condition only comes to light in later life. Septal defects that are diagnosed during pregnancy tend to be large, or are associated with other problems.

How a septal defect is diagnosed
Through ultrasound scans

Treatment
Small defects do not always require surgery. Larger defects are likely to require surgery.

Problems with flow of blood out of the heart

This can occur because the blood vessels have not joined up correctly or because the valves have not formed properly. Problems of this kind are often complex, and may be associated with septal defects (see above).

How blood flow problems are diagnosed
Through ultrasound scans

Treatment
Where connections are not in the right place, surgery is often successful. If the valves have not developed properly, surgery is more difficult and less likely to be successful in the long term. Many of these conditions are extremely complicated. As with any abnormality in a baby it is important for parents to talk to a specialist in the condition during pregnancy to discuss what the best treatment will be for the baby.

Problems with the spine or head
Neural tube defects
One of the most common developmental problems, a neural tube defect is the failure of the brain and spinal cord to develop properly during the first four weeks of pregnancy. This affects as many as 1 in 2,500 live births in the United Kingdom, and results in varying degrees of damage to the baby. Many more pregnancies are affected, but because of the severity of the condition most parents opt for termination when it is diagnosed early in the pregnancy.

Spina bifida occulta is the mildest form, in which one or two vertebrae are malformed. In spina bifida occulta, the spinal cord is covered with skin, so it usually causes no problems. Sometimes it is only discovered as the result of an X-ray in later life. Occasionally, there may be a tuft of hair or skin dimple over the affected site.

Myelo-meningocele is a more severe form of spina bifida. This involves a lesion on the spine, which can sometimes be the size of an orange, where nerve tissue, muscles and spinal fluid are exposed. The lesion causes nerve damage leading to problems with muscular control and bladder and bowel control. Hydrocephalus is also a related condition (see page 376).

Anencephaly is the most severe neural tube defect. An opening at the upper end of the tube results in portions of the skull and brain not forming. Babies with this condition can't survive after birth.

How neural tube defects are diagnosed
Spina bifida can be detected at 16 weeks by serum screening (see page 241), because it causes maternal alpha-fetoprotein levels to be very high. However, anomaly ultrasounds (see page 238) are very effective at picking up babies with significant neural tube defects.

Treatment
The treatment given will depend on the size and type of the neural tube defect and its severity. This

will be determined by ultrasound and magnetic resonance imaging (MRI) scanning after birth. If the baby has an open defect this will require an operation to close the spine. While this operation will close the defect, it cannot restore the nerves, which may have not developed properly. Hydrocephalus will also require an operation to relieve the condition after birth.

Prevention

Although the cause of neural tube defects is not clear, there is now good evidence that folic acid, a vitamin found in leafy vegetables, needs to be present in early pregnancy to allow the spine to close up properly. Because it is hard to achieve the recommended dose through diet alone, taking a folic acid supplement is now recommended three months before conception and up to the 12th week of pregnancy. Experts have suggested that all women of child-bearing age should have 400 micrograms of folic acid each day. Mothers who have had a previous baby with spina bifida or anencephaly, or are on certain drugs such as those used to treat epilepsy, need to take a higher-dose of folic acid – 5 mg. This can be prescribed or obtained from pharmacies and supermarkets.

Hydrocephalus

This is a build up of cerebrospinal fluid (CSF) in the head and is caused by an obstruction in the draining system around the brain. Sometimes the head of the baby becomes very large. Premature birth is the most common cause, because of a higher risk of bleeding into the brain, which may prevent absorption of CSF. It also can occur in babies with a congenital defect such as spina bifida; some cases are inherited, and some infections can have this effect. Babies known to have this condition may need to be delivered by Caesarean. How the baby will be affected depends on the underlying cause. Some babies will grow up to have a normal intelligence, while others can be profoundly disabled; however, this cannot be predicted before birth.

How hydrocephalus is diagnosed

During pregnancy, hydrocephalus can be diagnosed by ultrasound scan. After birth, the head measurement carried out on every newborn can indicate whether the condition exists. Early diagnosis and treatment improves the outcome.

Treatment

After birth, an operation is usually carried out to allow the CSF to drain, via a shunt, into the bloodstream. The shunt remains in place for life. An operation to insert a temporary shunt may sometimes be carried out before birth. A permanent shunt is then inserted after the birth. Some recent surgical techniques, in which an opening in the skull is made, are suitable for some forms of hydrocephalus.

Cerebral palsy

This term is used to cover a group of disorders affecting movement and posture. There may be associated learning difficulties in about one in four of affected children. The cause can be abnormal development of the brain before birth, oxygen deprivation, infection, bleeding in the brain, or physical injury during birth. Physical symptoms range from weakness and floppiness of muscles to spasticity and rigidity.

How cerebral palsy is diagnosed

A reliable diagnosis cannot usually be made until a child is at least one year old, because many parts of the nervous system have not fully developed before then. Diagnostic tests may include EEG, MRI and CT scanning and vision and hearing tests. In some cases blood tests may also be used to evaluate inherited conditions.

Treatment

There is no cure for cerebral palsy, but there are treatments that will help to minimize the effects and boost a child's abilities. These may include physical therapies, complementary therapies and drug treatments. Surgery may sometimes be helpful in dealing with limb deformities.

Genito-urinary problems
Urinary tract obstruction

This occurs when the flow of urine between the kidney and the bladder becomes partially or completely obstructed, leading to hydronephrosis (swelling of the kidney), which can cause loss of kidney function. This condition can be detected in a fetus as early as 15 weeks. Mild hydronephrosis – also known as renal pelvic dilatation – may get better spontaneously by the end of the pregnancy and need no treatment.

How urinary tract obstruction is diagnosed
Diagnosis during pregnancy is with ultrasound. In a newborn a renal scan will be performed to determine the severity of the blockage. Other tests may be necessary to assess how the baby's kidneys are functioning.

Treatment
Fetal surgery may be considered in very severe cases, usually when both kidneys are affected. For this to be effective it must be done before there is substantial damage to the developing kidneys. Once the baby has been born, surgical treatment may be needed to relieve the blockage. Antibiotics are prescribed to prevent the baby from getting a renal tract infection.

Multicystic kidney

When the body of the kidney does not successfully fuse with the drainage system this can lead to a poorly or non-functioning kidney, which appears large and cystic on an ultrasound scan. Everyone can manage with only one functioning kidney, and to develop in the uterus a baby does not need to have any functional kidney at all, as the placenta removes waste products. However, once born, a baby needs kidney function in at least one kidney. Sometimes abnormal development affects only one kidney, and the baby will usually have no serious problems, though sometimes the poorly functioning one has to be removed in childhood. But if both kidneys are affected, the amount of fluid around the baby will

decrease, and the baby's lungs will not grow adequately. At birth the baby would have difficulty breathing, as well as poor kidney function. For this reason bilateral multicystic kidneys (involving both sides) is a fatal condition.

A condition called adult polycystic kidney disease, can occasionally be seen in the fetus. It does not cause problems until later in adult life. Usually one parent will have this condition, although they may not know about it.

How kidney cysts are diagnosed
Diagnosis during pregnancy is with ultrasound. In a newborn a renal scan, or a CT scan may be used to check for kidney cysts.

Treatment
Depending on the severity of the problem, surgery may be required when the child is older. If there is a hereditary factor other tests may be done.

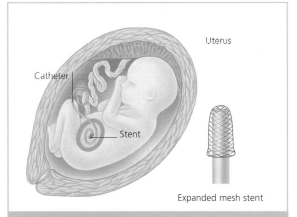

The latest treatment for urinary tract obstruction is carried out while the baby is in the uterus. A stent (right) is placed via a tiny hollow tube – catheter – through the mother's abdomen, into the fetal bladder to allow urine to escape.

Hypospadias

About 1 in 300 boys is born with this condition. The opening of the urethra, which is the tube bringing urine from the bladder to the outside, normally at the tip of the penis, develops in the wrong place, most commonly on the underside of the penis. This causes problems with urination and may also cause the penis to curve downwards, which may affect sexual performance when adulthood is reached.

How hypospadias is diagnosed
- Inability to pass a normal stream of urine
- Curved penis
- Hooded foreskin

Treatment
In very mild cases, no action will be taken. In more severe cases, surgery will be needed to extend the urethra. Children with hypospadias shouldn't be circumcised, as the foreskin will probably be used as part of the repair surgery.

Undescended testicle

Normally, during fetal development, the testicles pass from the abdomen through a canal into the scrotum. In some cases this doesn't happen prior to birth, and the exact cause usually isn't known. The condition occurs relatively frequently in premature babies, while full-term healthy babies are much less likely to have this problem. The testes usually descend by the 28th week of pregnancy, so if a baby is born prior to this time, the testes may not have had time yet to descend. Sometimes only one testicle descends or the descent is incomplete.

What to look out for
- Scrotum appears small or unevenly developed
- Testes cannot be felt in scrotum

Treatment
Usually the testicles will descend on their own during the first year. Sometimes a testis, which is sitting in the inguinal canal, is not truly undescended, and will drop spontaneously. If a testicle remains undescended, hormones may be given to help it to descend by itself or surgery may be required.

Left untreated, a baby will have a higher-than-average chance of being infertile and of developing testicular cancer as an adult.

Digestive tract problems
Intestinal obstruction

An obstruction can occur anywhere in the intestines, from the oesophagus to the anus. Blockages at the top can lead to an accumulation of amniotic fluid, and are usually diagnosed during pregnancy. A blockage just below the stomach is known as a duodenal atresia. This type of blockage is commonly found in babies with Down's syndrome (see page 249) and a test may be offered for this. Lower blockages may not be recognized until after birth.

How intestinal obstruction is diagnosed
Ultrasound scanning is used to identify the cause of the blockage.

Treatment
If a baby has an obstruction, surgery will be needed after birth to bypass the block to allow the baby to begin feeding.

Abdominal wall defects

These occur when part of the abdominal wall has failed to develop, leaving a hole. The contents of the abdomen can then escape outside the cavity. In some cases there is a membrane covering the contents. This is called an omphalocele or exomphalos and can be associated with other genetic problems in the baby, and testing may be offered. If the bowel is not covered, the condition is called a gastroschisis. This is not associated with any other developmental problems in the baby. If the baby remains healthy, a vaginal delivery should be possible. Sometimes, if the baby is unwell in other ways, or has a large exomphalos, a Caesarean section may be offered.

How abdominal wall defects are diagnosed

A baby with one of these conditions is likely to appear small, so close monitoring during pregnancy will be required. Abdominal wall defects can be picked up on ultrasound scanning.

Treatment

The baby will need an operation to close the defect. Usually this can be done at a single operation. Occasionally small amounts of bowel will need to be removed if damaged or blocked. Feeding is introduced slowly, and the baby will need to spend quite a long time – two to four weeks – in hospital until feeding is established.

Pyloric stenosis

This occurs when the pylorus (ring of muscle that links the duodenum to the stomach), becomes so enlarged with muscle that food can't pass. Symptoms usually start between 3 and 12 weeks. The condition is more common in boys and seems to run in certain families.

How pyloric stenosis is diagnosed

A physical examination is performed and ultrasound is used to confirm the condition.

Treatment

The condition is treated with minor surgery, where a small cut is made in the pylorus. After the operation your baby will feed normally and weight gain will be rapid.

Diaphragmatic hernia

The diaphragm is a muscle, which separates the organs of the abdomen from those of the chest. During the fetus' early development in the uterus, there is a hole in the diaphragm, which usually closes by the end of the third month. If the hole stays open, the contents of the abdomen, such as the intestines, can be pushed up into the chest cavity. If this happens, these organs can displace the heart and lungs and prevent them from growing normally.

How it is diagnosed

This condition will be detected using ultrasound. Babies with this condition frequently have breathing problems once they are born.

Treatment

A baby born with a diaphragmatic hernia can have an operation to have the defect in the diaphragm

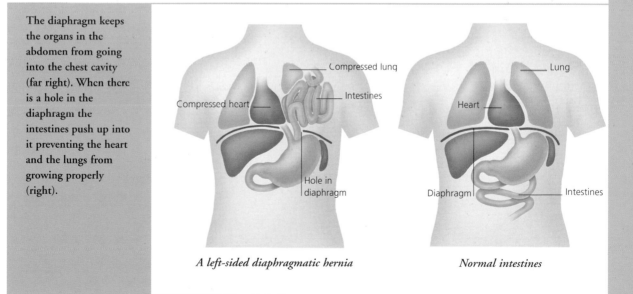

The diaphragm keeps the organs in the abdomen from going into the chest cavity (far right). When there is a hole in the diaphragm the intestines push up into it preventing the heart and the lungs from growing properly (right).

A left-sided diaphragmatic hernia　　　*Normal intestines*

closed. In severe cases, however, the lungs are not large enough to allow the baby to survive. There are no reliable ways of predicting which babies have adequate lung growth before birth.

Once a baby has had a successful operation on a hernia, he can expect to have a normal life. Sometimes diaphragmatic hernia is associated with a genetic problem, and a test will be offered to exclude this.

Musculoskeletal problems
Cleft lip or palate
These are among the most common defects affecting babies and may occur singly, or together. The defect occurs when the fetus' upper lip and/or roof of the mouth does not fuse properly before birth. In many cases, the cause is unknown, although in some the defect may be hereditary. If a baby is severely affected there may be some difficulty in feeding.

How cleft lip and palate are diagnosed
In most units with highly specialized ultrasound equipment, cleft lip or palate can be diagnosed prenatally in a mid-trimester scan. Otherwise it will be seen at birth.

Treatment
A cleft lip is usually repaired surgically by the age of 3 months. A cleft palate is repaired between 6 and 15 months of age. A plate may be fitted into the roof of a baby's mouth before this time if feeding is a problem. Plastic surgery produces good results (see picture, right) and allows speech to develop normally.

Club foot
Some babies are found to have a condition called talipes or 'club foot'. It affects about 1 in every 1000 babies. It means that one or both feet are turned away from the normal axis. Sometimes babies with this have a genetic condition. More usually it occurs either because the foot has been constricted in the uterus or because the bones of the foot have not developed properly.

How club foot is diagnosed
A routine ultrasound scan usually shows up any limb defects. This will be followed by further scans to check on the baby's development.

Treatment
If the condition is caused by restriction in the uterus all that may be required after birth are physiotherapy exercises to straighten the foot. If the bones of the foot have not developed properly a baby may need surgery in childhood.

Spinal problems
Occasionally one part of a vertebra may be missing or malformed, giving a misalignment of the spine. This can occur in some inherited conditions or where there are chromosomal problems. It is always difficult to judge what the effect will be in the long term.

How spinal problems are diagnosed
Spinal problems can be identified by an ultrasound scan.

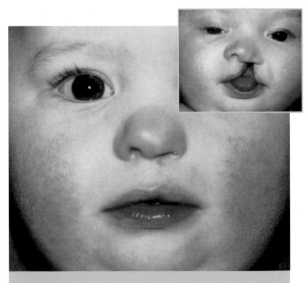

A cleft lip (top right) is usually repaired by surgery (above) when a baby is around 3 months. The outcome is usually very successful.

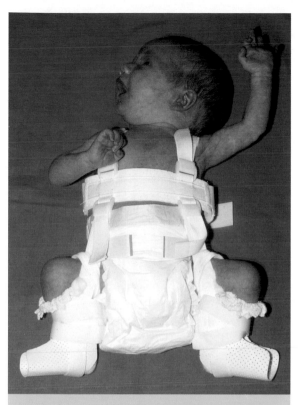

All newborns are checked for hip dislocation and, if found, a Palvick harness is often used to keep the hips in the correct position. The harness is worn for between 2 and 4 months and is very effective.

associated with other congenital conditions such as spina bifida or Down's syndrome. It is more likely to affect the left hip, although in 25 per cent of cases, it is found in both hips.

How congenital hip dislocation is diagnosed

During the standard neonatal paediatric check your baby's hips will be bent and flexed. A click could be a sign of congenital hip dislocation and a further test to confirm the condition is given at 6 weeks. Other symptoms may include asymmetric skin folds on upper legs and the inability to spread legs wide during nappy changes.

Treatment

Early treatment with a special harness (see left) increases the chances of normal hip development. The harness can be removed easily to change the baby's nappy and it does not interfere with feeding, bathing or sleeping. If treatment is needed after 6 months, a plaster cast may be used. Very rarely, surgery is carried out to enlarge the socket. This is usually done before walking begins.

Treatment

Treatment will depend on the severity of the problem. Some children can go on to have quite marked scoliosis (curvature of the spine), which may need surgery.

Congenital hip dislocation

Relatively common, hip dislocation occurs when an incorrectly formed hip joint allows the ball of the femur to slip out of the socket in the pelvic bone. The cause of hip dislocation is unknown; it may be hereditary. Hip dislocation occurs ten times more frequently in girls, and also more frequently in firstborns and breech babies. It is also more likely to occur in twins and may be

The loss of a baby

Whether parents lose a baby before the birth or afterwards, the loss is devastating. Coming to terms with the death of a much-wanted baby and being able to move on can seem an impossibility, but, as many couples have experienced, grieving is an essential part of the healing process.

It's natural to feel shock and denial after losing a baby. Many parents feel as if they're experiencing a bad dream, that what they're going through isn't real and when they wake up, their baby will still be with them.

As reality sets in, feelings of anger and deep sorrow can surface; tearfulness, loss of appetite, and sleeplessness are all part of this process. A woman's feelings are intensified by the massive fall in hormone levels, as her body returns to its pre-pregnancy state.

There's a desperate need to see and hold their baby, and many parents can be wracked with guilt that they didn't do enough for their child. Feelings of anger and the urge to blame the death on someone, anyone – the hospital, the medical staff, each other – can be overwhelming.

As the anger and deep sorrow subside, depression creeps in. What's the point in carrying on when life has been so unfair?

Acceptance is the final stage in the grieving process and will come with time. Acceptance doesn't mean that the pain and anger have disappeared, but that it's time to put the grief away and carry on with life. The death of a baby has changed everything forever, but it's possible to go on and be even stronger in time.

Support

Every parent's experience of loss is unique. For some, the healing will take a very long time, while others will be anxious to get back to 'normal' so that they can try to put the sad event behind them. The important thing is for every parent to experience whatever he or she is feeling, rather than feel that he or she has to act in the way others think appropriate.

Losing a baby also can put a huge strain on a relationship. Men have a tendency to internalise their emotions, so while a bereaved father will feel the loss as keenly as his partner he might not be able to express that grief openly. His partner might interpret this reticence as indifference and feel terribly hurt and isolated. The only way through this is for both parents to be as open and honest with each other as they can about the way they are feeling.

It's vital for both parents to accept as much help and support as possible. There are many support groups for families who have lost a baby, such as the Stillbirth and Neonatal Death Society (SANDS), and these can be very helpful.

Many parents have derived comfort from having a photograph of their baby or from holding the baby after the birth. Marking the baby's life, no matter how brief, through some sort of service, can also be very healing. Many hospitals arrange regular services of remembrance for all babies who die in pregnancy, at birth or in infancy. The hospital will offer to arrrange a funeral, burial or cremation free of charge, or you may choose to organise this yourself. You will need to register your baby's birth if he or she survived past 23 weeks.

Why babies die

Thanks to the advances in medical science, the number of babies who die before labour begins – referred to as stillbirths when the baby is more than 24 weeks gestational age – is exceedingly low (about 4,000 per year). When it does happen it is often not known why a baby has died before birth, but causes include abnormal development of the baby or a failing placenta. The mother may most often due to a lack of oxygen. There are a variety of reasons for this to occur including placental insufficiency, toxaemia of pregnancy and having the umbilical cord tightly around the neck.

When a newborn dies – neonatal death – it is most often due to breathing difficulties, especially if the baby is premature or with serious developmental problems.

If you or your caregiver think it important to ascertain the exact cause of death (though very often none will be found), it is possible to arrange a post-mortem. You may find one helpful for a future pregnancy.

Sudden infant death syndrome (SIDS)

Also known as cot or crib death (though only a small percentage of babies are found dead in their cot or crib), this is defined as the sudden unexpected death of an infant, under one year of age, that remains unexplained after a thorough case investigation, including an autopsy, examination of the death scene and review of the clinical history. Nine out of 10 deaths occur during the first six months of age (most between one and three months) and boys are more at risk than girls. The risks are also greater for babies who are born prematurely or with a low birth weight. The risk of unexpected infant death is greatly increased by both prenatal and postnatal exposure to tobacco smoke.

The causes of SIDS are multifactorial, but since parents have been advised to place their babies on their backs rather than on their tummies to sleep (see page 309), the number of deaths attributed to SIDS has plummeted. About 300 babies die from SIDS every year, making it the most common cause of death in babies over one month old but the incidence of has been declining steadily since the early 1990s. In the past 15 years, the number of SIDS deaths per 1,000 live births has fallen by 75 per cent. SIDS is still rare and the chances of a baby dying from it are small.

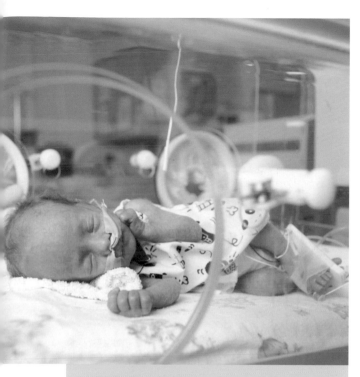

Occasionally in a multiple pregnancy, one baby does not survive. Losing a twin or triplet can be especially difficult. The parents are torn between grieving for their lost baby, and celebrating the life of the surviving one(s) – an emotional seesaw, which can test the strongest relationship. There's an unfortunate tendency for other people to diminish the loss, thinking that because there's still a living baby, the parents should be thankful. Bereavement doesn't work like that.

notice that something isn't right – the baby has stopped moving – or the healthcare provider is not able to hear the baby's heartbeat. An ultrasound scan will be used to check if the baby's heart is beating.

If a baby dies in utero, a mother has the difficult task of going through a normal labour knowing that her baby will not be alive at delivery. It is best to try and avoid Caesarean section as this could lead to more complications for the mother and affect future childbirth.

Very rarely, a baby dies during labour – this is called intrapartum death. When this happens, it is

Glossary

NB: words in italics have separate glossary entry

Afterbirth – the *placenta* and membranes that surround the *fetus*, which are delivered after the baby is born.

Afterpains – *contractions* of the uterus after the baby is born. These usually settle within a few days of the birth.

Amniocentesis – a diagnostic test usually carried out between 14 and 18 weeks of pregnancy in which a sample of fluid is withdrawn from the *amniotic fluid* surrounding a *fetus*. A needle is passed into the *amniotic sac* using *ultrasound scanning* for guidance. The fluid can be analysed to look for a number of conditions, including chromosomal abnormalities such as *Down's syndrome* and genetic disorders like *cystic fibrosis*.

Amnion – one of the two layers of the *amniotic sac* surrounding the *fetus*; the amnion is the inner layer, the *chorion* the outer.

Amniotic fluid – the fluid that surrounds the *fetus*.

Amniotic sac – the bag that contains the *fetus* and the fluid around it. The sac is made up of two layers, the *amnion* and the *chorion*.

Anaemia – a blood condition in which the concentrations of *haemoglobin*, the protein that carries oxygen around the body in the blood, are lower than they should be.

Analgesics – drugs taken to reduce the sensation of pain; some can be used during *labour*.

Anencephaly – a condition present at birth in which the brain has not formed and the top of the skull is missing. This is a severe *neural tube defect*. Babies with this condition may be *stillborn* or survive only for a few hours.

Anomaly ultrasound – a detailed scan, usually performed between 18 and 20 weeks of pregnancy, that checks for physical problems and shows where the *placenta* is positioned in the uterus.

Apgar score – a test given to all newborn babies that reflects how well they are at birth. A baby's colour, breathing, heart rate, muscle tone and response to stimulation are assessed at one minute after the birth and again at five minutes.

Atonic uterus – a condition in which the womb does not contract properly after the baby is delivered. If this is not treated effectively, there may be excessive bleeding.

Baby blues – the low mood and tearfulness that are common in the early days following childbirth.

Bacterial vaginosis (BV) – an imbalance of the bacteria usually present in the vagina that causes discharge. BV is not a *sexually transmitted disease*, but it is more common in those who are sexually active. The condition is treated with antibiotics.

Bilirubin – a brownish-yellow substance produced when the liver breaks down the *haemoglobin* in old red blood cells. High levels of bilirubin cause *jaundice*.

Birth canal – another name for the vagina, through which a baby passes during childbirth.

Birth plan – a list of wishes that a pregnant woman may prepare before she has her baby to let the midwives and doctors know how she would like her *labour* to progress. It may include, for example, the sort of pain relief she would like.

Blastocyst – the cluster of cells that develops from a fertilised egg and becomes the *embryo*.

Blighted ovum – when a fertilised egg attaches to the wall of the uterus, but does not develop. The condition may be picked up on an early *ultrasound scan* when an *amniotic sac* is seen, but no *embryo*.

Body mass index – a measure taking account of height as well as weight that indicates whether an individual is over- or under-weight or within the normal range for her height.

Braxton Hicks contractions – the painless *contractions* of the uterus that may be felt from around 20 weeks of pregnancy or sometimes earlier.

Breech presentation – when a baby is in a bottom-down rather than the usual head-down position at birth. Most babies will have turned into the head-down position by the time *labour* begins.

Caesarean section – delivery of the baby through an incision made in the abdominal wall. This operation may be elective (planned) or an emergency (performed urgently because there is a problem with the mother and/or *fetus*).

Candida albicans – also known as *thrush*, this common fungal infection commonly affects the vagina, often causing itching, a white discharge, and pain when passing urine.

Caput succedaneum – swelling of the scalp in a newborn baby usually caused by pressure on the head during a head-first delivery.

Carpal tunnel syndrome – a relatively common condition in pregnancy in which the median nerve that supplies the hand is squashed between the bones of the wrist and the strong band of tissue that overlies them. There may be tingling and numbness in part of the hand.

Cardiotocography – a method of monitoring a baby's heartbeat using an electro-fetal monitor.

Cephalhaematoma – a soft swelling on a newborn baby's head produced by pressure on the head during delivery or by the use of ventouse. The swelling, caused by bleeding between the skull and the tough sheet that overlies it (the periosteum), gradually disappears over days or a few weeks.

Cephalopelvic disproportion – when a baby's head is too big to pass through the pelvis during childbirth.

Cerebral palsy – a condition affecting movement that is caused by damage to a baby's brain during pregnancy or delivery or soon after birth.

Cervical cerclage – stitching of an *incompetent cervix,* which aims to prevent a miscarriage or premature birth.

Cervical dilatation the widening of the neck of the womb that occurs during *labour* to allow the baby to pass through.

Cervical ectropion – a common condition in which the inner lining of the cervix protrudes from the cervical opening so that it can be seen from the vagina.

Cervical incompetence – a weakness of the cervix that may result in a *miscarriage* or *premature labour* if the cervix begins to widen during pregnancy as the pressure exerted by the *fetus* above increases. *Cervical cerclage* may be advised.

Chadwick's sign – a bluish colouration of the cervix, vagina and *vulva*. It can be seen from early in pregnancy.

Chignon – small mark left by a ventouse on a baby's head.

Chlamydia – a bacterial infection that is usually symptomless in women but can affect the *Fallopian tubes* and cause fertility problems.

Chloasma – a fairly common condition in pregnancy in which pale brown patches appear on the forehead, nose and cheeks. The patches usually fade with time but may recur.

Chorion – the outer layer of the *amniotic sac* surrounding the fetus; the *amnion* is the inner.

Chorionic villi – the small finger-like projections extending from the *chorion* at the edge of the *placenta*.

Chorionic villus sampling – a diagnostic test in which tiny pieces of *chorionic villi* are removed and examined for chromosomal and genetic abnormalities in the *fetus* such as *Down's syndrome* and *cystic fibrosis*. (The villi and fetus have the same *chromosomes* and genes.) Usually performed around 11 weeks of pregnancy.

Chromosomal disorders – conditions that result from the presence of too many or too few copies of a certain *chromosome* or an abnormality in the structure of a chromosome (part of the chromosome may be missing or may be attached to another).

Chromosomes – the tiny structures in our cells that carry all our *DNA* in the form of genes. We have 23 pairs of chromosomes, two being the *sex chromosomes*, which determine whether we are male or female.

Cleft lip and palate – conditions present at birth in which there is a gap in the lip and/or roof of a baby's mouth.

Colostrum – the breast milk first produced by the mother.

Combined screening – a blood test and *nuchal translucency ultrasound* performed between 8 and 14 weeks of pregnancy to give the risk of *Down's syndrome* and other *chromosomal disorders*.

Congenital abnormalities – conditions present at birth.

Congenital varicella syndrome – birth defects caused by chicken pox contracted while pregnant.

Conjoined twins – twins connected at some part of their bodies, for example the head, chest or abdomen. Increasingly sophisticated surgical techniques enable more of these twins to be separated so they can live independently. However, shared organs make separation a complex and difficult process.

Conjunctivitis – inflammation of the conjunctiva (the membrane that covers the white of the eye). The condition may be caused by an infection.

Contractions – tightenings of the muscular walls of the uterus that occur during *labour* and push the *fetus* down and out through the neck of the womb.

Cord compression – pressure on the *umbilical cord* during *labour* that may impair the oxygen supply to the baby.

Cord prolapse – when the cord comes out through the cervical opening before the baby. This is potentially very serious as it can cause *cord compression*.

Cordocentesis – removal of a sample of blood from the *umbilical cord* during pregnancy. Carried out under *ultrasound scanning*, the procedure is also known as *fetal blood sampling*.

Corpus luteum – a small patch of tissue that develops in the ovary from the ruptured egg follicle after *ovulation* has occurred. The corpus luteum secretes the hormone *progesterone*, which causes the lining of the womb to thicken ready for a fertilised egg. If the egg is not fertilised, the corpus luteum shrinks away.

Cradle cap – a harmless condition in which thick whitish-yellow patches appear on a baby's scalp.

Crowning – when the widest of a baby's head can be seen emerging through the vaginal opening.

Crown-to-rump length – the length of a baby in early pregnancymeasured from the top of the head to the buttocks.

CVS – abbreviation *for chorionic villus sampling.*

Cystic fibrosis – a *genetic disease* in which body secretions become thick and sticky and affect the lungs and absorption of food in the gut.

Cystitis – inflammation of the bladder, which may be caused by a bacterial infection.

Cytomegalovirus – a usually symptomless viral infection that an infected woman may pass on to her baby, which may result in birth defects.

Dating ultrasound – the *ultrasound scanning* procedure, usually performed between 8 and 14 weeks, that measures the *fetus* to confirm how far along a pregnancy is and so provide the *estimated date of delivery.*

Deep vein thrombosis – when a clot forms in one of the deep veins – usually in the leg – that carry blood back towards the heart. There may be swelling, warmth and redness of the affected limb. Treatment should be prompt as there is a risk of clot fragments travelling in the blood vessels to the lungs or brain (see *embolism*).

Developmental delay – a term used when a child achieves developmental 'milestones', such as crawling and walking, later than expected from what generally occurs in childhood.

Diaphragmatic hernia – when a weakening in the diaphragm, the muscular sheet that lies between the chest and the abdomen, allows abdominal organs to push upwards into the chest.

Diphtheria – a bacterial infection that can cause a fever and sore throat. Diphtheria may also cause potentially serious complications, so *immunisation* against the disease is part of the recommended childhood *immunisation schedule.*

Dizygotic twins – non identical twins that develop when two separate eggs are fertilised. They have separate *placentas* and their *DNA* is no more alike than a normal brother and sister.

DNA – deoxyribonucleic acid, the structure that carries all our genes and is arranged into *chromosomes* in our cells.

Dominant disorders – conditions that are caused by a *dominant gene* overriding an equivalent *recessive gene*. Only one dominant gene is needed for such a condition to develop, whereas both genes in a pair need to be recessive for *recessive disorders* to develop.

Dominant genes – our genetic material is passed down in the form of gene pairs – with one gene in each pair being inherited from each parent. The genes can either be dominant or recessive. A dominant gene will override the directions given by an equivalent *recessive gene.*

Doppler ultrasound – a scanning technique that measures fetal blood flow, for example in the *umbilical cord*. The findings are used to assess a baby's wellbeing during pregnancy.

Down's syndrome – a *chromosomal disorder* in which there are three copies of chromosome 21 rather than two, as there should be. (The syndrome is also called Trisomy 21.) Children with Down's syndrome have a characteristic appearance. They have learning difficulties and are at increased risk of certain conditions, including heart problems.

Ductus arteriosus – the blood vessel that helps divert oxygen-rich blood derived from the placenta from the fetal heart to the aorta (the main artery that carries blood away from the heart to the body) bypassing the fetal lungs. During pregnancy, oxygen from the maternal circulation is added to the fetal blood via the placenta so the blood does not need to travel to the fetal lungs. The ductus closes soon after birth.

Dystocia – when a baby's shoulders become stuck when the head has been delivered. This is very uncommon but serious and urgent treatment is needed.

Eclampsia – a rare complication of *pre-eclampsia* that occurs during late pregnancy, *labour* or shortly after delivery. The woman's blood pressure is very high and seizures can occur. Urgent treatment is required.

Ectopic pregnancy – when a pregnancy does not develop in the uterus at it should, but in another part of the abdomen or pelvis. The commonest site for an ectopic is the *Fallopian tube*.

EDD – abbreviation for *estimated date of delivery*.

Edward's syndrome – the condition that is caused by the presence of three number 18 chromosomes in the cells instead of the usual two. The syndrome is also known as trisomy 18. Babies with Edward's syndrome have low birth weight as well as other serious difficulties including kidney and heart problems. Many babies with the condition don't survive for more than a few days.

Effacement – the thinning of the cervix that occurs during early *labour*.

Embolism – when a fragment of tissue, often from a blood clot in the deep veins of the legs, travels in the circulation and blocks a blood vessel in another part of the body, such as the lungs (pulmonary embolism).

Embryo – the term used for the developing baby in the first eight weeks of pregnancy. After this the term *fetus* is used.

Endometritis – inflammation of the lining of the uterus.

Endometrium – the lining of the uterus.

Endorphins – pain-relieving substances released naturally by the body.

Engagement – when the *fetus* moves down into the pelvic cavity.

Engorgement – when the breasts became swollen and tender in the early days of breastfeeding.

Epidural anaesthesia – an injection of drugs into the space around the membranes that surround the spinal cord, which relieves pain below the level of the injection.

Episiotomy – a cut made in the tissues next to the vaginal opening that creates more room for the baby to pass through at delivery.

Erythema toxicum – a rash that is common in newborn babies. Red blotchy spots with tiny white or yellowish spots in the centre appear within a couple of days of the birth. Most are found on the baby's trunk.

Estimated date of delivery – the day the baby is expected worked out from the first day of the last menstrual period.

Expressing milk – drawing milk out of the breasts by hand or using a pump.

External cephalic version – the method used by doctors of massaging a woman's abdomen to turn a baby in a breech position into the head-down position ready for the onset of *labour*.

Failure to progress – when the *labour* is long and the cervix is dilating very slowly so that the baby cannot pass through.

Fallopian tubes – the tubes that extend from each side of the uterus. At the outer end of each tube lies an ovary. Eggs released by the ovaries travel along the Fallopian tubes to the uterus.

False labour – when *contractions* are mistaken for the onset of *labour*. In false labour, contractions do not become regular or stronger as time passes. The cervix is not dilating.

Fasting blood sugar – glucose levels measured in the blood after eight hours without any food or drinks other than water.

Fertilisation – when a sperm and egg unite.

Fetal alcohol syndrome – a range of birth defects that can be associated with drinking too much alcohol in pregnancy.

Fetal anomaly – a malformation of the *fetus*.

Fetal blood sampling – see *cordocentesis*.

Fetal distress – when fetal well-being is compromised. Changes in fetal movements and in the fetal heartbeat are possible signs.

Fetal monitoring – continual or frequent assessment of the baby's heart and movements to check all is well.

Fetus – unborn baby from nine weeks of pregnancy until birth.

Fibroids – noncancerous swellings in the wall of the uterus.

Folic acid – a vitamin supplement shown to reduce the risk of *spina bifida* and other *neural tube defects*. It should be taken for the first 12 weeks of pregnancy, as this has been

Follicle stimulating hormone – the female hormone, produced by the *pituitary gland* that causes an egg follicle to start developing in the ovary.

Fontanelles – the 'soft' spots between the bones of a baby's skull. These gaps gradually close.

Footling breech – when a baby's foot is the presenting part (closest to the cervix).

Forceps delivery – an assisted delivery in which forceps (like tongs) are used to help deliver the baby down through the vaginal canal.

Frank breech – when the baby's bottom is the presenting part (closest to the cervix).

Fundal height – the distance from the pelvic bone to the top of the uterus. This can be felt by gently palpating the abdomen and is measured to assess the size of the *fetus*.

Gas and air – this is breathed in through a mask or tube in the mouth and is used as *analgesia* during *labour*.

General anaesthesics – drugs to relieve pain in the body and induce unconsciousness.

Genetic diseases – diseases caused by an abnormality of a gene, e.g. *cystic fibrosis*.

Genetic mutation – an abnormality of a gene that may cause a *genetic disease*.

German measles – also known as *rubella*, this viral illness can cause serious fetal abnormalities if a woman catches it when she is pregnant. For this reason, rubella *immunization* is offered routinely as part of the childhood *immunization schedule*.

Gestational diabetes – a form of diabetes that develops during pregnancy, where the body cannot make enough insulin to cope with the increased blood sugar levels.

GIFT (gamete intra-fallopian transfer) – a fertility treatment suitable for women with normal *Fallopian tubes* as the sperm and egg are placed in one of the tubes in the hope that *fertilisation* will occur and the fertilised egg pass into the uterus and attach to the wall normally.

Glucose tolerance test – blood tests used to look for *gestational diabetes*. Two blood samples are taken, the first following a night with no food or drinks other than water, the second two hours after a special sugary drink.

Gonorrhoea – a *sexually transmitted disease* that can cause serious problems in the *fetus*.

Glycosuria – sugar in the urine; this may indicate diabetes.

Grasping reflex – an early normal reaction, when a baby grips an object placed in her hand.

Gravida – the term used for a pregnant woman. A *primigravida* is a woman in her first pregnancy, a multigravida has had at least one.

Group B streptococcus – a bacterial infection that is present in the vagina of many women and is usually harmless, but can cause serious illness if the infection is passed on to the newborn during delivery.

Haemoglobin – the protein that carries oxygen in red blood cells.

Haemophilia – an inherited disorder in which one of the substances that is needed for normal blood clotting is lacking. Haemophilia results from a genetic abnormality and excessive bleeding is a problem.

Haemophilus influenza type B (Hib) – a bacterial infection that can cause serious illnesses in childhood including meningitis. *Immunization* against Hib is part of the recommended childhood *immunization schedule*.

Haemorrhoids – swollen veins in the lining of the anus. They are a common in pregnancy.

Heartburn – burning discomfort in the chest caused by stomach acid in the oesophagus (gullet). This is common in pregnancy as the one-way valve between the stomach and oesophagus may be leaky, allowing stomach acid to travel back up the oesophagus. The problem tends to worsen later in pregnancy.

HELLP syndrome – a serious variant of *pre-eclampsia* in which red blood cells are broken down excessively, liver enzymes are raised and the level of platelets (for normal blood clotting) is low. This condition requires urgent delivery of the *fetus*.

Hepatitis B – inflammation of the liver caused by a viral infection.

Hernia – the bulging of an organ or tissue through a weakened area of muscle.

Herpes simplex virus – a viral infection which can come in two forms: type 1 that tends to cause cold sores around the lips and type 2 that affects the genitalia.

Hip dislocation – a *congenital abnormality* in which the ball of the hip joint (the top of the femur) skips out of the cup-shaped socket of the pelvis.

HIV (human immunodeficiency virus) – a viral infection that may lead to AIDS (acquired immuno-deficiency syndrome) in which there is reduced immunity, so the body has problems fighting infections and certain types of cancer. An HIV test is offered to all pregnant women in the UK.

Hole in the heart – also known as a *septal defect*, this is when there is a hole in the wall that separates the upper or lower chambers of the heart.

Human chorionic gonadotrophin (hCG) – a hormone produced by the *placenta* to help maintain pregnancy, which can be detected in home pregnancy tests.

Human genome – the full *DNA* sequence in a human being.

Human placental lactogen – a hormone produced by the *placenta* that breaks down maternal fats to provide nutrition for the growing *fetus*.

Huntington's disease – an inherited disorder caused by a defect on chromosome 4. There is a slow degeneration of cells in the brain with symptoms including memory impairment, confusion, and uncontrolled movements starting after the age of 30 years.

Hyaline membrane disease – also known as respiratory distress syndrome is where immature lungs (say, of a premature baby), do not produce enough surfactant, a substance needed for the lungs to function normally.

Hydatidiform mole – see *molar pregnancy*.

Hydramnios – an excessive amount of fluid contained in the *amniotic sac*.

Hydrocele – a soft scrotal swelling caused by the accumulation of fluid in the space around the testis.

Hydrocephalus – an excessive amount of fluid within the skull. The condition can affect premature babies or be associated with some conditions, including *neural tube defects*.

Hydrops fetalis – a life-threatening condition of severe *oedema* (accumulation of fluid) in a *fetus* or newborn, which may have a number of causes including *rhesus disease* and *chromosomal disorders*.

Hyperemesis gravidarum – severe vomiting in early pregnancy.

Hypertension – persistently elevated blood pressure.

Hypoglycaemia – an abnormally low blood sugar level.

Hypospadias – an abnormality of the penis in which the opening is on the underside rather than the end as it should be. Surgery may be performed to correct the problem.

Identical twins see *monozygotic twins*.

Immunisation – the process used to protect against infectious diseases. It may be passive, in which ready-made antibodies are given, or active when substances are given to trigger the formation of antibodies by the immune system. Most immunisations are given by injection.

Immunisation schedule – a programme of *immunisations* given to protect against one or more infections. The childhood immunisation schedule includes immunisations against *diphtheria*, *pertussis* and *tetanus*.

Implantation – when the fertilised egg becomes attached to the wall of the uterus.

Incompetent cervix – see *cervical incompetence*.

Incomplete miscarriage – see *miscarriage*.

Incontinence – involuntary passing of urine or – less commonly – faeces. Stress incontinence, which occurs when the pressure in the abdomen increases (e.g. when laughing), is particularly common after a vaginal delivery.

Incubator – a plastic cot for the care of premature and unwell babies. Oxygen can be given as required and the temperature is kept at an optimum level.

Indigestion – pain or discomfort in the upper abdomen and chest usually after eating. Indigestion is common in pregnancy, particularly in the later part.

Induction of labour – the use of methods to trigger the onset of *labour*. A pessary may be inserted in the vagina that causes the cervix to dilate (widen) or, if the cervix is open, an instrument may be used to break the waters. The drug form of the hormone *oxytocin* may also be given to trigger *contractions* of the uterus.

Intrauterine contraceptive device – a small device that is passed through the cervix into the uterus with the aim of preventing *implantation* of embryos.

Intrauterine growth retardation (IUGR) – slow growth of a *fetus*.

Iron deficiency – lack of iron in the body. This is one cause of *anaemia*.

IVF (In vitro fertilisation) – a fertility treatment in which eggs and sperm are put together outside the body in the hope that *fertilization* will take place and it will be possible to transfer an *embryo* into the uterus.

Jaundice – yellow colouration of the skin and whites of the eyes caused by a build-up of *bilirubin* in the blood. Jaundice is often caused by liver problems. It can affect infants who may not be able to process bilirubin fast enough. In most cases it is temporary and can be treated with light treatment (called *phototherapy*).

Karyotype – a 'picture' of an individual's *chromosomes* – number, size and shape.

Kegel exercises – exercises that aim to strengthen the *pelvic floor* muscles in order to reduce continence problems.

Kick chart – a record of the number of fetal movements felt by a pregnant woman. The chart may help to monitor the wellbeing of the *fetus*.

Labour – the process of childbirth. Labour comprises three stages: the first ends in full dilatation of the cervix; the second is delivery of the *fetus*; and the third is delivery of the *placenta*.

Lanugo – the fine hair that appears on the body of a *fetus* from about 15 weeks' pregnancy.

Latching on – a term used in breastfeeding to describe when a baby takes the nipple and most of the areola tissue around it into her mouth and a tight seal is formed.

Linea nigra – a dark line running from the pubic bone to the navel that may appear in pregnancy.

Listeriosis – a bacterial infection that may be found in certain foods, such as unpasteurised milk and cheese. Severe cases in pregnancy can result in complications, including a *miscarriage*, *stillbirth* and *meningitis* in the newborn.

Luteinising hormone – the hormone that triggers *ovulation*.

Macrosomia – a medical term for a large baby.

Mastitis – inflammation of the breast tissue.

Measles – a viral infection that causes a fever and a rash. A number of complications may develop, including a rare but life-threatening condition when the brain is affected. Measles *immunisation* is part of the recommended childhood *immunisation schedule*.

Meconium – thick, dark, and sticky faeces passed by newborn babies for a day or two after birth. Meconium can also be passed by the *fetus* in late pregnancy and this can be associated with *fetal distress*.

Membrane sweep – during a vaginal examination, a midwife will use her finger at the neck of the womb to try to separate the membranes from the cervix, in order to encourage the release of prostaglandins and bring on the start of labour.

Meningitis – inflammation of the membranes that overlie the brain and spinal cord (the meninges). The cause may be bacterial or viral.

Meningocele – a form of *spina bifida* in which the meninges (the layers of membranes that cover the spinal cord) protrude through a defect in the vertebral column.

Meningomyelocele – a form of *spina bifida* in which there is a malformation of the spinal cord and cord tissue is exposed.

Menstrual cycle – the monthly cycle in women which involves, due to the changes in various hormones, thickening of the *endometrium*, release of an egg, and then shedding of the endometrium and the egg if *fertilization* does not occur.

Milia (milk rash) – tiny whitish-yellow spots on a baby's face, particularly on the nose.

Miscarriage – loss of a baby before 24 weeks of pregnancy:

- Complete – when the uterus has expelled the entire pregnancy and an ultrasound scan shows an empty uterus.
- Incomplete – when the uterus does not expel the entire pregnancy and pieces of tissue are left behind.
- Missed – when the *fetus* has not developed and an empty pregnancy sac can be seen on the scan.
- Threatened – when there is vaginal bleeding but the ultrasound scan shows a fetus with a beating heart.

Molar pregnancy – a rare disorder in which the *placenta* develops into a clump of abnormal tissue, so that a normal *fetus* cannot develop.

Mongolian spots – bluish patches found on a baby's skin. They are more common in dark-skinned babies.

Monozygotic twins – identical twins that develop when one fertilised egg divides. They share a *placenta* and the same *DNA*.

Morning sickness – nausea and sickness that are common in pregnancy, particularly early on. The symptoms can occur at any time of the day.

Moro reflex – the natural startle reaction of a young baby to a loud noise or sudden movement.

Morula – the ball of cells formed when the fertilised egg divides.

Moulding – the abnormal shaping of a baby's head that occurs due to pressure on the head during childbirth.

Mucus, cervical – the fluid produced by the cervix that changes consistency during the *menstrual cycle*.

Mucus plug – the plug that blocks the cervix during pregnancy.

Mumps – a viral illness that causes swelling of one or both of the parotid glands on either side of the face and a number of possible complications including viral *meningitis*. Mumps *immunisation* is part of the recommended childhood *immunisation schedule*.

Nappy rash – a rash in the nappy area that mainly develops when there is prolonged contact with urine or faeces.

Natural childbirth – giving birth without drugs and other invasive procedures.

Natural pain relief – ways of relieving the pain of *labour* without using prescribed drugs.

Neonatal – in the first month following a delivery.

Neonatal jaundice – *jaundice* in the first four weeks of life.

Neonate – a newborn baby in the first four weeks of life.

Neonatologist – a *paediatrician* who specializes in the care of babies in their first four weeks.

Neural tube defects – abnormalities resulting from the failure of the brain and spinal cord to develop normally in early pregnancy. *Anencephaly* and *spina bifida* are both forms of neural tube defect.

Non-identical twins – see *dizygotic twins*.

Nuchal translucency screen – this test, performed by *ultrasound scanning* between 8 and 14 weeks of pregnancy, assesses the thickness of an area at the back of the baby's neck. The results are used to assess the risk of *Down's syndrome*.

Oedema – accumulation of fluid that can cause swelling, sometimes around the ankles.

Oestrogen – female sex hormone essential for the normal functioning of the female reproductive system.

Oligohydramnios – when there are insufficient amounts of *amniotic fluid* around the *fetus*.

Omphalocele – a rare condition in which part of the baby's gut, covered by a layer of membranes, protrudes through the *umbilicus* at birth. The condition is caused by a weakness in the abdominal wall and requires surgery.

Ossification – the formation of hard bone.

Ovulation – release of an egg from the ovary, which then passes along the *Fallopian tube* to the uterus.

Oxytocin – a hormone that is released from the pituitary gland, a pea-sized structure at the base of the brain, and stimulates the *contractions* of the uterus for *labour* and the release of milk when breastfeeding.

Palmar erythema – reddening of the palms caused by a number of medical conditions, but also occurring during pregnancy.

Parvovirus – a virus that causes the illness Fifth disease. Mainly affecting children, Fifth disease can cause a rash, bright red cheeks, and a mild fever. Occasionally, adults that are affected suffer prolonged pain and swelling of the joints.

Patau syndrome – a chromosomal disorder in which there are three copies of chromosome 13 rather than two, as there should be. A number of problems may be present, including low birth weight and deformities such as a *cleft palate*, as well as abnormally developed organs (heart defects are one example).

Pelvic floor – the muscles that make up the pelvic floor run from the pubic bone at the front to the bottom of the spine at the back. They support the bladder and urethra, the tube that carries urine away from the bladder.

Pelvic floor exercises – see *Kegel exercises*.

Pelvimetry – measurements taken from the pelvis to assess whether it is likely to be wide enough to allow the baby to pass through during *labour*.

Percentile charts – charts that show national averages for weight, head circumference and length. Your baby will be measured during her first year and the numbers plotted on these charts to see whether her measurements are within the average range.

Percutaneous umbilical blood sampling see *cordocentesis*.

Perinatal – the time around the birth of a baby.

Perineum – the area between the vaginal opening and the anus.

Pertussis – another name for whooping cough, which affects infants and young children, causing bouts of coughing and other complications including pneumonia and seizures. Pertussis *immunisation* is part of the recommended childhood *immunisation schedule*.

Pethidine – a painkiller given by injection that may be used during *labour*.

Phenylketonuria – an inherited disorder in which the enzyme that enables the amino acid phenylalanine to be converted into the amino acid tyrosine does not work properly. Phenylalanine needs to be excluded from the diet or it accumulates, resulting in learning difficulties.

Phototherapy – the use of light to treat *neonatal jaundice*.

Pica – cravings for non-food substances. This can occur during pregnancy.

Pigmentation changes – alterations in skin colouration, which can occur in pregnancy, for example *linea nigra*.

Piles – see *haemorrhoids*.

Pituitary gland – a pea-sized structure at the base of the brain that produces many hormones.

Placenta – the organ that is attached to the wall of the uterus on one side and the fetus via the *umbilical cord* on the other, which connects the maternal and fetal circulations.

Placental abruption – when the *placenta* becomes partially or fully detached from the wall of the uterus before delivery.

Placenta accreta – when the *placenta* grows into the deeper layers of the wall of the uterus.

Placenta praevia – when the *placenta* is positioned low down in the uterus. It may partially or completely cover the cervix.

Poliomyelitis – a viral infection that tends to be mild, but has the potential to affect the brain and spinal cord, causing paralysis and even death. Polio *immunisation* is part of the recommended childhood *immunisation schedule*.

Polyhydramnios – excessive amounts of *amniotic fluid* surounding the *fetus*.

Port wine stain – a permanent purplish-red mark on the skin.

Possetting – small amounts of milk brought up after feeding.

Postnatal depression – persistent low mood and other symptoms of depression that begin in the first six months after childbirth.

Postpartum haemorrhage – excessive bleeding after childbirth.

Post-term pregnancy – a pregnancy that continues beyond the *estimated date of delivery*.

Pre-eclampsia – a condition in pregnancy in which there is high blood pressure, *oedema* of the feet and legs and protein in the urine.

Pregnancy test – a urine or blood test carried out to see whether a woman is pregnant.

Pre-implantation genetic diagnosis – IVF treatment is carried out to isolate then implant embryos free of a genetic condition such as the inherited form of breast cancer.

Premature baby – a baby born before 37 weeks of pregnancy.

Premature delivery – the birth of a baby before 37 weeks of pregnancy.

Premature labour – *labour* that starts before 37 weeks of pregnancy.

Primigravida – a woman in her first pregnancy.

Progesterone – a hormone normally present in women but at greatly increased levels during pregnancy. Progesterone has a number of key roles in maintaining a pregnancy, including keeping the *placenta* working effectively.

Prolactin – a hormone that prepares the breasts for breastfeeding.

Prolapsed cord – when the cord comes down into the vaginal canal before the baby.

Prolapsed uterus – when the womb descends into the vagina.

Prolonged labour – a long *labour* in which there is slow or non-existent progress.

Prostaglandins – substances produced by the body that have a number of actions, including stimulating uterine *contractions*.

Pruritis gravidarum – itchiness in pregnancy, which tends to affect the palms and sometimes the soles of the feet if it occurs. Occasionally, itching is a sign of a liver problem called cholestasis.

PUBS – abbreviation for *percutaneous umbilical cord sampling*.

Pudendal block – a type of analgesia given at the delivery by a needle passed up the vagina. The pain is numbed locally so that *contractions* can still be felt but discomfort that may be associated with a forceps- or vacuum-assisted delivery will be reduced.

Pyloric stenosis – thickening of the pylorus (the ring of muscle at the outlet of the stomach) that narrows the outlet and prevents food from passing from the stomach into the duodenum.

Quickening, the – the first fetal movements felt by a pregnant woman.

Recessive disorders – disorders caused by a defective *recessive gene*. Two copies of the gene must be present for the disorder to occur.

Recessive genes – one gene in our gene pairs is inherited from each parent. A recessive gene will be overridden by a *dominant* one. Two copies of an abnormal recessive gene can produce a *recessive disorder*.

Regional anaesthetics – drugs given to numb or reduce pain in a particular area while the person stays awake. Examples include *epidural anaesthesia*.

Relaxin – this hormone relaxes the pelvic ligaments and helps prepare the uterus for *labour*.

Respiratory distress syndrome – see *hyaline membrane disease*.

Retained placenta – when the *placenta* remains attached to the uterine wall after a baby's delivery and cannot be removed as usual.

Retinopathy of prematurity – an eye disorder that occurs in *premature babies* that may result in visual impairment or blindness.

Rhesus disease – a condition in which antibodies in the blood of a rhesus-negative woman attack the blood cells of her rhesus-positive baby (see *rhesus incompatibility*).

Rhesus factor – a protein that may be present on the surface of red blood cells (if it is present, a person is said to be rhesus positive; if it is absent, rhesus negative).

Rhesus incompatibility – when a pregnant woman is rhesus negative and her fetus is rhesus positive. It does not usually cause problems in a first pregnancy, but if the woman comes into contact with the fetal rhesus-positive cells she gets sensitised, developing antibodies to them. These antibodies may cross the *placenta* in a subsequent pregnancy and attack the red blood cells of another rhesus-positive fetus causing a serious condition called haemolytic disease of the newborn.

Rheumatic fever – an uncommon condition in which inflammation in the body, particularly in the joints and affecting the heart valves, follows a bacterial infection.

Ripening of the cervix – the thinning and softening of the cervix that occurs as *labour* approaches.

Rooting reflex – the automatic response in early life in which a baby will turn towards a breast or bottle if her cheek is tickled.

Round ligaments – bands of fibrous tissue on either side of the uterus.

Rubella – see *German measles*.

Rupture of membranes – when the *amniotic sac* that surrounds the *fetus* breaks, releasing the amniotic fluid inside.

Salmon patches – red patches present on the face that fade as babies get older.

Salmonellosis – food poisoning caused by the salmonella bacteria; which can be present in poultry or eggs.

Screening in pregnancy – tests that look for certain disorders in the mother or *fetus* or that identify those at increased risk.

Septal defect – see *hole in the heart*.

Serum screening – a blood test that measures three or four pregnancy-associated blood chemicals to give a woman her individual statistical chance of having a baby with Down's syndrome. Normally performed at 16 weeks of pregnancy.

Sex chromosomes – the *chromosomes* that determine a person's sex (females have two Xs, males an X and a Y).

Sexually transmitted diseases – infective diseases that are passed on during sexual intercourse.

Show – the passing vaginally of the mucus plug that blocks the cervix during pregnancy.

Sickle cell disease – an inherited abnormality of red blood cells.

SIDS abbreviation for *sudden infant death syndrome*.

Sonogram – an image produced by *ultrasound scanning*.

Speculum – instrument that is used to separate the walls of the vagina to enable the examiner to get a clear view of the cervix.

Spider angiomas – tiny red spots on the skin, also known as spider naevi.

Spina bifida – a form of *neural tube defect* in which the spinal

cord does not develop properly. The lesions vary in severity.

Startle reflex – see *Moro reflex*.

Station – a term used to describe how far down the *fetus* is positioned in the pelvis during childbirth.

Sticky eye – a common condition present at birth in which there is yellow discharge around the eyelids.

Stillbirth – when a baby dies before *labour* begins after the age of 24 weeks.

Stork mark – a red mark on the back of a baby's neck caused by a collection of dilated blood vessels.

Strawberry mark – a raised red mark on a baby's skin caused by a collection of capillaries (tiny blood vessels).

Streptococcus B – see *group B streptococcus*.

Stretch marks – lines caused by the rapid stretching of the skin of the abdomen that occurs during pregnancy.

Sucking reflex – the baby's natural reaction to suck things put in her mouth.

Sudden infant death syndrome – also known as cot death, when a baby dies suddenly for no apparent reason.

Swaddling – a way of wrapping a baby which may soothe her when she is crying.

Syntocinon – a synthetic form of *oxytocin* that may be given to help progress *labour* by increasing the strength of *contractions*. It can also be given after the delivery to keep the uterus contracted.

Tay-Sachs disease – an inherited disorder in which harmful chemicals build up in the brain causing severe – and eventually fatal – brain damage.

Tear – damage to the perineal tissue that occurs during delivery.

TENS (transcutaneous electrical nerve stimulation) – method of pain relief that uses low-voltage electrical pulses delivered by a machine applied to an area.

Teratogenic – something that can cause abnormalities in the developing *embryo* or *fetus*.

Termination of pregnancy – to stop a pregnancy by means of medical or surgical treatment.

Tetanus – a serious and potentially fatal infective disease that affects the nervous system. *Immunisation* against the bacteria

is offered routinely as part of the childhood *immunisation schedule*.

Thalassaemias – inherited disorders in which *haemoglobin* is not produced correctly, resulting in *anaemia*.

Thrombophlebitis – inflammation of the surface veins of the skin that can cause redness and soreness.

Thrush – see *candida albicans*.

Thyroid disease – conditions in which the thyroid gland produces too much or too little of its hormones, and/or in which the gland is enlarged. Thyroid hormones regulate many processes in the body, so abnormal production can cause a variety of symptoms affecting, for example, energy levels, body weight, bowel function, and the condition of the skin.

Tocolytic agents – medicines used to suppress premature labour.

Tocophobia – fear of giving birth.

Toxoplasmosis – an infection that can cause fetal abnormalities if passed on by the mother during pregnancy. The infection can be caught by eating undercooked meat and unwashed vegetables.

Transducer – that part of the equipment used in *ultrasound scanning*, which is moved over the skin, or against the vaginal wall in *transvaginal ultrasound*. It emits sound waves and receives echoes that are passed back from the area being examined and then used to form images.

Transition phase – the period of a *labour* when the cervix fully dilates, widening from 8 to 10cm.

Translocations – when a piece breaks off two different *chromosomes* and the genetic material is exchanged.

Transvaginal ultrasound – ultrasound where the *transducer* is put in the vagina.

Transverse lie – when a *fetus* is positioned sideways across the abdomen.

Trimester – one of the three time periods of a pregnancy.

Triple test – blood test that measures three substances, used to assess the risk of *neural tube defects and* chromosomal abnormalities.

Triplets – three babies born from one pregnancy. Triplets occur naturally about 1 in 6,400 births.

Trisomies – *chromosomal disorders* in which there are three copies of a particular *chromosome* rather than the normal two. The commonest example of this is *Down's syndrome*.

Ultrasound scanning – sound waves and echoes are used to make pictures of the uterus and the developing *fetus*.

Umbilical cord – the connection between the *fetus* and placenta that carries blood between the mother and the *fetus*.

Umbilicus – navel or tummy button; the point where the *umbilical cord* enters the *fetus*.

Urinary tract infections – infections that affect the bladder, ureters or urethra, for example, *cystitis*.

Uterine inversion – a rare but potentially life threatening condition in which the *placenta* does not separate from the wall of the uterus at it should after the baby has been delivered and the uterus is pulled inside-out when attempts are made to deliver the placenta. The top of the uterus may come through the cervix or the whole uterus may come through.

Uterine rupture – a tear of the wall of the uterus occurring during pregnancy or *labour*.

Vacuum extraction – a method by which the woman is assisted in delivering her baby by suction applied through a soft cup applied to the baby's head.

Varicose veins – dilated veins that are visible just under the skin. They tend to affect the leg veins and may develop in pregnancy as a result of pressure exerted by the growing *fetus* on the pelvic veins.

Vernix – the thick, white, greasy substance that covers the skin of a newborn baby. Vernix protects and insulates the skin.

Vertex position – when a *fetus* is in the head-down position in the womb.

Vulva – the external part of the female genitalia.

Whooping cough – see *pertussis*.

Winding – methods used to encourage a baby to burp during or after feeding.

X-linked disorders – inherited disorders caused by an abnormal X chromosome. *Haemophilia* is one example.

Yeast infections – another name for fungal infections, such as *candida albicans*.

Zygote – formed when a sperm fertilises an egg.

Some common chart abbreviations

ALB (urine) – albumin, a protein that may be detected in urine.

ARM – artificial rupture of the membranes.

BP – blood pressure.

Br – breech position; baby's bottom is lying near cervix.

Ceph – baby's head is nearest the cervix.

CTG – *cardiotocography*.

FHH – foetal heart heard.

FMF – foetal movement felt.

H – fetal heart heard.

Hb – haemoglobin; this is tested for in blood to check for anaemia.

IOL – *induction of labour*.

LMP – last menstrual period.

LSCS – lower segment Caesarean section.

NAD – nothing abnormal found.

NIL – nothing abnormal found.

P G O (urine) – indication of whether protein, glucose or any other substance is present in urine sample.

PP – presenting part.

SROM – spontaneous rupture of the membranes.

Tr – trace.

USS – ultrasound scan.

UTI – urinary tract infection.

Vx – vertex position; baby's head is nearest the cervix.

Index

Fish 101, 103, 112
FITT principle 121
Flu 77
Fluid: intake 103, 115, 332
    retention 53, 70, 73, 112, 239,
        273
Fluorescent in Situ
    Hybridisation (FISH) 245
Flying, safety 82
Folates 106
Folic acid 24, 106, 252, 376,
    389
Follicle stimulating hormone 10,
    389
Fontanelles 283, 389
Food *see* Diet
Food: cravings 27, 99
    hazards 81, 110
    hygiene 111
    poisoning 77, 81
Foot: club 380
    massage 127
Footling breech 226, 389
Forceps delivery 187, 229, 389
Formula milk 303, 304
Fragile X disease 249
Frank breech 226, 389
Friends, support from 153
Fruit 101, 107
Full blood count 90
Fundal height 91, 389
Furniture, nursery 195

G

Gas and air 180, 389
Gastroenteritis 77
General
    anaesthetics 180, 230, 389
    practitioners (GPs) 177
Genetic
    diseases 240, 243, 246, 389
    mutation 249, 389
Genetics 12, 17
Genitals, baby's 284, 313
German measles 89, 240, 258,
    390
Gestational diabetes 89, 93, 241,
    253, 390
GIFT 390
Glucose, in urine 89
Glucose tolerance test 241, 390
Gluten intolerance 105

Glycosuria 390
Gonorrhoea 390
Grandparents 165, 191, 353
Grasping reflex 291, 390
Gravida 390
Group B strep 260, 363, 390
Growth, babies 261, 292, 295
Gums, bleeding 61, 132

H

Haemoglobin 390
Haemophilia 18, 240, 248, 390
Haemophilus influenza type B
    (Hib) 310, 370, 390
Haemorrhage 321, 356
Haemorrhoids 69, 255, 322,
    390
Hair: baby's 36, 45, 50, 283, 314
    mother's 28, 63, 130, 325
    removal 134
Handedness 145
Hands: carpal tunnel syndrome
    260
    itchiness 66
    newborn baby's 284
    skin care 134
    swollen 73
Hazards: everyday 78
    food 110
    work 80
Head, baby's: after birth 282–3
    crowning 56, 222, 224
    engagement 210
    measurement 367
    moulding 56, 215, 233, 282
    and pelvis size 230, 251
    position in pelvis 204
Headaches 61, 180, 273
Health visitor 86
Hearing, baby's 41, 142, 288
Heart: congenital problems 249,
    374
    exercise 120, 338
    pre-existing disease 265
    resuscitation 372
Heartbeat: baby's 185, 208, 217,
    237
    mother's 62, 115, 121
Heartburn 29, 61, 70, 210, 390
HELLP syndrome 254, 390
Hepatitis B 90, 240, 267, 286,
    370, 391

Herbal remedies 74, 208
Hernia 379, 390
Herpes simplex virus 267, 390
Hiccups 288
High blood pressure *see*
    Hypertension
Hip dislocation 381, 390
HIV 90, 191, 240, 256, 268,
    391
Holding babies 311
'Hole in the heart' 375, 391
Home births 174
Homeopathy 74
Hormonal bleeding 275
Hormones: breastfeeding 297,
    299
    during pregnancy 60
    placental 141
    pregnancy tests 15
    preparation for birth 148
    see also Oestrogen; Oxytocin;
        Progesterone
Hospital birth 174, 213
    active management of labour
        215
    discharge 286
    packing bag 206
    pain relief 178
    postnatal care 286
    when to go to 213
Hot spots 204
Household products 78
Housework 94, 194, 327, 344
Human
    chorionic gonadotrophin
        (HCG) 15, 20, 21, 60, 240,
        274, 391
    genome 391
    placental lactogen 61, 391
Hunger 62
Huntington's disease 18, 240,
    243, 248, 391
Hyaline membrane disease 391
Hydatidiform mole 256
Hydramnios 262, 391
Hydrocele 391
Hydrocephalus 375, 391
Hydrops 245, 374, 391
Hyperemesis gravidarum 257,
    391
Hypertension 89, 253, 265, 391
Hypnosis 181

Hypoglycaemia 366, 391
Hypospadias 378, 391

I

Identification, babies 176
Illegal drugs 75
Illness 77, 264
Immune system 49, 264, 370
Immunisation: baby 286, 310,
    370, 391
    foreign travel 82
    pregnant women 77
    rubella 89, 256, 258
    schedule 370, 391
Implantation: bleed 275
    embryo 14, 15, 20, 391
Implants, breast 134
Incisions, Caesarean section 232,
    324
Incompetent cervix 279, 391
Incontinence 29, 68, 359, 392
Incubators 373, 392
Indigestion 29, 204, 392
Induction 185, 228, 392
Infantile eczema 364, 365
Infections: food safety 111
    newborn babies 362
    postnatal 356
    pre-existing 269
    in pregnancy 257
Inherited diseases *see* Genetic
    diseases
Insecticides 78
Insects 82
Insomnia 71
Insulin 61, 253, 269, 392
Integrated test 241, 392
Intensity levels 121
Internal examinations 21, 214
Intestinal obstruction 378
Intrauterine contraceptive
    devices 88, 352
Intrauterine growth retardation
    (IUGR) 392
Intravenous (IV) lines 214, 227,
    230, 324
Invasive tests 241
Iodine 108
Iron: deficiency 62, 252, 392
    sources of 90, 108, 332
    supplements 90, 95, 252
    vegetarian diet 104